Clinical Nutrition

FOR

DUMMIES®

A Wiley Brand

by Michael Rovito, PhD

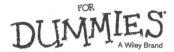

FOR

DUMMIES®

A Wiley Brand

Clinical Nutrition For Dummies®

Published by
John Wiley & Sons, Inc.
111 River Street
Hoboken, NJ 07030-5774
www.wiley.com

For general information on our other products and services, please contact our Customer Care Department within the U.S. at 877-762-2974, outside the U.S. at 317-572-3993, or fax 317-572-4002. For technical support, please visit www.wiley.com/techsupport.

Wiley publishes in a variety of print and electronic formats and by print-on-demand. Some material included with standard print versions of this book may not be included in e-books or in print-on-demand. If this book refers to media such as a CD or DVD that is not included in the version you purchased, you may download this material at http://booksupport.wiley.com. For more information about Wiley products, visit www.wiley.com.

Library of Congress Control Number is available upon request

ISBN 978-1-118-66546-6 (pbk); ISBN 978-1-118-66576-3 (ebk); ISBN 978-1-118-66581-7 (ebk); ISBN 978-1-118-66588-6 (ebk)

Manufactured in the United States of America

10 9 8 7 6 5 4 3 2 1

Contents at a Glance

Table of Contents

Part I
Getting Started with Clinical Nutrition

getting started
with
clinical
nutrition

In this part. . .

✔ Discover the basic concepts of nutrition and how new approaches seek to address both individual and global healthcare issues

✔ Recognize the components of a career in clinical nutrition and identify which area interests you most

✔ Understand how nutrition is increasingly being integrated into educational and clinical applications to promote wellness of groups and individuals

✔ Become familiar with the different nutrients, the recommended intake levels, and how diet promotes or hinders optimum heath

✔ Discover strategies that help you change behaviors to make your life, or your patients' lives, longer and healthier

Chapter 16: Caring for Kids, from Infancy through the Teen Years 249

Chapter 17: Making Sense of Middle Age 271

Introduction

The notion that you can eat your way to a healthier, longer life is an awesome concept. Think about it: Within your power is the opportunity to control one of the biggest factors impacting your health: your diet. Through diet, you can prevent, treat, and even cure diseases. Even more amazing is that the diet that promotes good health isn't difficult to follow. It's quite simple, actually: You simply eat high-fiber, low-fat foods, choose lean proteins, limit junk food, and watch portion sizes.

Still, changing lifestyle behaviors can be very difficult psychologically. Even though some will tell you that losing weight is a simple matter of math — eat fewer calories than you burn — the reality is much different. Eating isn't merely a way to fuel your body; how people react to foods also has emotional and social components as well. On top of that, you have to factor in food addictions, dietary allergies, and the thousands of other factors that influence how and what a person eats. Well, you can see how a simple concept — that you can improve your health by improving your diet — gets a bit more complicated. Eating right for your health is more than a physical challenge; it's a mental challenge as well.

Clinical nutrition is both an art and a science, and the primary goal of clinical nutritionists is to help people make healthy dietary choices. To do so requires doing the following:

- Understanding the connection between food and health and incorporating that information into an action plan for patients
- Developing effective ways of explaining that connection to people to inspire them to make changes that can improve their health

This method — mastering the data and finding compelling ways to communicate that data to patients — helps people get healthy. This is clinical nutrition.

About This Book

This book is a compilation of concepts and information that are thousands of years old. As far back as recorded history, people have been extolling the virtues of eating right and exercising. What we have on our side today is lots of hard data and scientific research that lets us know why, for example, oranges and other citrus fruits prevent scurvy, or that uncovers connections between certain kinds of food and cancer prevention. But the general ideas are the same.

This book shares the hard data with you and gives you the tools you need to communicate this information to others in an effective and persuasive manner. My hope is that the content here not only empowers you to eat right for a great cause — living a long, healthy life — but also inspires you to find out more about clinical nutrition or become a clinical nutritionist yourself.

Sometimes people don't realize that the power to change health for the better lies within, not without. And clinical nutrition gives you a way to improve health and prolong life that doesn't rely on medications. Eating for health is one way you can claim ownership over your life. Eat on, I say!

Conventions Used in This Book

This book is designed so that you can easily find the information you need. Here are some conventions I've used throughout the book:

- ✔ The illustrations and tables are included to help you understand the general concepts being explained. In other words, I didn't include pictures just because I thought they were pretty; every one can help you more easily grasp the material.

- ✔ The units of measurements for food material are in grams (g) and milligrams (mg), which is the industry norm.

- ✔ The word *serving* refers to the United States Food and Drug Administration serving size regulations. Most other Western nations have similar, if not identical, serving size rules.

- ✔ I've made nonessential information easy to recognize. Look for the Technical Stuff icon and the shaded boxes of information. This isn't vital to your understanding of clinical nutrition, but those who like the nitty-gritty details will definitely find these bits worthy of note.

In addition, you may note that some web addresses break across two lines of text. If you're reading this book in print and want to visit one of these web pages, simply key in the web address exactly as it's noted in the text, pretending as though the line break doesn't exist. If you're reading this as an e-book, you've got it easy — just click the web address to be taken directly to the web page.

Foolish Assumptions

Maybe you're a college student looking for some extra help in an introductory course to clinical nutrition. Maybe you're a retiree who is just interested on how to make sure you're eating right to increase your chances of living a healthier, longer life. Maybe you just picked this book up randomly at a bookstore because you wanted some quick tips on eating responsibly for better health. Whoever you are, I've made some assumptions about the kind of information you want:

- ✔ You're interested in nutrition, either personally or because you're considering it as a career choice.
- ✔ You want to know how diet can help prevent, treat, and maybe cure certain diseases.
- ✔ You don't want overly technical or jargon-laden explanations.
- ✔ You're busy and want information that you can reference easily.

If this list describes you, you've picked up the right book. That said, here's one more thing I am assume about you: You are a responsible person who, after reading this material but before changing your diet based on this information, will consult a physician.

Icons Used in This Book

I use several icons in this book to help you identify certain kinds of information so that you can easily find the information you seek. They're all worth reading (even the Technical Stuff, which I included specifically for nutrition geeks — people who, like me, really like the details of what's going on behind the scenes). Here's what the different icons mean:

This icon highlights information that can help you make responsible choices in your life to improve your health. I also use this icon when I share shortcuts, timesavers, or tricks that can help you grasp a concept.

Certain information is absolutely vital for anyone interested in nutrition. When you see this icon, you know you've come across one of these nuggets. Keep these very important facts in your head.

Clinical nutrition is all about using diet to produce beneficial health outcomes. But some behaviors — like over- or under-consuming certain vitamins, minerals, fats, carbs, and so on — put you at risk for negative health consequences, some even severe enough to kill you. Pay special attention when you see this icon because it alerts you to these dangers.

As I mention earlier, this icon highlights the info you don't have to read. Skipping these tidbits won't impair your understanding of clinical nutrition. But I recommend you read them, of course. Some are fun facts, some are esoteric details, some are behind-the-scenes looks, but *all* are interesting.

Beyond the Book

In addition to the material in the print or e-book you're reading right now, this product also comes with some access-anywhere information on the web. How convenient! Clinical nutrition can be complicated, and you may need to access resources when you're away from your text, and that's what this online content provides: super convenient, super quick access to interesting info. For additional content related to clinical nutrition, be sure to check out the free Cheat Sheet at `http://www.dummies.com/ cheatsheet/clinicalnutrition`. I've also provided lots of bonus material at `www.dummies.com/extras/clinicalnutrition` that goes beyond the content in both the print and e-books.

Where to Go from Here

This book is modular, meaning that you can start anywhere you want to find the information you need. You don't have to read from beginning to end because I've written each chapter as a stand-alone element, and if a discussion somewhere else would be helpful, I add a cross-reference to tell you where to go to find the information.

Still, if you're new to clinical nutrition, I recommend that you begin reading through Part I, which lays the foundation for the discussions in the rest of the book. Beyond that, head to the table of contents or the index to find a topic that interests you, or thumb through the pages until something catches your eye. Wherever you land, you'll find information you can use.

Chapter 1

Getting Clinical about Nutrition

· ·

In This Chapter

▶ Conceptualizing clinical nutrition

▶ Understanding the fundamentals of clinical nutrition

▶ Becoming aware of the growing international focus on proper nutrition

· ·

The fact that you are reading this book means that you are at least partially tuned into the connection between what you eat and how it affects your health. Congratulations! Either through a course you are taking or through your own personal curiosity, you are choosing to get better acquainted with the study of diet and how it influences your overall status of health and wellness.

The relationship between what you eat and how healthy you are can be complex, but it's not impossible to understand. In fact, this text focuses on a few simple guidelines:

✔ You must eat fruits, vegetables, and whole grains.

✔ You must moderate your fat, salt, and sugar intakes.

✔ You must exercise.

If you follow all these guidelines, you'll find yourself more healthy than not and will realize the truth behind the adage that you are what you eat.

This chapter takes you on a quick tour of the fundamental principles related to the study of clinical nutrition. Retaining a basic understanding of the concepts I introduce you to here is a great foundation for all the chapters that follow.

Pillars of the Practice: Recognizing the Links between Nutrition and Health

To state the obvious, food is essential for human survival. Since humans — or some form thereof — first started to walk the earth, the human body has evolved to benefit from the foods available in a given environment.

Generations of trial and error, in which we sampled literally tens of thousands of different species of potential food, enabled us to obtain from nature the nutrients needed for life. Our bodies adapted over thousands of years to both the bounty and the scarcity of what existed in the environment — what we were able to gather, hunt, and farm.

Recently, however, that relationship has been altered, and along with that change is a realization that modern eating habits aren't necessarily better. From that realization have sprung efforts to return to a healthier way of eating.

Revisiting traditional views of food and health

Just up until the middle of the last century, people ate a variety of foods that were in balance with the major food groups. Through the process of evolution, humans naturally gravitated toward a diet that was relatively in tune with what the body needed to survive. The availability of — and our preferences for — food were naturally balanced in a way that provided a healthy diet. Whether the available diet and the human body's needs evolved together is uncertain, but one thing we do know for sure is that, back then, humans didn't overeat as much.

A snapshot of the past

Before industrialization, globalization, and modern farming and transportation techniques, food was scarcer than today. You ate what you needed — not what you wanted — and what was available.

Convenience stores selling all kinds of processed foods didn't dot every city corner. Nor were there gigantic supermarkets holding thousands of items to choose from. If you wanted a grape grown in Chile or an apple grown in New Zealand, you needed to live in (or pretty darn close to) those countries, because systems for transporting fresh food around the globe didn't exist.

Basically, you had yourself to rely on: You had to grow and harvest your own food, and prepare it yourself — all tasks that involve lots of manual labor. Of course, hunger was an issue (as it still is for too many people today), but the overabundance of food that's common today simply did not exist back then.

Fast forward to today

Today, the food landscape is very different. You can walk into a supermarket and buy almost any fresh product from any corner of the world. You can swing by a convenience store for a quick snack and a mega-gulp. You can go to a fast-food restaurant and buy a meal packed full of a day's worth of calories and gobble it down within 15 minutes of walking in the door. You have the world at your culinary disposal.

Ample quantities of food are available, and you don't have to exert much physical labor to procure it. Before, if you wanted a special type of walnut from some distant land, you'd probably have to go there yourself, or order it and wait four months for it to arrive at the dock. You wouldn't be able to find it prepackaged in plastic in aisle 10 of your local megamart.

Never has such a scenario existed in the course of human history. Consider yourself lucky — and then recognize the health trade-off that's occurred due to the abundance of unhealthy, highly processed foods.

Diets that are high in fat, salt, and sugar have become more commonplace. Public health and nutrition researchers theorize that this phenomenon has promoted epidemic levels, perhaps even *pandemic* (worldwide) levels, of adverse health effects. Whereas the rates of obesity, heart disease, and diabetes (and even some type of cancers) occurred at drastically lower levels before the mid-20th century, today those conditions occur at an alarming rate.

With the discovery of the direct relationship between the foods we eat and these (and other) health conditions, people are beginning to return to a more simplistic, healthier, and, dare I say, natural way of eating food. (For details on the relationship between diet, nutrition, and a variety of conditions and diseases, head to Part II.)

Introducing the key tenets of clinical nutrition

Clinical nutrition is the study of the connection between your body's overall state of wellness and the foods you eat each day. What's so interesting about this field is that, if you go beyond the details (how particular nutrients do particular things or what proportion of what kinds of foods produces optimal results, for example), you realize that *it really matters:* Because of this awareness, clinical nutrition, in a sense, seeks to re-establish the connection people used to have with food, in which their diets provide the nutrients necessary to ensure adequate nourishment and to build and maintain healthy, strong, and resilient bodies.

If you took all the tips and tricks mothers, fathers, grandparents, and others have passed down about what to eat to maintain healthiness or to prevent disease, and distilled those nuggets into a science, you would end with many of the key tenets of clinical nutrition. Here are some things that Grandma may have said and what modern science shows (I delve into these tenets in more detail throughout this book):

✔ **You are what you eat:** If you eat too much fat and calories without being active, you'll put on weight. If you eat healthy foods, you'll be healthy. If you eat lots of carrots, you'll be . . . okay, well this one doesn't quite work, but interestingly you can get beta-carotene poisoning, which makes your skin turn orange . . . like a carrot! Silly example aside, the point is still a good one: What you put *into* your body has a direct affect *on* your body and your health.

✔ **An apple a day keeps the doctor away:** The quality of the food you eat has a direct impact on your health. (I cover the role of diet in a variety of diseases in the chapters in Part II).

Ask yourself this question: Would you put sand into the fuel tank to make the vehicle run? Of course not. Not unless you want to irreparably damage the inner workings of your car. A car needs gasoline, not sand, just as your body needs healthy, whole foods for better health outcomes. Both need the best sources of fuel to optimally perform.

✔ **Don't eat anything you don't recognize as food:** Your body evolved to digest food, not food products, to maintain health. You want to eat as many simple, whole foods as possible. Eating oranges is better than drinking orange juice, and drinking orange juice is better than eating orange popsicles.

Here's a tip to help you avoid foods that are overly processed: Avoid or find alternatives for food that

  • Has more than five ingredients

  • Has ingredients you cannot pronounce

  • Contains high-fructose corn syrup or hydrogenated oils

If a food falls into two of these three categories, it may be processed and not one your ancestors would have recognized. Steer clear as much as possible from these products.

✔ **To lengthen your life, shorten your meals:** One key to a healthy life is to eat in moderation. Research suggests that, on average, the more energy (calories) you consume, the worse health outcomes you have compared to people who eat a moderate amount of food. I delve more deeply into this concept in Chapter 2.

✔ **A little dirt never hurt anybody:** Did you ever hear your mother or father say, "Germ him up!" Maybe not, but my father said it numerous times about me to my mother. They knew that children, and adults, benefit from certain bacteria in dirt and other external sources. Being exposed helps train your body to become resistant to these microbes in the future. In other words, food doesn't have to be sterile to be good for you.

Now, don't take this advice too far and eat random, dirty objects. That is *not* the best thing to do. You will get sick. (Head to Chapter 10 for information on food contaminants you need to protect yourself from.) Still, as the phrase suggests, a little dirt will never hurt. Many beneficial microbes vital to the human body are ones that you can only get through external sources — your food and things on your food. Be sure to check out Part III for more information on specific diets and how they benefit specific systems of the body.

Although clinical nutrition is a comprehensive, advanced science, a simplified version of the tenets of clinical nutrition can be learned from talking to older members (grandparents or even great-grandparents) of your family. Ask them how or what they used to eat, their exercise habits when they were younger, and how they eat now. You'll be surprised at the similarities between what your older family members used to eat (or maybe still do) and what the most advanced clinical nutrition research suggests for a healthier life. The terms may be more complicated on the clinical nutrition side, but the premises are very similar.

Taking a New (-ish) Approach to Medical Care and Public Health

Clinical nutrition is mainly concerned with two overarching goals — disease prevention and therapies used to treat particular diseases — which it seeks to achieve by focusing on the following areas:

✔ **Dietetics:** *Dietetics* is the study of food and its regulation, and proper nutrition, and how these factors influence health outcomes in both behavioral settings (public health, community-wide applications) and clinical settings (laboratory or hospital-based applications).

✔ **Nutritional genomics:** Nutritional genomics is an expanding field in clinical nutrition. Professionals are placing more and more emphasis not only on the immediate effects of a poor diet on the body but also on the long-term effects, including those passed through generations. *Nutritional genomics* studies how your diet affects your genes and how possible differences in genetic components of the human body can affect your health. Essentially, nutritional genomics is the study of how your ancestors ate and how their diets possibly affect *your* health outcomes. It is interesting — maybe even alarming — to think that what you're eating now could have an impact upon your great-great-grandchildren's health!

In this section, you get a general look at how the field of clinical nutrition helps prevent disease and can be used to improve treatment therapies. For detailed information on the connection between diet and disease, head to Part II; Part III explores the role nutrition plays on the organ systems in the body.

Preventing disease

Most dietary recommendations from the majority, if not all, governing health bodies aim to prevent the following three major conditions and the diseases associated with them:

✔ **Obesity:** Obesity is caused by eating more calories than the body burns, a situation that leads to increases in body fat. Research suggests that weight gain is at the root of many of the risk factors leading to a variety of different diseases, including heart disease, diabetes, sleep apnea, arthritis, hypertension (high blood pressure), gout, and certain types of cancers, to name just a few.

People who are obese tend to have other diseases associated with obesity, a situation referred to as being *comorbid*. Clinical nutritionists are working with public health officials to alter public dietary behaviors by providing individual counseling, promoting policy changes (such as banning, or limiting, trans-fats in foods), and modifying school lunch programs to offer more fruit and vegetable choices in place of processed carbohydrate-dominated foods (like pizza and french fries), to name a few.

✔ **Heart disease:** Heart disease is the number one cause of death worldwide, and it is largely the result of poor dietary choices and physical inactivity. Research suggests that people who live sedentary lives and eat high-fat, low-fiber foods have a higher risk for developing heart disease than those who are active and eat a low-fat, high-fiber diet. Clinical nutritionists work with individual patients and public health officials to help promote heart-healthy behaviors, like exercising regularly and eating low-fat diets.

✔ **Malnutrition:** The World Health Organization (WHO) currently emphasizes malnutrition as one of the most important public health concerns the world faces today. According to WHO, malnutrition consists of *undernutrition* (chronically not getting enough nutrition through food or supplements, or the body's inability to process certain nutrients to support normal bodily functions) and overweight/obesity — both major global health concerns. Clinical nutritionists are implementing various educational campaigns aimed at raising awareness and limiting the spread and effects of these diseases.

Devising therapeutic measures to treat disease

As I note earlier, clinical nutrition is the study of how foods you eat each day impact your body's overall state of wellness, and it's yielded all sorts of information that health professionals can use to design more effective treatment programs for those suffering from disease. Specifically, clinical nutrition has made possible a therapeutic approach for treating health conditions and their associated symptoms by using a therapeutic, or specialized, diet.

A *therapeutic diet* is specifically designed to promote optimum wellness for an individual, based upon that individual's immediate dietary needs. This tailored diet is based upon the patient's entire medical history profile. Such treatments aim to reduce the risk of developing complications for conditions such as diabetes and to ameliorate the effects of conditions like high cholesterol.

Many of these modern-day recommendations stem from knowledge our ancestors had about different foods and their potential curative properties. Following are some examples of folk wisdom that research has shown to be effective:

✔ **Orange juice assists immune system response.** Orange juice is high in vitamin C, an antioxidant that helps protect your body from cell damage and plays a key role in your immune system.

✔ **Honey can be used as an antiseptic.** Honey has antimicrobial qualities and forms a protective barrier over a wound to prevent other microbes from getting into the cut. To find out more about the medicinal and antibacterial properties of honey, check out the article "Honey: its medicinal property and antibacterial activity," by Manisha Deb Mandal and Shyamapada Mandal at `http://www.ncbi.nlm.nih.gov/pmc/articles/PMC3609166/`.

✔ **Fiber and whole grains help gastrointestinal tract issues.** Excess fat and cholesterol bind to fiber in the intestines, which then excrete the waste out of the body instead of recycling it back into the blood. Further, fiber promotes bacterial growth in the intestines to aid in digestion. For more on the ins and outs of the excretory system, head to Chapter 14.

✔ **The BRAT diet (bananas, rice, applesauce, and toast) is good for diarrhea.** If you are experiencing an overactive gastrointestinal tract, like diarrhea, for instance, you should eat low-fiber foods that are bland, which is what the BRAT diet proposes. In addition to keeping you feeling full, the BRAT foods provide nourishment without further upsetting your already sensitive stomach and intestines.

These recommendations stem from more traditional sources that have been used for generations. What clinical nutritionists are doing now is perfecting the science and attempting to understand the physiologic components of the relationship between those foods and overall health. Bottom line: Our ancestors knew these treatments worked; nowadays, we want to know why.

Some food remedies can actually cause more harm than good. Most people know to be wary of products that claim to bring about rapid weight loss, strength gain, longevity, and so on. But you must also be extremely cautious about the supplements you take. Some situations — the presence of existing health conditions, negative interactions with medications you're already taking, and more — can make taking the supplement dangerous. For example, some research suggests that taking calcium supplements may actually raise your risk for heart disease. Check out this website for more information on the topic: `http://www.health.harvard.edu/blog/link-between-calcium-supplements-and-heart-disease-raises-the-question-take-them-or-toss-them-201205304813`

Addressing nutritional needs throughout your lifespan

Healthy dieting and maintaining wellness is a lifelong effort, not a temporary distraction. As you work to maintain a healthy diet throughout your life, you must be aware that your diet will change. Nutritional requirements are not static. As you age, your needs shift, and your diet must change to fulfill those needs.

Clinical nutrition helps individuals transition their dietary and lifestyle behaviors throughout life. Clinical nutritionists give patients information to help them choose and eat the right foods at the right times of their lives. This field is expanding and becoming a main contributor of scientific advancements related to aging and diet.

I discuss how nutritional needs change throughout life in Part IV. Head there to find details and suggestions for ensuring that your diet matches your nutritional needs.

Increasing Visibility (and Abbreviations) through Key Organizations

The dramatic rise in chronic diseases stemming from nutritional deficiencies and/or excesses, poor quality food supply, and other diet-related issues has spurred a flurry of research and outreach from a number of levels. Governmental, nongovernmental, academic, and international agencies have all joined the fight in combatting health risks by promoting wellness and disease prevention through lifestyle change and nutritional therapy. The following sections introduce you to a few of the different kinds of organizations involved. For a list of ten specific organizations combatting diet- and nutrition-related problems around the globe, head to Chapter 23.

Walking the hallowed halls: Clinical nutrition in academia

Globally, many colleges and universities now provide training and credentialing services for clinical nutrition sciences. This attention is prompted primarily by the increasing incidence of chronic diseases around the world and the number of clinical care facilities offering dietary services. These two primary driving factors create a demand for trained professionals who can provide those services.

Currently in the United States alone, scores of institutes of higher learning provide some type of degree or certificate in clinical nutrition sciences — a figure that doesn't include the colleges and universities that offer courses on the topic but don't provide credentials of training. If those institutions were included, the number of facilities offering education in the field would be in the hundreds.

Globally, thousands of institutes of higher learning may offer some type of training in the field of clinical nutrition. Although exact numbers aren't known, one thing is clear: In recent decades, clinical nutrition is becoming a more and more popular field.

When you choose a program, make sure you receive your training at facilities or institutions that are certified, endorsed, and/or accredited by professional organizations such as the following:

- **American Clinical Board of Nutrition (ACBN, www.acbn.org):** This organization establishes education, examination, experience, and ethics requirements for certification in the field of nutrition.

- **Academy of Nutrition and Dietetics (www.eatright.org):** Formerly known as the American Dietetic Association, this organization is committed to improving the nation's health and advancing the profession of dietetics through research, education, and advocacy. The organization empowers its members to become national and global nutrition leaders.

- **International & American Association of Clinical Nutritionists (IAACN, www.iaacn.org):** This organization aims to enrich the curriculum offered in clinical nutrition training programs through competency and practice. The IAACN helps establish education programs for clinical nutritionists in order to ensure the highest quality standards and processes for those who practice in the field.

- **International Nutrition Consultant Association (www.in-ca.org):** This body upholds professional standards in the field for practicing clinical nutritionists.

These governing bodies' strict guidelines regarding the quality of clinical nutrition education offered are intended to dissuade any unqualified entities from training future practitioners in the field. Sometimes, however, facilities that are not endorsed by these organizations offer very high-quality training but are new and in the process of being accredited; others are not worth the investment. Do your homework before entering a specific program!

Getting better: Clinical nutrition in healthcare settings

More and more clinical health facilities worldwide offer services designed to reconnect diet and health for their clients and patients. These facilities, a few of which I list here, offer services ranging from dietetic therapy to nutritional counseling:

✔ **Hospitals:** Hospitals employ clinical nutritionists to offer nutritional treatment for certain health issues on an in-patient basis (that is, to patients admitted to the hospital). These nutritionists use food and supplements to assist with a patient's therapy, based on the particular health concern.

✔ **Health clinics:** Health clinics offer access to nutritional counseling or to dietary supplements. This type of service is primarily provided on an out-patient basis.

✔ **Outreach programs:** These programs provide services that help clients navigate health systems for dietary treatment; they may offer free services for nutritional counseling, for example. Outreach programs also offer programs that improve access to fresh and safe sources of food for disadvantaged and needy populations.

Selling wellness: Clinical nutrition as a business

The private sector is also staking claim to the expanding interest in clinical nutrition sciences. Everywhere you look nowadays, you are likely to see advertisements selling the idea of the diet-health connection and claiming that a dream diet can help you achieve your ideal weight with minimal effort or that a dietary supplement can rid your body of toxins. You probably see ads for new medical practices that offer dietary services, as well as ads for health coaches, life coaches, and diet coaches who promise to help you become a healthier person through healthier eating. Even spas, resorts, community centers, and gyms often claim to have services that can reconnect you with the knowledge and tools to improve your health.

Do your homework to ensure you are getting the best quality from a qualified professional. Try these suggestions:

✔ Look for diplomas on the walls of the professionals providing advice and make sure the diplomas come from reputable universities or training facilities.

✔ Go online to find reviews written by the business's other clients or patients.

Make sure that you obtain information about nutrition and health from credible sources. Take special care with open-source information, like blogs and other sites that allow anyone with an opinion to state thoughts on any given topic without verification of facts. The easy flow of information gives you the opportunity to find information efficiently, but you must vet the information you find. Anyone can post material online, even content that is full of errors or misinformation.

✔ Ask about the business's accreditation. Is the professional organization that accredited the business reputable? Refer to the earlier section "Walking the hallowed halls: Clinical nutrition in academia" for a list of reputable organizations.

Affecting public policy: Governmental organizations

Governments are taking a more active role in helping their citizens eat healthier, gain better access to healthy foods, and live healthier lifestyles. In this section, I provide examples of governmental organizations from around the world that seek to address the nutrition needs of their respective populations.

USDA

Working with the First Lady of the United States Michelle Obama, the United States Department of Agriculture (USDA) introduced ChooseMyPlate.gov. The goal of this program is to help Americans make better, more informed choices about what they eat.

ChooseMyPlate, shown in Figure 1-1, was unveiled to take the place of MyPyramid, the pyramid-shaped food guide that most people found more confusing than helpful. The MyPlate graphic and the persuasive and educational messaging that accompanies it (head to `www.choosemyplate.gov` to see) aim to demonstrate not only what to eat, but also how much to eat.

National Institute for Health and Clinical Excellence

The National Institute for Health and Clinical Excellence (NICE), part of the U.K.'s National Health Service (NHS), seeks to promote good health and prevent diseases through evidence-based medicine. NICE puts forth an array of guidelines to help combat health issues stemming from improper nutrition. These guidelines — such as promoting breastfeeding to expectant and new mothers and offering ways to prevent stroke or decrease hypertension — set the standard for high-quality healthcare services while simultaneously promoting healthy living for a longer life.

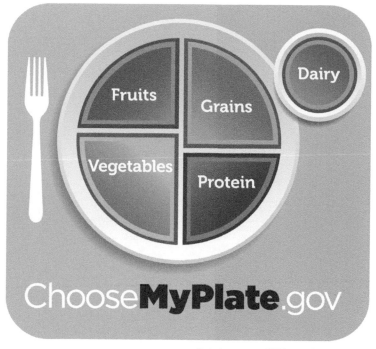

Figure 1-1:
Choose-
MyPlate
seeks to
simplify
healthy
eating
guidelines.

Illustration courtesy of USDA, www.choosemyplate.gov

Canadian Nutrition Society/la Societe canadienne de nutrition

The Canadian Nutrition Society/la Societe canadienne de nutrition (CNS/SCN) promotes health and preventative services through clinical nutrition science and continuing education programs. One primary objective of CNS/SCN is to integrate academic, clinical, private sector, and governmental agencies involved with dietetic education and nutritional counseling. One such effort is the Canadian Malnutrition Task Force (CMTF), which aims to improve nutrition care across the country to help all Canadians achieve optimal nutrition.

National Health and Medical Research Council

The Australian National Health and Medical Research Council (NHMRC) supports health and medical research used to develop health education and awareness campaigns across the country. A primary goal of NHMRC is to provide disease prevention and therapy through the use of healthy diets and exercise. The NHMRC provides an entire library of research and policy statements on health and wellness issues. For more information on NHMRC programs, be sure to check its website: http://www.nhmrc.gov.au/about/committees-nhmrc.

Chapter 2

Nutrition 101

Can eating to ensure a longer life and higher quality of life be as simple as A, B, C? Pretty much, yes. Despite the abundance of confusing and often misleading or incorrect information circulating in the media, the best diet is a basic, common-sense diet.

No magic bullet can guarantee that you will live longer or healthier. The key to building a healthy lifestyle is to ensure proper dietary habits. Fortunately, doing so isn't complicated. The formula is simple and easy.

In this chapter, I provide an overview of basic nutritional concepts and body functions related to how your body digests, transports, and uses nutrients. This information is vital to your understanding of major diseases and organ systems and of how proper nutrition is essential to a healthy, vibrant lifestyle. (For detailed discussions of the impact of nutrition on major diseases and organ systems, head to Parts II and III, respectively).

The ABCMVs of Eating

Here's a fact that many people have a hard time believing: Eating more like your ancestors did (fresh, seasonal varieties of fruits and vegetables, lean meats, whole grains, and yes, even saturated fats) is actually better for your health and well-being than dining on some power smoothie chock-full of synthetic vitamins. (Apparently Mom and Grandma really did know best!)

Research and current thinking indicate that individuals need to adopt such a diet in order to produce positive health outcomes. I delve more into that topic in Part II, which is devoted to the link between diet and disease, and Part III, which covers the connection between nutrition and the function of major body systems. Here, I start with the basics.

Most of the time, the simplest food is also the healthiest. For example, are hard-boiled eggs a better source of fat and protein for you than a synthetic protein powder blend with some form of hydrogenated oil? You betcha.

Introducing a common-sense diet

The answer to living longer and healthier is actually as simple as A, B, C, with a couple of other letters thrown in:

- **Adequacy:** Are you getting sufficient vitamins and minerals from your food? The key here is to eat foods that are packed with nutrients rather than foods that offer nothing other than empty calories. An easy way to do this is to eat colorful fruits and vegetables, whole grains, and lean meat.

- **Balance:** Are you getting enough food from each food group? For most of your meals, you want to have more vegetables and fruits on your plate than any other type of food, such as bread, meat, or dairy.

- **Calorie control:** Are you consuming the right amount of calories — not too many or too few — per day? A great way to control calories is to limit the amount of high-sugar and high-fat foods you eat, like soft drinks, candy, cookies, and other baked goods.

- **Moderation:** Are you sure that you're not getting too much of one thing over another? When it comes to moderation, you also want to limit the amount of highly processed food you eat, like fried snack foods, fast food, and prepackaged prepared meals.

- **Variety:** Are you eating a varied diet and not the same thing over and over again? Try eating something different for breakfast, lunch, and dinner every day. Don't be hesitant to eat something you never tried before. Remember: Variety is the spice of life!

If you can answer "yes" to the preceding questions, your diet is probably one that gives you the nourishment necessary to help prevent illness and early death. That's it. Nothing spectacular. No pills. No bells. No whistles. Just plain, old-fashioned common sense.

Be wary of any product or regimen that guarantees you can live a longer, healthier life by taking a pill or supplement alone. The key to living longer and living healthier is a healthy diet and a lifestyle that incorporates regular exercise and refrains from tobacco use, alcohol abuse, or any other risky behavior.

Well, don't I have egg on my face!

You've probably heard plenty of tall tales on what you need to eat to live long and prosper. Take for, example, the information you've probably heard about eggs:

✔ **Myth:** The well-meaning but misguided mandate says that you shouldn't eat eggs because of all the cholesterol and saturated fat they have; after all, we've known since the 1960s that saturated fat and cholesterol are the heart's main enemies.

✔ **Fact:** True, eggs do contain cholesterol and saturated fat. It's also true that both can be bad for your heart. But that doesn't mean

that you need to cut out any and all amounts of fat or cholesterol in your diet. And eggs, eaten in moderation — say one small egg a day — are actually *good* for you.

The fact is that you can eat foods containing saturated fat and cholesterol and still be healthy. The key is controlling how much you're eating. Later in this chapter, I explain how you can have the foods you like, including eggs and other foods higher in saturated fats and cholesterol, and not have to worry so much.

Determining whether your diet is adequate

In the context of diets and nutrition, *adequacy* essentially means that your food choices provide all the essential nutrients, calories, and other mainstays of a healthy diet, including fiber and water. In other words, are you getting what you need from your diet to maintain a healthy lifestyle?

What's important to note about adequacy is that not everyone has the same nutritional demands. What is adequate for one person is not necessarily adequate for another. Usually gender, age, activity level, and body composition determine individual adequacy levels. Part IV explains the varying nutritional needs at different stages in life. For general guidelines for the average adult, see Table 2-1.

Table 2-1	Nutritional Needs for the Average Adult
Nutrient	*Percentage of Daily Diet*
Protein	15–20%
Fat	25–30%
Carbohydrates	50–60%
Water	Men: 3 liters (13 cups) per day Women: 2.2 liters (9 cups) per day

To determine whether your diet is adequate, simply track what you eat over the course of a week; then break down your meals into the main nutrient categories (carbohydrates, fats, proteins, vitamins, minerals; see the later section "Knowing Your Nutrients" for details). Also keep track of how much water you drink.

To help you track your food intake, try one of the following strategies:

✔ Look up the items on a database. The USDA National Nutrient Database at `http://ndb.nal.usda.gov/` is a good place to start.

✔ Create a profile in the SuperTracker section of the MyPlate website (`http://www.choosemyplate.gov/`).

If you see that you are consistently getting too much or too little of one of those categories, your diet may be inadequate.

Balancing your diet

Usually, the more variety in the foods you eat, the more balanced your diet will be. By eating a balanced diet, you ensure that you get the appropriate amounts of nutrients in the right proportion. Doing so allows for optimum health outcomes and helps you avoid any type of toxicity (too much) or deficiency (too little) of one type of nutrient or another.

The term *balance* also relates to variety, in the sense that you should balance your diet according to a nutritional guideline. Varying guidelines exist, and each gives you a sense of what you should be eating and in what amount in order to achieve balance. Many nations, including the following, have some form of governmental guideline for their citizens to follow:

✔ **MyPlate (United States):** `http://www.choosemyplate.gov/food-groups/`

✔ **Food for Health (Australia):** `http://www.nhmrc.gov.au`

✔ **Health Canada's Food Guide (Canada):** `http://www.hc-sc.gc.ca/fn-an/index-eng.php`

✔ **Food-Based Dietary Guidelines (European Union):** `http://www.fao.org/ag/humannutrition/nutritioneducation/fbdg/en/`

If not, the United Nations provides some dietary recommendations for select countries on each continent via its Food and Agriculture Organization's (FAO) Agriculture and Consumer Protection Department. Go to `http://www.fao.org/food/en/`.

In the context of ABCMV (refer to the earlier section "Introducing a common-sense diet"), eating a balanced diet ensures that the types of foods you eat are in balance, and it safeguards you from having too much of one nutrient over others. Many dietary guidelines and professional recommendations go beyond this and state that you shouldn't eat too much (overconsume) fat, sugar, and/or alcohol. They suggest you eat these foods in moderation.

Keeping caloric intake in check

Your recommended caloric intake is dependent upon your sex, age, and level of activity or exercise. For example, a healthy male in his 20s who exercises ten hours a week requires a higher caloric intake than an elderly female who is bedridden.

Depending on what your health goals are (weight gain, weight loss, or maintaining your current weight), you need to adjust your energy consumption and expenditure to achieve that goal. Monitoring how much you're eating, what you're eating, and how much physical activity you get in a given day is important to maintain optimum health. Use this equation to estimate how many calories you should be consuming in a given day and to determine whether you need to adjust how much you're eating:

> Energy In (calories consumed) – Energy Out (calories expended) =
>   Change in energy stores (excess/loss/equilibrium)

If you end up with a value above 0, you are eating more energy than you are burning, which means that you are building up energy in your body and thus gaining weight. If the value is below 0, you are burning more energy than you are consuming, and you are losing weight. If the value is at 0, you are neither building up energy nor losing it. You reached an energy equilibrium, which is how you maintain your current weight.

Here are some tips to help you figure out how many calories you consume:

- ✔ **Look on the food label and count them up.** If there is no food label, use this website to help keep track of the energy you eat per day: `http://foodcaloriescounter.com/`.

- ✔ **To measure energy out, a general rule is to take your body weight in pounds and multiply it by 12.** That product is approximately the number of calories your body burns in a given day from your basal metabolic rate, assuming a moderate amount of physical activity.

Your basal metabolic rate is simply the amount of energy your body burns to fuel its processes (breathing, blood circulation, digestion, temperature regulation, and so on) when you are at rest.

The Energy In (calories consumed) and Energy Out (calories expended) values are dependent on very important demographic variables such as age, exercise level, gender, and daily physical demands. Remember, not everyone needs the same amount of calories per day.

Many people struggle with maintaining a healthy weight, and one of the main reasons is excess calories (the Energy In component of the equation). Here are a few things to watch out for to avoid eating too many calories:

- Snacking while watching television
- Eating too many high-fat foods
- Consuming too much sugar in soft drinks

Following the "everything in moderation" rule

To avoid excesses or shortages not only in caloric intake but also in nutritional levels, the rule is to do everything in moderation. When you do things in moderation, you avoid excess or extremes. Dietary moderation refers most commonly to moderating the consumption of sinful culinary pleasures like sugar, salt/sodium, fat, and alcohol. The focus on these items in particular is due to the fact that chronic overindulgence in any of them can result in adverse health outcomes, including obesity, high blood pressure, and other health issues.

Spicing up your life with variety

The world we live in provides a bountiful harvest of foods to eat. Yet, even though literally tens of thousands of foods are available, people usually confine themselves to eating no more than maybe a hundred or so, and the diets of the vast majority of people are created from about 20 or fewer of all the items available.

If you sit down and tally what *you* eat, you'd probably be surprised at the simplicity of your own diet. Think about it. What do you normally eat? Chicken, beef, and/or pork? Wheat, rice, soy, and/or corn? A few other fruits and vegetables? Perhaps some fish?

People's diets tend to be very plain and boring. Chances are you know at least one person, maybe a few (maybe even you), who goes to a restaurant and orders the same thing or makes the same meals time and time again at home. Perhaps Tuesday night is pot roast night, and Friday night is pizza or take-out Chinese night.

But opting to put different condiments on a pot roast isn't really diversifying your diet. To change things up, add something truly different. Try a new protein source, opt for fruits and vegetables you don't generally eat, experiment with new-to-you herbs and spices. In addition to your pot-roast-and-potato mainstay, for example, go for the tilapia with creamed kale or roasted duck with mango salsa once in a while. *That's* diversity.

People often opt for a non-diverse diet because of convenience and familiarity. Whipping up something familiar for dinner is less time-consuming, and choosing the same things when you eat out eliminates the possibility of being disappointed in your selection. Yet your diet's diversity depends on the availability of exotic foods and your willingness (and ability) to add them to your dinner plate. By varying the foods you eat, you ensure that you're getting the appropriate amount of nutrients from your food source.

A quick and easy way to broaden your dietary regimen is to try something different — a new food you've never had before or a menu selection you don't generally make — for each meal for a week. For example, eat some star fruit (found in most grocery stores) with oatmeal in the morning instead of strawberries. Or for lunch, opt for the grilled vegetable panini with a side salad instead of the usual burger and fries. For dinner, go ahead and eat a vegetable you may have distanced yourself from when you were a child. You still may not like it after all these years, but you may get lucky and discover your next favorite food!

Knowing Your Nutrients

Nutrients are chemical compositions that your body uses as building blocks in order to function properly. You need nutrients to breathe, to smile, to watch television — to live healthily and well. Nutrients fall into several classes:

- **Proteins:** Proteins are an organic energy source, and they provide the raw materials necessary to build body tissues, such as muscles and organs.

    Four out of the six types of nutrients — proteins, fats, carbs, and vitamins — are organic compounds, meaning they contain the element carbon and are derived from living things.

- **Fats:** Fats are another source of energy for the body. This organic compound helps with many different functions in the body, including vitamin absorption, hormone production, and normal cell functioning.

- ✔ **Carbohydrates:** Carbs are the primary source of energy for most organisms. This organic compound is essential for normal brain and gastrointestinal activity and functioning.

- ✔ **Vitamins:** The fourth and final organic nutrient, vitamins are vital to a large number of bodily functions. Needed in small amounts, they are found in almost all whole foods you eat.

- ✔ **Minerals:** Solid, inorganic compounds found in most of the foods you consume, minerals are crucial to basic body functions. The range of processes that minerals help regulate and maintain is nearly endless.

- ✔ **Water:** *The* nutrient, the giver and sustainer of life, water is a fundamental element of all foods you eat, and it is the most important nutrient. The majority of the foods you eat are mostly made of water, you are constantly in need of water due to its continuous excretion, and your body is always looking to replace lost water.

You obtain the majority of your nutrients from the foods you eat, but your body can manufacture some as well. For example, your body can create human proteins from the plant or animal amino acids you consume during dinner, and it can create fatty acid chains from an excess of glucose (a building block of carbohydrates) in your diet. Nutrients that you must get from your food because your body cannot manufacture them are called *essential nutrients,* which I explain in more detail in the later section "Examining the essentials — essential nutrients, that is."

Energizing nutrients: Proteins, carbs, and fats

Every single thing you do (walk, laugh, or pick up sticks) or your body does without your direction (breath, regulate internal temperature, and so on) requires energy, and that energy comes from certain food sources: carbohydrates, fats, and proteins. In other words, the energy required for you to read these words came from the bacon and eggs you may have eaten this morning for breakfast; this energy allows you to open this book, turn the pages, read the text, and comprehend the material.

All carbs are just chains of glucose molecules held together by chemical bonds. When those bonds are broken down by digestion, they release energy, called *food energy.* Fats (three fatty acid chains connected into a triglyceride), proteins (chains of amino acids connected by peptide bonds), and carbs all have this property; thus, they are the *energy nutrients*. Here are the things you need to know about these nutrients:

- Carbs should supply 50 percent to 60 percent of your daily caloric needs, by far the largest supplier. Fats are the next highest supplier of energy for a healthy diet; they should provide approximately 25 percent to 30 percent of your daily energy needs. Proteins are the lowest supplier and should provide around 15 percent to 20 percent of your needed daily calories.

- A diverse and balanced diet provides a rich source of energy from foods like wheat (carbs), beef (protein), cheese (protein and fat), and so on. Having too much of one source is unhealthy and can pose adverse health problems in the future.

- When you eat too much energy, your body stores it as fat. Even fat-free foods may be high in calories (think of soft drinks) and can contribute to weight gain if you eat them in excess. Refer to the earlier section "Keeping caloric intake in check" and the formula for caloric intake and expenditure for information about keeping your body weight stabilized. Bottom line: Try not to overconsume energy nutrients.

You may have heard, or perhaps believe, that vitamins, particularly the B vitamins, are a good source of energy. Don't believe the hype. Many energy supplements claim that they can give you hours and hours of "natural" energy via B vitamins. The problem is that B vitamins *metabolize* energy; they don't *provide* energy. If you don't eat energy nutrients (carbs, fats, and proteins), the B vitamins do little to give you that boost you paid for.

Aiding in body function: Vitamins and minerals

Vitamins and minerals act as managers of the body by aiding in pretty much every function your body performs, such as tissue formation, muscle movement, digestion, waste excretion, and more. They are not, however, a source of energy for the body, as I explain in the preceding section.

Vitamins and minerals are present in almost every food in varying proportions, and you must eat a diverse diet to obtain the appropriate amount of these nutrients.

Distinguishing between water-soluble and fat-soluble vitamins

Vitamins come in two classifications:

- ✔ **Water-soluble (vitamins B and C):** With water-soluble vitamins, your body metabolizes what it needs, and then you urinate the rest out. Because your body doesn't store these vitamins in any large capacity, toxicity is rare. However, because your body easily excretes water-soluble vitamins, you have to make sure you get enough in your diet.

  The exception is vitamin B$_6$, which your body does not excrete as easily. Be careful not to exceed the upper limit of this nutrient.

- ✔ **Fat-soluble (vitamins A, D, E, and K):** Fat-soluble vitamins are stored in the liver and fatty tissues and are not as easily excreted by the body as water-soluble vitamins. For these reasons, taking supplements is not necessary unless your doctor directs you to do so. If you're not careful about how much of the fat-soluble vitamins you are ingesting, they can become toxic.

  You need fat in your diet to metabolize fat-soluble vitamins. If you take a supplement and eat fat-free foods, you're wasting your money because your body won't be able to use those expensive fat-soluble vitamin supplements.

Understanding what a precursor vitamin is

Some vitamins are *precursor* vitamins; think of them as "raw material" vitamins. Just as crude oil must be refined into the gasoline/petrol that powers your motor vehicle, precursor vitamins must be refined into *active vitamins* that your body can use.

Any fruit or vegetable you consume contains a good amount of precursors. Examples of inactive precursor vitamins include the following:

- ✔ **Beta-carotene:** Beta-carotene makes a carrot orange and is a precursor form of vitamin A (no plant food contains an active form of vitamin A). When you eat a carrot, the beta-carotene is activated by the liver into a usable form of vitamin A, which is then utilized by your eyes to ensure healthy retina and cornea functioning.

- ✔ **Subcutaneous cholesterol:** Cholesterol in skin transforms into precursor vitamin D when ultraviolet rays hit your skin. The inactive precursor vitamin D then travels to the liver and kidneys to become activated.

- ✔ **Tryptophan:** Tryptophan is an amino acid found in eggs, fish, or — my favorite — turkey. It is a precursor form of niacin, a B vitamin, or it can be converted to serotonin, a neurotransmitter with a calming effect.

Vitamins don't cure diseases (other than diseases caused by vitamin deficiencies, of course). For example, drinking orange juice to obtain vitamin C won't cure a cold. The vitamin C may assist in healthy immune-system functioning, but the vitamin alone doesn't cure the disease. On the other hand, drinking orange juice does help cure scurvy, a disease caused by the lack of vitamin C.

Minding your minerals

Minerals — solid, inorganic compounds found in food — are crucial to basic body functions and make up about 5 pounds (2.27 kilograms) of your body weight. The majority of your body's minerals lies in your bones and consists of calcium and phosphorus. Here are the details on these and other key minerals:

- **Calcium:** Found in milk and dairy products and leafy, green vegetables, calcium is crucial for bone development, blood vessel health, and brain activity.

- **Phosphorus:** Found in dairy products, beans, and various fruits and vegetables, phosphorus assists with bone and teeth development, DNA/ RNA health, and blood lipid creation.

- **Potassium:** Found in sources such as honeydew melons, citrus fruits, potatoes, and bananas, this mineral is central to healthy cell functioning and blood pressure regulation.

- **Sodium:** By balancing fluids in the body and assisting in proper sensory nerve and muscle contraction functioning, sodium is highly influential on raising blood pressure. Because salt is the major source of sodium, you must be careful not to overconsume high-salt foods.

- **Sulfur:** Used for treating skin conditions and essential for amino acid manufacturing, this mineral is found in eggs, onions, garlic, and cabbage.

- **Chloride:** Chloride is crucial for digestion, serving as a fundamental element in the creation of stomach acid. It's found in salt, tomatoes, lettuce, celery, and other vegetables.

- **Magnesium:** Essential in metabolism and blood pressure regulation, magnesium is found in whole grains and beans.

The *minor* (or *trace*) minerals consist of iron, zinc, manganese, iodine, copper, and selenium. (Your body is made up of other minerals, as well, but they are in minute amounts.) Each mineral has a specific role to play in the proper functioning of your body. To ensure that you get the right amount of minerals, eat a balanced diet.

As with all nutrients, you must be keenly aware of the risks associated with having too much (toxicity) or too little (deficiency) of a particular mineral. Some common and serious adverse health outcomes resulting from mineral deficiency or toxicity include the following:

 ✔ **Calcium deficiency — osteoporosis:** Reduced bone mineral density leading to increased risk of fractures and falls

 Young women (teenagers to women in their 30s) should get plenty of calcium to lessen the risk of adult bone loss (osteoporosis) later in life. Unfortunately, many young women are unaware that they need adequate amounts of calcium while they are younger to avoid major bone issues when they reach menopause.

 ✔ **High sodium intake — hypertension:** High blood pressure, which increases risk of heart disease

 ✔ **Iodine deficiency — goiter:** Enlargement of the thyroid gland and possibly hyperthyroidism

 ✔ **Iron deficiency — anemia:** A decrease in red blood cells and/or hemoglobin in the blood, which can lead to extreme fatigue, pale skin, and chronic body chills

Water: The most important nutrient

Thirsty? Grab a cold one. That's right. A nice, tall, cold glass of water. Water is *the* nutrient of all nutrients. You need it to live. Water is so essential that you can't live much more than three days without it. You can live for a month or so without food but not even a week without water.

Other than slaking thirst, your body needs water to perform these functions:

 ✔ Regulate body temperature

 ✔ Cushion the joints (knee, shoulder, elbow, and so on)

 ✔ Remove bodily waste

 ✔ Protect your spinal cord

How much water you need depends on your activity level, your age, and what you're eating. Ideally, in a given day, you should drink the same amount of water that you lose. Figuring out precisely how much that is is pretty difficult, given that you lose water in many different ways. You even lose water when you exhale! As a general rule, if you drink a glass or two of water with every meal, you'll be fine.

The most obvious way to get the water you need is to drink it. However, you also get water from the foods you eat. That apple you may have eaten for lunch is mostly water. And that bottle of soda you drank last night is mostly carbonated water. You even get water from the turkey sandwich you may be eating right now reading this book.

Having a diet full of fruits and vegetables, drinking water with your meals, and making sure to drink water before, during, and especially after exercising ensures you're staying hydrated! One way to tell that you're staying adequately hydrated is to look at the color of your urine. It should be a pale yellow color. If it's dark yellow, increase your water intake.

Make sure you drink enough fluids throughout the day. Dehydration can lead to many health problems, like dizziness and exhaustion, but if it's persistent, it can lead to kidney failure, coma, and death. Also keep this in mind: When you feel thirsty, you're already dehydrated. So get drinking!

Examining the essentials — essential nutrients, that is

An *essential nutrient* is a nutrient that the body cannot process and therefore must obtain from an external source (that is, your diet). The six nutrient classes (carbohydrates, fats, proteins, vitamins, minerals, and water) all include, or are themselves, essential nutrients.

Here's a list of some essential nutrients and, where appropriate, the classes they come from:

- ✔ Glucose, from the carbohydrate class

- ✔ Omega-3 (from fish oil, for example) and omega-6 (from vegetable oil), from the fats class

- ✔ Nine out of the 22 primary amino acids (valine, lysine, leucine, tryptophan, and so on), from the proteins class

- ✔ Various vitamins from both water- and fat-soluble classes

- ✔ All minerals

- ✔ Water (of course)

Sometimes a nonessential amino acid can act as an essential amino acid when your diet is lacking in some regard or your body cannot process the essential amino acid. This amino acid is then called a *conditionally essential*, or *conditional*, amino acid. For example, if your diet is low on phenylalanine (an essential amino acid) or you are diagnosed with phenylketonuria (an inherited disease where your body cannot process phenylalanine), tyrosine (a nonessential amino acid) becomes an essential amino acid because the body makes tyrosine from phenylalanine, meaning you would then need to obtain it from your diet.

Exploring Nutrient Mobility and Use

Your gastrointestinal/digestive system (mouth, esophagus, stomach, intestines, colon, pancreas, and so on) is the main mechanism that breaks down and absorbs nutrients. From your saliva to your rectum, your digestive system continually transforms proteins, carbohydrates, fats, and all the other nutrients into usable elements.

Your body employs a number of methods to break down the minerals for use. Which method it uses depends on the "toughness" of the nutrient:

- **Carbs:** Carbohydrates are the easiest nutrient for your body to break down. Glucose (the building block of carbs) starts to break down in your mouth from your saliva.

- **Amino acids:** Amino acids (proteins) are broken down in your stomach. The peptide bonds that hold amino acid chains together are strong, and saliva is no match for them. You need stomach acid to break those up.

Stomach (gastric) acid has a pH of 1.5 to 3.5 and is primarily made up of hydrochloric acid — which is one reason why heartburn is so uncomfortable. Imagine how painful dumping acid on your hand would be. That's what your esophagus feels like when gastric acid is refluxed into it. If the reflux persists over a few years, you run the risk of developing some very serious adverse health outcomes, including cancer.

- **Fats, vitamins, minerals, and water:** Fats are broken down and absorbed in your small intestine, as are vitamins, minerals, and water. Your liver is an essential tool in fat digestion because it secretes bile to assist in breaking down fats. They, along with vitamins, minerals, and water, are then absorbed through your intestinal walls into the bloodstream for transport to your cells.

Chapter 3

Determining Whether You're Eating Correctly

*A*s you begin to understand the influence of nutrition in health outcomes (either good or bad), you also begin to understand that knowing what foods are healthy for you can be confusing. Further, determining how much of any particular food to eat on a given day to ensure proper nutrition can be even more daunting. Although these tasks are difficult, they're not impossible.

As I explain in Chapter 2, the ABCMVs of nutrition can help you understand *how* you should be eating. However, the question of *what* you should be eating and *how much* is a bit more specific. Quite a bit of research has been done — and continues to be done — in this area to help people make the best dietary decisions for the best health outcomes. In addition, nutrition research organizations and governments around the world have published guidelines to help their citizens choose appropriate foods.

In this chapter, you discover some universal nutritional guidelines to help you choose a healthy diet. This chapter also introduces to you some international nutritional policy organizations that are instrumental in developing and cheerleading some of these guidelines. Finally, I provide some tips and tricks on how to investigate what foods are best for you to eat.

The Dietary Reference Intakes: An Alphabet Soup of Recommendations

The *dietary reference intakes (DRI)* are the standards used in the United States and Canada to assist in nutritional planning; these standards outline recommendations regarding how many calories (energy intake), how many and what kinds of nutrients, and how much water an average person needs to ingest daily.

A committee of nutrition experts — consider it the DRI Committee — establishes the DRI and consists of clinicians and health professionals who use clinical studies in nutrition to provide the goal values for fats, carbohydrates, water, proteins, vitamins, minerals, and energy expenditure. The committee's recommendations tell you how much of each type of nutrient a person needs daily, based on the amount of energy that person expends, and these values are based on scientific studies.

Four lists of values make up the core of the DRI, which you can read more about in the following sections:

- ✔ **Recommended dietary allowances (RDA) and adequate intakes (AI):** These guidelines set recommended intake values of nutrients that people should get from their diets. These recommendations satisfy the needs of 97.5 percent of healthy individuals.

- ✔ **Estimated average requirements (EAR):** These guidelines set nutritional policies at local, state, and federal levels that would satisfy 50 percent of healthy individuals.

- ✔ **Estimated energy requirements (EER):** These requirements indicate the number of calories you must consume to maintain your current weight.

- ✔ **Upper Intake levels (UI):** These guidelines determine nutritional safety and indicate the highest amount that can be ingested daily without causing side effects.

The purpose of these lists is to provide accurate guidelines and responsible goals to help individuals achieve optimum health status, to define limits of safety for dietary intake, and to prevent chronic disease.

The units used for the dietary reference intakes guidelines are International Units (IU) and milligrams (mg). Some nutrients are more commonly expressed as either one or the other. You can find more information on IUs at the following website: http://nutritionovereasy.com/2011/08/how-much-is-an-international-unit/.

The RDA: Setting recommended intake values

The *recommended dietary allowance (RDA)* is the amount of a nutrient that meets the needs of 97.5 percent of all healthy individuals within a group of people. Why aren't these recommendations good for 100 percent of the population? Because some individuals may need more or less, depending on their specific medical needs or issues. The general guidelines, for example, aren't suitable for someone on an elemental diet (a form of strict nutritional therapy).

Here are some things to keep in mind about RDAs:

- ✔ The RDA is the official recommendation the DRI Committee sets for the population. These values are defined after rigorous experiments and are the values that the vast majority of the population should follow to help ensure optimum health.

- ✔ RDAs are the foundational information that Americans can use to guide their nutrient intake. All the other recommendations about what nutrients you should eat and in what amounts stem from the RDAs. These guidelines encourage healthy outcomes by giving individuals the information they need to establish responsible dietary patterns.

- ✔ An established RDA is a generous value, covering almost all individuals in a population with enough of a given nutrient to prevent deficiency diseases. Not everyone needs as much of a nutrient as the RDA specifies, but the human body does a fantastic job at managing the excesses to prevent toxicity issues. (Refer to Chapter 2 for more on the differences between water- and fat-soluble vitamins and minerals and the risks associated with toxicity.)

Looking at how the values are derived: EARs

The RDA values don't just appear out of nowhere. They are based on rigorous scientific research and experiments that help researchers determine what daily intake level is safe and healthy.

In the quest to establish a specific RDA, the DRI Committee conducts numerous experiments on a nutrient, and the results from each of these preliminary experiments establish an estimated average requirement (EAR) value for that nutrient. An *EAR* is the average daily intake of a nutrient that meets the nutritional needs of half the individuals in the group.

The EAR value is temporary because the available information isn't strong or because it isn't reliable enough to define the actual RDA. Along the way to developing RDAs, a series of adequate intake (AI) values are defined with the assistance of determined EARs; an AI serves as a temporary guideline from which to suggest daily allowances of specific nutrients. Only when scientists feel comfortable with the existing evidence do they formally define RDAs.

Just like the RDA, the EAR is expected to meet or exceed the nutritional needs of almost everyone in the group. However, the EAR is an estimate based on preliminary experiments and is not a defined calculation, as is the RDA. In other words, EARs serve as recommendations until nutrition experts feel comfortable that the level of evidence is strong enough to establish the RDA.

In addition to helping establish the RDA, EARs also provide nutritional guidance to subgroups in a population. Subgroups are clusters of people who, although part of a larger population, are defined by some unique characteristic, usually a demographic identifier, like sex, race, age, or ethnicity. For example, the DRI Committee establishes EARs for different age groups (seniors or teenagers, for example) or racial or ethnic groups (white, black, Asian, or Hispanic). Other EARs are produced for other subgroups.

Estimated energy requirements (EERs): Monitoring your energy intake

You need a certain amount of calories per day to encourage the best possible health outcomes, and the *estimated energy requirements (EER)* are guidelines that indicate how many calories (energy) an individual should consume. The purpose of EERs is to help individuals not overconsume calories and to discourage improper weight gain. Table 3-1 lists EERs for 30-year-old men and women, based on their activity level.

Table 3-1	Estimated Energy Requirements for Men and Women 30 Years of Age				
Height (inches)	**Physical Activity Level**	**Men (kcal/day)**		**Women (kcal/day)**	
		BMI of 18.5	**BMI of 24.99**	**BMI of 18.5**	**BMI of 24.99**
59	Sedentary	~1,850	~2,080	~1,625	~1,760
	Low activity	~2,010	~2,270	~1,805	~1,955
	Active	~2,215	~2,505	~2,025	~2,200
	Very active	~2,555	~2,900	~2,290	~2,490

Height (inches)	Physical Activity Level	Men (kcal/day)		Women (kcal/day)	
		BMI of 18.5	BMI of 24.99	BMI of 18.5	BMI of 24.99
65	Sedentary	~2,070	~2,350	~1,815	~1,980
	Low activity	~2,254	~2,565	~2,015	~2,200
	Active	~2,490	~2,840	~2,270	~2,480
	Very active	~2,880	~3,300	~2,570	~2,810
71	Sedentary	~2,300	~2,635	~2,015	~2,210
	Low activity	~2,515	~2,885	~2,240	~2,460
	Active	~2,780	~3,200	~2,519	~2,770
	Very active	~3,225	~3,720	~2,855	~3,140

Source: Food and Nutrition Board, Institute of Medicine, National Academies

As I note earlier, RDAs of vitamins and minerals can be generous because your body has a way to remove excess amounts through excretion. Energy intake recommendations, on the other hand, cannot be generous because the body doesn't have an easy way to get rid of excess calories. In fact, the primary way to remove excess energy is to exercise more — an act that many people are loathe to do. For that reason, people have to be careful about how much they consume.

Factors like gender, age, and activity level impact the optimum number of calories a person consumes in a day. To determine how many calories you should eat in a given day, you need to factor in your height, your weight, your age, your activity level, and any medical conditions that you may have. Although the EER is set up for the average man or the average woman, the amount of calories that you need in a given day is specific to you, based on the listed criteria.

The foods you choose need to be primarily nutrient-dense, not energy-dense. In other words, you need to eat more fruits and vegetables (nutrient-dense) and less french fries (energy-dense). The good news, however, is that you can enjoy energy-dense food as part of a healthy diet.

The term *discretionary calories* refers to the energy you can consume daily in excess of the energy you need for healthy body function. Say, for example, that you need 2,000 calories a day per your EER; approximately 1,700 of those calories should come from nutrient-dense, lower energy-dense foods. But you have approximately 300 discretionary calories that you can consume from a range of different sources to fulfill your EER. You can choose a soft drink, pizza, celery, whatever. What you choose is up to you. As long as you don't go above your EER, which would cause you to gain weight, you can get your discretionary calories from any food source you like.

You can find more information on how to determine how many discretionary calories you should consume at the following website, which shows the section on discretionary calories in the USDA's publication *Nutrition and Your Health: Dietary Guidelines for Americans:* `http://www.health.gov/dietaryguidelines/dga2005/report/HTML/D3_DiscCalories.htm`.

For every 3,500 calories you consume in excess of your EER, you put on one pound of body weight. Add it up: A bottle of soda contains approximately 220 calories. If you consume five bottles a week in excess of your EER, you're consuming an extra 1,100 calories per week. If you continue at that rate, in less than a month, you may put on one pound of body fat just from extra soda consumption alone.

Upper intake levels (ULs): Determining nutritional safety

Upper intake levels (ULs) provide information on the maximum amount of a nutrient you should consume. If you consistently consume an amount of a given nutrient above the UL, toxicity of that nutrient can result.

Can there be a tolerable lower intake level? Sure. It's the value that represents the minimum amount of a nutrient you should consume. Consistently consuming an amount of a nutrient below this level can produce a deficiency disease.

Although ULs provide information about how much of a nutrient is safe to consume, keep in mind that gray areas between healthy levels and toxicities or deficiencies exist. In other words, these levels don't work like switches, in that once you get below or above the safety intake levels, you'll get sick immediately. Instead, individual tolerances to lower or higher intakes of a certain nutrient exist and can result in a variety of responses to over- or underconsumption of a nutrient. If both a child and a healthy adult eat above the recommended level of a certain nutrient, for example, the child's response would probably be different from the healthy adult's response because, as a group, children usually are a more vulnerable population.

When trying to understand RDAs and ULs, keep in mind that the response between healthy and unhealthy levels is definite, but gradual. You don't often experience an automatic or immediate adverse response as soon as you cross the threshold. Taking a view that is too simplistic can lead you to erroneously assume that you don't need to worry about regularly exceeding or going below the ULs. A better view is one that acknowledges a transition zone between safe and dangerous levels, as Figure 3-1 illustrates.

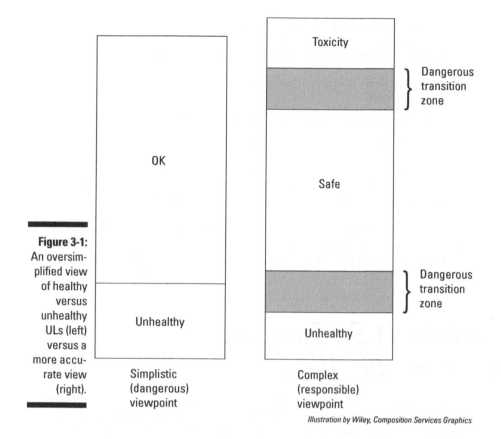

Illustration by Wiley, Composition Services Graphics

Figure 3-1:
An oversimplified view of healthy versus unhealthy ULs (left) versus a more accurate view (right).

Although the RDA is generous with nutrient levels, don't automatically assume you can consume as much as you want without the risk of adverse health outcomes resulting from that overconsumption. You really need to be careful with what and how much you put in your body. To be safe, consult with a physician on any major dietary change.

Acceptable macronutrient distribution ranges (AMDR): Preventing disease

The end goal of all these guidelines and recommendations is to make you healthier. Simple as that. In Chapter 4, I explain how chronic diseases are now becoming *pandemics* (worldwide epidemics, or outbreaks of diseases) and that the majority of these diseases stem from unhealthy behaviors, like tobacco use, alcohol abuse, unsafe sex, a lack of exercise, or, most pertinent to this book, improper nutrition. To combat this trend, the DRI Committee produces *acceptable macronutrient distribution ranges (AMDR)*.

The purpose of the AMDR values is to help prevent chronic disease by presenting lifelong nutritional goals of energy intake, including guidelines on daily carbohydrate, protein, and fat consumption. According to the AMDR,

- ✔ 45 percent to 65 percent of daily energy should come from carbohydrates
- ✔ 20 percent to 35 percent of daily energy should come from fats
- ✔ 10 percent to 35 percent of daily energy should come from proteins

If you follow the simple dietary guidelines outlined in the AMDR, your risk of becoming obese or developing diabetes, heart disease, and many other diseases linked with improper nutrition is dramatically reduced.

The values set by the DRI Committee are meant for healthy individuals only and are not applicable to people who need very specific dietary regimens. Those with special dietary needs should consult with a physician, who can help them determine what their individual guidelines should be.

Beyond the U.S.: Standards from around the World

A misconception of nutritional guidelines is that the majority stems from an internationally accepted or even U.S.-driven standard. For some nutrients, perhaps this is true, but other nations, particularly other Western nations — Australia, the U.K., Canada, the European Union, and so on — have their own unique approaches to presenting dietary recommendations for health and wellness. In this section, I outline some of these initiatives.

The European Food Safety Authority

In much the same way that the DRI Committee establishes RDAs for Americans and Canadians, the European Food Safety Authority (EFSA) establishes *dietary reference values (DRVs)* for the European community. The end goal is to produce healthier outcomes for EU citizens by providing scientifically sound research on what is good to eat and in what amount, and by whom it should be eaten.

The EFSA guidelines are similar to the American/Canadian DRI recommendations, with the main differences being the official labels given to the recommendations. For example, the DRI produces RDAs, while the EFSA produces DRVs.

The thing to remember about both RDAs and DRVS (and most other such recommendations) is that they apply to healthy individuals but don't apply to people who have specific health issues or special dietary needs — an approach that is the standard when making dietary recommendations meant to meet the needs of the majority of a population.

You can find more information on the EFSA at the European Food Safety Authority website: `http://www.efsa.europa.eu/en/topics/topic/drv.htm`.

Australia's Food for Health

Australia's Food for Health produced the *Dietary Guidelines for Australians* to provide tips and recommendations for how Aussies should be eating to promote optimum health outcomes. The guideline offers tips for adults and children on how to prevent unwanted weight gain and how to prepare food properly, as well as other helpful information on how to be healthier by eating and living well.

To get more specifics on each of these guidelines, along with many others, visit the National Health and Medical Research Council website at `http://www.nhmrc.gov.au/guidelines/publications/n55`.

The UN's World Health Organization

The World Health Organization (WHO) of the United Nations (UN) has a rich history on publishing guidelines for proper dietary intake. The WHO produces a wide range of information — from special issues on the prevention of chronic disease (you can see more about this topic in Chapter 4) to actual food-based dietary guidelines — for billions of people.

Because hunger and obesity are worldwide problems, the WHO's efforts are multinational and comprehensive and include guidelines on the following:

- Calcium and other supplementation in pregnant women
- Recommendations on wheat and corn flour fortifications
- Iron supplementation for school-age children
- Sodium intake for adults and children
- Protein-energy malnutrition for females and children

You can find the WHO guidelines on nutrition at this website: `http://www.who.int/publications/guidelines/nutrition/en/index.html`

Vetting Nutrition Information

You may be wondering why you need help determining what constitutes optimal nutrient and energy intakes. Chances are that, without the guidelines mentioned earlier in this chapter, you wouldn't know how much of any particular vitamin you should get in a given day or how much to recommend as a future dietary health professional to a client or patient.

Even if you did know how much to consume (if you'd taken an introductory nutrition class or researched the topic), you may wonder how trustworthy those recommendations are. After all, did you conduct a randomized controlled trial (the highest standard for clinical trials) to determine proper levels? Probably not. But the organizations and agencies that produce the guidelines do.

Whether you're pursuing a career as a clinical nutritionist or are just someone who wants to ensure you're eating a healthy diet, you need to know how to vet the information and guidelines you hear or read about. This info can come from a variety of sources, ranging from bulletins posted by governmental health agencies to the claims manufacturers make on their products. In this section, I tell you what things to pay attention to as you vet your sources of information.

Going to expert sources

We all search for advice from those who are more knowledgeable about a given topic or have more experience in a given situation. For example, do you know what prescription medication to take in what doses at which time for whatever ailment you have? Probably not. You rely on guidelines provided by physicians or pharmacists/chemists, whose advice you consider valid and reliable because of their professional training, education, and/or experience.

Similarly, there are experts in the field of nutrition, and reliable sources of nutrition information include college professors, researchers, and governmental agencies. Their expertise and research are trusted sources of nutrition information. Remember, no one knows everything, especially about proper nutrition. It's a collective endeavor.

Judging the quality of online information

Posting or publishing information on the Internet is relatively easy. Many times, health information posted on the web isn't based in evidence and/or it doesn't come from trusted sources who are qualified to provide such information. The problem is that thousands, perhaps millions, of people read — and too often make health decisions based on — these thoughts and opinions.

Trust only the information that comes from qualified physicians, health professionals, or governmental agencies. Here's how you can (usually) tell reliable online sources from unreliable ones:

- The post identifies the author of the work and lists recognized credentials.

- References are provided from peer-reviewed journals.

- Websites should end with .gov, .edu, or .org. These suffixes indicate that the site is the product of a governmental, educational, or institutional entity and is not simpy commercial.

- Look for financial claims, motivations, or relationships mentioned on the website or in any publications produced by the sponsor of the site. Usually, you can tell when the goal of the site is to sell something. One indication is the suffix .com. Although these sites may contain accurate information, be aware that the claims made often have a commerical bias tied to the business's financial interests.

Bottom line: Always check your sources of information regarding health and wellness advice or guidelines, especially if you find it online.

Evaluating the usefulness of the study findings

As you find nutritional information in magazines, books, and websites, or hear stories from friends and family, keep in mind that only information from evidence-based sources can be trusted and adopted. Use this list, arranged from most trustworthy to least trustworthy as a guide:

- **Randomized controlled trials:** In a randomized controlled trial, researchers experiment with different exposures (a nutrient; a certain risk factor, like nicotine; or any other element) to determine which one is the most responsible for producing a stated outcome or a certain health effect, such as a decrease in blood cholesterol, an increase in sodium levels, and so on.

  Most scientific disciplines use randomized controlled trials because they are the gold standard of scientific inquiry. A randomized controlled trial is the best way to conduct an experiment for these reasons:

  - The subjects are divided into two groups: one that receives the nutrient (or treatment) being tested, and one that doesn't. Having a comparison group allows the researchers to make accurate comparisons across the experimental groups.

- They use a random sample of subjects. Random test subjects eliminates most errors in sampling or measurement. By using random groups, the researchers ensure that the groups are identical in all ways except for the factors introduced during the study.

- ✔ **Cohort studies:** A study that compares two or more groups (cohorts) of participants, each of which differs on some exposure. The researchers follow the cohorts over time and make observations about the differences that occur in each cohort's specific outcomes (that is, wellness and/or disease status).

- ✔ **Case series and reports:** These look in depth at a particular health status or exposure report for a specific person (a case report) or small group of people (a case series).

- ✔ **Opinion:** An opinion is subjective piece of research commentary about a particular health topic or a set of data. Anyone can state an opinion: a world renowned nutrition expert or your Uncle Clyde.

As you can see, randomized controlled trials are the most-trusted sources, and opinions are the least-trusted sources.

Assessing Your Lifestyle Choices

Governments and health organizations around the world have put decades of research and tons of money into developing nutritional guidelines so that people can make dietary choices that will help them live longer, healthier lives. After you know what the guidelines are, it's up to you to read them and then (hopefully) follow them.

Simple, right? Not really. Barriers to following these recommendations exist and include the following major hurdles:

- ✔ **Money issues:** Sometimes fruits, vegetables, and healthier protein sources (lean meats, chicken, and seafood) are more expensive than more unhealthy foods, such as processed and convenience foods, like prepackaged meals and fast foods.

- ✔ **Lack of knowledge:** Perhaps you have no idea what foods have omega-3 fatty acids in them, for example, even though the guideline tells you to eat some daily. (By the way, foods that are high in omega-3s include salmon, mackerel, and flaxseed oils, which makes them a good place to start!)

- ✔ **Personal or cultural food preferences:** Individuals haven't acquired a taste for healthier foods as much as unhealthy ones. Your body evolutionarily learned to view salt, sugar, and fat — and foods that contain them — as delicacies. As a result, your body craves them, and cultures evolved around creating dishes made with them.

The reason your body craves sugar, salt, and fat and wants to eat as much of these foods as possible is because of its evolutionary drive to prepare for famine. These foods are very energy-dense, which is great for building body fat. Of course, back when these kinds of foods were luxuries — expensive to buy, time-consuming to make, and only occasionally available — and people expended much more energy in their everyday lives, sweets weren't a problem. Now, however, these foods are readily available, our lives are more sedentary, and, ironically, our busy schedules make planning *healthy* meals a greater challenge. Yet we still crave those salty, fatty, and sugary treats.

✔ **Personal challenges:** This obstacle is perhaps one of the most common. Many individuals lack the willpower to make changes, even though they want to eat a healthier diet; others lack the time to fully follow the guidelines. Changing the way you eat has a pretty steep learning curve. Until the information becomes second nature, meal planning, grocery shopping, and meal preparation all take more time and energy to incorporate into your life.

Whether you struggle to overcome any of these challenges yourself, know someone who wants to get healthy but is stuck, or are treating a patient whose ability to follow the guidelines is being undermined because of these difficulties, you can try or suggest a few simple tips and tricks, which I outline in this section.

Keeping track of your habits

Being able to change a behavior requires knowing what behaviors you want to change. Therefore, the first tip is to keep track of your habits. Here is a list of things you should pay attention to and write down:

✔ **When you get hungry, have an appetite, or just feel like eating:** Note the time (upon rising, mid-morning, and so on), as well as your mood. You may discover that your eating is triggered by more than actual hunger. Although you may be eating because you are really hungry, your urge to eat may be triggered because you're bored or stressed. Perhaps you simply want to eat because it's part of your routine; you always have lunch between 11:30 a.m. and 12:30 p.m, whether you're hungry or not, for example.

Your body tends to get hungry periodically throughout the day, usually when you wake up (perhaps 7 a.m.), around 1 p.m. to 2 p.m., and then again around 6 p.m. Notice that those are the times we normally associate with breakfast, lunch, and dinner. Of course, when you get hungry depends on your activity level throughout the day. If you are more active, you may get hungrier at earlier times. But when you are sedentary, bored, or both, be careful not to confuse lack of stimulation with feelings of hunger. You may just have an appetite and not actually be hungry. You need to learn the difference in how your body craves food and distinguish between when your body actually needs nourishment and when it's just bored and wants to snack.

✓ **What you eat:** You need to pay attention not only to when and how much you eat, but also to what you eat. What foods do you tend to gravitate toward? When you want a snack, what kind of food do you reach for? What generally makes it on your meal menu, both when you have time to prepare and when you're on the run and need to grab something quick?

Everyone falls into bad habits that undermine the ability to foster healthy outcomes, and bad habits related to food are particularly hard to break. Favorite foods, no matter how bad they may be for you, make you feel good (at least in the short run), taste delicious, help you fit into a group, and so on. In some cases, food preferences can even become an addiction.

All hope isn't lost, thankfully. You can break the cycle. The first thing to do to achieve any goal is recognize your limitations and acknowledge your habits. Doing so is a very good first step to overcoming your challenges. To find a detailed discussion on motivation and changing your attitude about healthy dieting, head to Chapter 19.

Giving yourself a bit of leeway

You don't have to have a militaristic mindset when following nutrition guidelines. They are exactly what they say they are: *guidelines!*

So go on, have a can of cola. Eat pizza with extra cheese. You want to have chips and cheese? Be my guest. Just don't eat too much or indulge too frequently. You can have a sense of healthy portions of fat and adjust your diet accordingly.

"Blasphemy!" you exclaim. "Nonsense!" I reply. Life would be completely boring without the flavor of fats, salt, and sugar. Enjoy them. But enjoy them responsibly.

And don't worry about measuring. Having to measure every milligram, ounce, liter, or teaspoon of your food is tedious, and quite frankly, utter misery. Success doesn't require that you ensure you get exactly one cup of vegetable matter at every meal. Just eat a nice, moderate portion of vegetables and have a little bowl of fruit with a meal, and you're fine.

Life isn't meant to be so rigid. It's meant to be fun, enjoyable, and tasty. So lighten up with that calculator and notepad full of dietary measurements. With enough training and discipline, you'll be able to manage a healthy diet without measuring too many items. It just takes practice with the guidelines.

Reading food labels

One skill you really do need to learn is to be able to read food labels. Figure 3-2 shows an example of a nutrition label. Follow these guidelines to make sense of the information:

✔ **Pay attention to the serving size and the number of servings per package.** The package may have multiple servings even though the calories, fat, and other nutrients listed are *per serving*. For example, if a serving has 40 calories, and the package includes four servings, you'll actually ingest 160 calories if you eat the entire package.

Be especially careful to look at number of servings in packages that seem to be single servings (a can of soda, for example, or small bag of chips). These often include more than one serving. Also be aware that some manufacturers use the confusion about serving sizes in a way that's less than forthcoming about how much fat, sodium, sugar, or calories a single serving contains. A bratwurst package, for example, may list a serving size as 2 ounces, even though a single link has 3 ounces.

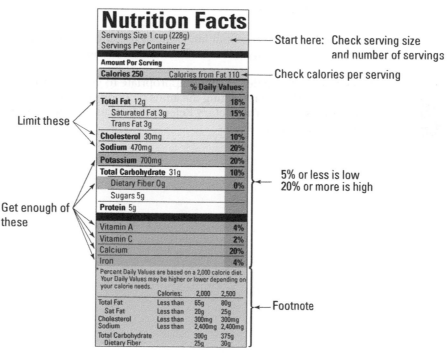

Figure 3-2: Reading a food label.

Illustration by Wiley, Composition Services Graphics

✔ **Food labels always list vitamins A and C, calcium, and iron.** In addition, the Daily Value amounts are determined for the normal, average, healthy human. Is that you? Talk to a physician to find out.

✔ **The ingredients are listed from largest to smallest in terms of weight by proportion.** For example, in a bag of pretzels, the first ingredient listed is probably some form of wheat product because wheat, by weight, is the primary ingredient in pretzels. You can bet that salt is the second or third ingredient. Use this information to check just how big a porportion the healthy ingredients are in a product. For example, if the first ingredients listed in something labeled "Fruit Snack" are sugars and refined flours, and fruit appears way, way down on the list, you know that the heathly ingredients don't count for much.

✔ **Watch out for hidden forms of sugar, salt, and fat.** These ingredients come in many guises and can make something seemingly healthy into something very unhealthy. Ingredients to be on the lookout for include

- Oils (fats)

- Sweeteners and anything that ends in *-ose,* like *glucose, sucrose, fructose,* and so on (all types of sugars)

- Sodium (salt)

In a nutshell, you want to limit fat, cholesterol, and sodium, and make sure you get enough carbohydrates and vitamins and minerals.

Always consult the guideline that is appropriate to your age, weight, and activity level to ensure that you're eating the kinds of foods you should be eating. Refer to the earlier section "The Dietary Reference Intakes: An Alphabet Soup of Recommendations" for details.

Chapter 4

The Grim Reality of Worldwide Wellness

In This Chapter

▶ Defining chronic disease

▶ Discussing global, nutrition-related health disparity issues

▶ Getting familiar with diets and supplements

*L*ike it or not, you live in a global society. But even before international communication, technology, travel, and finance became commonplace, researchers and people in general have always had a sense of the impact the spread of infectious diseases had on global health and wellness. From the bubonic plague pandemics of the Middle Ages to the smallpox eradication efforts of the 1970s to the HIV/AIDS pandemic of the last three decades, some attention has been paid throughout history to global health.

Most of the past discussions on global health have focused primarily on *infectious disease* (transmissible diseases resulting from an infection of a pathogen), not *chronic disease* (conditions that are usually non-transmissible and last longer than three months). Yet an interesting new twist is being unveiled in international health and wellness debates: mass increases in global chronic disease. Even more interesting is that many of these discussions focus around the notion that the rise in worldwide chronic disease often stems from improper nutrition and exercise.

In this chapter, I explain how, over the past century, the main causes of sickness and death in the world shifted from infectious diseases (pneumonia, influenza, infections, and so on) to chronic diseases (like cancer, obesity, and diabetes) and how diet and exercise are at the heart of this sea change in health and wellness. Finally, I discuss dieting as a response to this shift, introduce some popular diets, and tell you which ones to steer clear of.

From Infectious to Chronic Diseases: A Global Transformation

If you take a look at the top ten causes of death in 1900 in the United States, listed in Table 4-1, you can see that most were infectious diseases, like pneumonia and diphtheria; cancer came in eighth, and heart disease ranked fourth. In 2010, the leading two causes of deaths were heart disease (in first place) and cancer (second place), and influenza/pneumonia, which came in ninth place, was the only infectious disease on the list. This pattern is mimicked in most, if not all, other developed nations today and is becoming more and more evident in the developing world as well.

Table 4-1	Top Ten Leading Causes of Death in the U.S. in 1900 and 2010			
	1900		*2010*	
	Cause of Death	*Number per 100,000*	*Cause of Death*	*Number per 100,000*
1	Pneumonia or influenza	202.2	Heart disease	192.9
2	Tuberculosis	194.4	Cancer	185.9
3	Gastrointestinal infections	142.7	Chronic lower respiratory diseases, like COPD and bronchitis	44.6
4	Heart disease	137.4	Cerebrovascular disease	41.8
5	Cerebrovascular disease	106.9	Accidents	38.2
6	Kidney diseases	88.6	Alzheimer's disease	27.0
7	Accidents	72.3	Diabetes	22.3
8	Cancer	64.0	Kidney diseases	16.3
9	Senility	50.2	Pneumonia or influenza	16.2
10	Diphtheria	40.3	Suicide	12.2

Source: U.S. Centers for Disease Control and Prevention

Making the epidemiological transition

The term *epidemiological transition* refers to the phenomenon wherein the main health problems plaguing a society go from infectious to chronic disease. This phenomenon has three core concepts:

- During the transition, the primary source of *mortality* (death) and *morbidity* (sickness) in societies changes from infectious diseases to chronic diseases.

- As infectious diseases give way to chronic diseases, the primary source of diseases also changes. Whereas infectious diseases stem from pathogens (that is, bacteria, viruses, and parasites), chronic diseases stem from behaviors (poor nutrition, lack of exercise, tobacco use, and alcohol abuse).

- Each society will eventually make the transition, at least theoretically. Sometimes, chronic economic or social obstacles, like financial depressions or even wars, can prevent the long-term, sustained development of a nation, which would forestall the transition.

Observing the forces that drive the transition

The primary forces driving each society through the epidemiologic transition from infectious to chronic disease are technological, scientific, and industrial advancements, such as the following:

- Advances in mathematics and the sciences

- Advances in public sanitation and public works projects like roads and bridges

- Advances in transportation technologies, like high-speed rail and air travel.

These achievements, either directly or indirectly, spur medical and public health discoveries, which then lead to more effective treatments and prevention measures to help stem the burden of infectious diseases. Such advancements, for example, led to the discovery of vitamins and allowed scientists to learn how trans-fats increase risks of heart disease through the hardening of arteries.

Noting the phases of the transition

The epidemiological transition occurs in four stages, outlined in Table 4-2. As you can see, socioeconomic development, life expectancy, and morbidity/ mortality are all intricately connected.

Table 4-2	Phases of the Epidemiologic Transition		
Phase	*Socioeconomic Development*	*Average Life Expectancy*	*Morbidity and Mortality Trends*
1 — Age of pestilence and famine	Pre-developed	~ 30 years	Infections and nutritional deficiencies
2 — Age of receding pandemics	Developing countries	30–50 years	Improved sanitation, improved diet (safer food sources from increased sanitation), life expectancy rising
3 — Age of degenerative and man-made diseases	Countries in transition	50–55 years	Improving economy (more money), continuing rise in life expectancy, improved sanitation and workplace safety, and large increase in chronic diseases from behavior choices
4 — Age of delayed degenerative diseases	Developed countries	~70 years	Reduced risky behaviors in the population (due to prevention and health promotions) and an increase in new treatments

Looking at the outcomes of the transition

Although making the transition from infectious to chronic disease has many positive outcomes — who can argue against the benefits of preventing infectious diseases or the scientific and industrial advancements that brought us cellphones, computers, and reality TV? — the transition also brings with it some possible negative consequences:

✔ **Sedentary lifestyles:** People don't perform manual labor as much now, nor does everyday life require regular physical exertion; thus, physical activity declines in developed nations. In addition, the changing economy and the pace of the modern life doesn't leave much free time for physical activity, like playing sports or exercising.

✔ **Highly-processed foods stemming from the industrialization of the food industry:** Essentially, people switch from growing their own food to buying their food in a grocery store. As reliance on processed foods grows, diets become exponentially higher in salt, fat, sugars, and preservatives — all bad things from a nutrition standpoint.

A case in point: Watching as the transition occurs in China

Currently, diets high in fat and calories, combined with inactive lifestyles, have set in motion a chain of events leading to the dramatic rise in morbidity and mortality rates among all societies across the globe. Shifts toward high-fat, energy-dense diets and sedentary lifestyles first occurred in industrial regions; more recently, they've been occurring in developing countries.

Take a look at present-day China, for example. Once a predominantly agrarian society (mostly made up of farmers who lived in rural areas), China now is a bustling, industrializing nation that is becoming highly urbanized as many more people move to the cities. With this industrialization come more chronic diseases.

Although the Chinese aren't dying as much from tuberculosis and pneumonia as they were 50 years ago — an improvement due to medical and public health advancements — the Chinese population is now on the verge of obesity and diabetes epidemics. Because of its citizens' increasingly sedentary lifestyle — compliments of the mass production and sale of automobiles, personal computers, and instantaneous, reliable communication media (such as cellphones and social media interfaces) — as well as the growing popularity of a highly processed, less traditional diet, China is in transition to become burdened with primarily chronic, not infectious, diseases.

What is happening in China is happening in most nations around the world. Today, poor diets and sedentary lifestyles are a global problem.

Getting familiar with chronic disease: Public Enemy Number 1

Take another look at the 2010 list from Table 4-1. How many of the health problems do you think are nutrition related? Heart disease? Of course. Diabetes? Surely. Cerebrovascular disease (stroke)? Yep, again. Cancer? Yes, to some degree. In later chapters, I talk about the ways you can use diet and nutrition to lessen your chances of developing these diseases: Lowering your intake of high-sugared foods, for example, can lower your risk of diabetes, and eating a diet high in fiber can lessen your risk of getting colorectal cancer, for instance. The thing I want you to notice now is the trend here: The majority of these present-day chronic diseases, experienced globally, stem from poor diets.

Chronic diseases are noncontagious and are many times incurable, meaning you have them for years, perhaps even the remainder of your life. Some examples of chronic disease are obesity, cardiovascular disease, arthritis, cancer, diabetes, osteoporosis, and others. The majority of chronic diseases may stem from diets consistently high in fat, calories, salt, and sugar. Furthermore, these diseases also result from a lack of exercise, as well as engaging in risky behaviors like using tobacco or abusing alcohol.

Disabilities associated with chronic diseases

Because people with chronic diseases usually live with them for sustained periods of time, they tend to have associated disabilities stemming from the disease. Consider these examples:

- **Many obese people develop musculoskeletal problems.** The mechanics of walking, bending, and other body movements are compromised, or altered, due to the excess body fat. Obese individuals, for example, tend to sway side to side when they walk, which is an unnatural movement. Over time, this swaying motion causes lasting back, knee, joint, and/or muscle pain.

- **People with diabetes who do not effectively monitor their condition tend to have worse cases of the disease than those who manage the condition better.** If left unmanaged, diabetes can lead to amputations of the toes, feet, legs, and other extremities due to poor blood circulation and nerve damage.

Now accounting for over 60 percent of deaths worldwide (with approximately 50 percent of these deaths attributed to cardiovascular disease), chronic disease is now Public Enemy Number1 in the eyes of many, if not most, medical and public health professionals. Not only are they seeing an increasing number of people becoming sick from these diseases globally, but they are also seeing these diseases in younger and younger generations.

When morbidity and mortality from infectious diseases decrease, morbidity and mortality from chronic diseases increase. Why? The longer you live (meaning that you aren't succumbing to an infectious disease early in life), the higher your risk of developing a chronic disease. Simply stated, as the body ages, it wears down. As the body wears down, the risk of developing cancer, diabetes, heart disease, and most other chronic disease increases.

Although you can largely prevent chronic diseases by implementing healthy habits into your lifestyle, once developed, these diseases can be debilitating and, many times, deadly. One major problem that prevents many from taking steps to reduce their risk is that chronic diseases take a long time to develop. If, for example, your primary sources of nutrition are fried foods with little nutritional value (french fries, hamburgers, potato chips, and so on), years may pass before you become obese or develop heart disease or some other disease related to a high-fat, high-salt diet. After you develop any of those diseases, however, they are difficult, perhaps even impossible, to cure.

Chronic diseases going global

A large misconception is that chronic disease affects only industrialized, developed nations (the United States, Europe, Australia, Japan, Canada, and so on). However, the World Health Organization (WHO) indicates that 79 percent of all chronic disease deaths occur in industrializing nations (Southeast Asia, Latin American, Sub-Saharan Africa, and South Asia). Chronic diseases are now a global issue.

Factoring in large population growth, increasingly worsening nutrition patterns attributed to high-salt, high-sugar, and high-fat foods, and, ironically, more efficient and effective healthcare treatment (that is, pharmaceuticals), many people in the industrializing world are now living longer but sicker.

Garbage In, Garbage Out: Why What You're Eating Is Killing You

In the past few decades, the link between poor diet and poor health outcomes (chronic diseases, like obesity, diabetes, heart disease, cancer, and so on) has become well known among researchers. An exhaustive amount of research has been done, identifying which health behaviors and other factors increase the risk of developing chronic diseases. These factors include the following:

✔ Unhealthy diet

✔ Physical inactivity

✔ Tobacco use

✔ Alcohol abuse

✔ Genetic inheritance (that is, metabolic disorders such as insulin resistance and cholesterol processing abnormalities)

✔ Socioeconomic factors (inconsistent access to food or medical care, poor working conditions, and poor education opportunities)

Making a link between diet and disease

As I explain in Chapter 2, the more a person eats and the less he or she exercises, the more weight that person puts on. Hence, a poor diet can cause obesity. However, poor nutrition is the cause of many more diseases than just obesity.

The following disease and health conditions are linked with improper nutrition (for detailed information about other specific diseases and organ systems affected by poor nutrition, head to Parts II and III):

- ✔ Cancer (gastrointestinal, pancreatic, and other types of cancer)

    One in ten cancers in the United Kingdom stem from improper nutrition. Cancers of the gastrointestinal tract and breast cancer and many others have links to eating poorly.

- ✔ Obesity

- ✔ Diabetes

- ✔ Cardiovascular disease (heart disease) and cerebrovascular disease (stroke)

- ✔ Tooth and gum disease

- ✔ Kidney disease

- ✔ Liver disease

Considering that most cancers have long latency periods that can last years and, in many cases, decades, what you're eating now can have a profound impact on your health 20 years from now. Alarming, but true. ***Note:*** The *latency period* is the time between exposure to a cancer-causing substance and the clinical appearance of the cancer.

Say you're a 20-year-old whose diet is high in fat and low in fiber. You eat burgers and fries — or something similarly high in salt and calories but lacking in nutrients — three times a week for dinner. You eat little or no vegetables, and your fruit consumption is rare, if not nonexistent. You regularly consume more than your fair share of soft drinks, and you occasionally smoke a cigarette when you go out with friends for a pint or two (or three) at a local pub.

If you continue this behavior into your 30s and perhaps even beyond, your risk of developing colon cancer in your 50s is markedly higher than it is for a person of the same age who ate a high-fiber, low-fat diet, refrained from smoking, and limited his or her alcohol consumption. Even if you don't smoke now and limit or eliminate alcohol from your diet, continuing to eat a fatty diet still puts you at greater risk.

A diet that includes lots of colorful fruits and vegetables and whole grains, is low in fat and added sugars, and incorporates lean meat can actually prevent many cancers, as I explain in Chapter 6. Following the guidelines I outline there can improve your chances of enjoying many years of cancer-free, healthy living! Here are a couple of tips to get you started:

✔ **To ensure that you are getting enough vegetables and fruits on your plate,** make the vegetable and fruit portion of your dinner plate the main focus and treat the meat as a side dish.

✔ **To ensure that you're getting the proper amounts of nutrients from the proper sources,** try to make your plate the colors of the rainbow. The color of the fruit or vegetable indicates the presence of different phytochemicals (antioxidants, cancer-fighters, and other types of health benefactors). Bell peppers, for example, come in green, yellow, orange, and even purple colors. Therefore, the more colorful your dish is, the more likely you're eating a diverse diet, which probably means you are getting the proper amounts from the proper sources.

Taking its toll on your mental and cognitive health

Not only are the effects of improper nutrition something *physical,* but a poor diet can also affect *mental* health status. In a 2011 study, Australian researchers linked dietary choices and the development of depression and anxiety. They suggest that better nutritional choices lead to better mental health in adolescents. In studies conducted in 2013, American researchers found that eating breakfast regularly increases IQ scores in kindergarten children.

Even before these studies, people recognized that nutritious meals improve mood and performance. Think about how you feel when you skip a meal. Chances are you feel weak, tired, lethargic, or even irritated. And how often did your mother tell you to eat a good breakfast before school? Now we have the benefit of plenty of research proving that eating a healthy meal, particularly breakfast, before an exam can help boost test-takers' abilities. But eating just one good meal isn't enough. If you incorporate healthy meals in your regular dietary regimen, your chances of doing better on exams are increased dramatically.

Tackling Nutrition Head On: Common Strategies

For the most part, people want to be healthy, however they define that term. For some, getting healthy means taking the newest supplement on the market. For others, it means going on a drastic diet or combining a mix of dieting and weight-loss drugs. Others take a different approach, making gradual, but long-term healthy changes to their diet and increasing their levels of activity. In this section, I discuss these and other strategies that people have employed to improve their health.

Many people around the world are now living longer but sicker, with the majority of that sickness stemming from poor nutrition. Because chronic diseases are largely preventable, a global strategy to improve diets, increase physical activity, and promote health is needed. However easy solving the problem may seem — after all, all people need to do to decrease their risk of chronic disease is simply alter the way they eat and to start exercising — getting people to change their habits is very difficult. Take a look at Chapter 19 for more information on what's being done to help people modify their health behaviors.

Is there a pill for that? Taking supplements

Magazines, television commercials, daytime talk shows, late-night infomercials, roadside billboard signs . . . all are trying to sell you, the consumer, one thing or another. This "thing" may be an idea, a product, a behavior, or something else that you can consume, buy, or adopt. Many of these ads boil down to a simple promise: Take (or do) this product, and all your problems will easily go away! Right now! With minimal effort! It's that simple!

Wouldn't being able to reverse five years of aging by simply drinking a glass of juice be fantastic? Who wouldn't want to get rid of wrinkles by taking a tablet with breakfast or lose weight by sprinkling a powdery substance on their food? Before taking this route, you need to know a couple of things about supplements.

In this section, I don't focus on simple multivitamins that you see at your local drugstore, but other types of supplements, like ones that claim to alleviate discomfort or improve performance, stamina, mood, cognition, and so on. Still, even with multivitamins, you must do your homework about which ones to buy and how to take them.

Getting familiar with popular supplements and their dangers

People have a staggering number of choices to instantly cure what ails them, and supplements are one of the primary ways people attempt to get healthy. You can find supplements to strengthen your knee cartilage, to increase your sex drive, to boost your energy levels, to help you lose large amounts of weight without exercise or dieting, and more. These supplements aim to treat everything from back pain to psoriasis to cancer to sunburn and to produce those results *now*.

In every corner of the globe, many cures for many ills are being sold every day. Do these cures work? Some may. Others do not. Some are harmless additives. Others can kill you. Remember ephedra? That supplement caused cardiac arrest among consumers, and many died, leading the U.S. Food and Drug Administration to ban it in 2004. Two reasons to be wary of supplements:

- ✔ Most of them are not regulated by a governing body of trained, legitimate researchers and lack significant testing for safety and effectiveness.

- ✔ They usually don't include an ingredient list, and the source of their ingredients is unknown at worst and ambiguous at best.

So how do you know which supplements work and who makes sure they work? How do you find out what the supplements actually do, whether they work as advertised, or what happens if they're dangerous? If you're considering taking a supplement, discuss your options with your healthcare provider. He or she can give you the best guidance and information.

Determining the safety and efficacy of supplements

Researchers from various governmental and academic institutions conduct studies to answer many of the questions about supplement safety and effectiveness. The Food and Drug Administration in the United States, the Medicines and Healthcare Products Regulatory Agency in the United Kingdom, the Health Products and Food Branch of Health Canada, and the Therapeutic Goods Administration in Australia all take part in the research. Most nations around the world have their own version of these agencies, testing the safety, quality, and effectiveness of drugs and supplements.

Most countries' testing or oversight procedures are not nearly as rigorous or thorough as developed nations' testing procedures. Furthermore, even though these tests may be conducted and the deleterious effects shown to be significant, some governments fail to act upon the recommendations for various reasons (mainly economic). In some cases, the recommendations aren't acted upon due to national instability, lack of funding, and so on. Bottom line: Make sure that whatever supplement you are taking has been approved by a legitimate governmental research organization.

Thankfully, some health agencies and research organizations are keeping tabs on all these products and their safety, or lack thereof. A recent report published in the *Natural Medicines Comprehensive Database, Professional Version*, June 2010, and reported by CBS news, identified a number of supplements that can lead to an array of adverse health effects, including major organ failure and possibly even death. Table 4-3 lists these supplements.

Table 4-3	Supplements Linked to Adverse Health Outcomes
Supplement	*Adverse Health Reaction*
Aconite	Toxicity, nausea, vomiting, low blood pressure, respiratory system paralysis, heart rhythm disorders, death
Bitter orange	Fainting, heart rhythm disorders, heart attack, stroke, death
Chaparral	Liver damage, kidney problems
Colloidal silver	Bluish skin, mucous membrane discoloration, neurological problems, kidney damage
Coltsfoots	Liver damage, cancer
Comfrey	Liver damage, cancer
Country mallow	Heart attack, heart arrhythmia, stroke, death
Germanium	Kidney damage, death
Greater celandine	Liver damage
Kava	Liver damage
Lobelia	Fast heartbeat, very low blood pressure, coma, death (at high dosages)
Yohimbe	High blood pressure, rapid heart rate (at usual dosages); severe low blood pressure, heart problems, death (at high dosages)

Source: http://abcnews.go.com/Health/AlternativeMedicineSupplements/ consumer-reports-dirty-dozen-12-risky-supplements/story?id=11309450

In addition, the following supplements may damage your liver:

- ✔ **Green tea extracts:** Ingesting more than the maximum recommended amounts of green tea extracts can raise your risk of acute liver failure.

- ✔ **Niacin:** Although necessary for good health, this B vitamin can lead to liver disease if chronically taken above recommended amounts.

- ✔ **Pennyroyal:** The oil in pennyroyal can cause liver damage when taken chronically or in large doses. Further, it can make existing liver disease worse.

- ✔ **Red yeast:** When taken in combination with acetaminophen (that is, the class of pain relievers that includes Tylenol), red yeast can exponentially increase your risk of liver damage.

- ✔ **Sassafras:** Sassafras oil has a highly toxic carcinogenic material, called *safrole*. Taken in large doses, it can irreparably damage the liver.

Many supplements are available that do wonders for many people. The point I want to make in this section is not to avoid supplements at all costs. Instead, consult your physician or healthcare provider about whether a particular supplement is one you should consider taking. You may find that it is very beneficial for you. Or you may discover that the supplement is not only dangerous in its own right, but that it could also be deadly in combination with another drug you're taking. Bottom line: Be careful and talk to your doctor.

Dieting: What is it and who should be doing it?

Many people, instead of taking supplements, go on a diet. As a clinical nutritionist, you need to be aware of what a diet actually is. Technically, a *diet,* also called a *therapeutic diet,* is an extremely regimented intake of nutrients designed to make a sickly person healthy. Individuals with cancer, HIV/AIDS, morbid obesity, vitamin or mineral processing issues, and other diseases go on therapeutic diets. These individuals need a specific diet to achieve certain health outcomes in a certain amount of time.

You may be wondering, "Isn't losing weight a specific health outcome?" Well, technically, yes. However, people who are slightly above normal weight (say, a body mass index of 26) and decide to lose a few pounds aren't on therapeutic diets, per se. Instead, they're altering the way they eat — and hopefully their lifestyle — to achieve long-term weight loss.

A diet in the world of clinical nutrition is a medical regimen initiated by clinicians, which, if not followed properly, could have serious consequences. So when a client or patient is discussing a diet, you should treat it as a strict dietary regimen. Joe Smith, however, who is trying to lose ten pounds isn't going on a diet. Joe is altering his eating. Although some researchers argue this distinction, you need to start thinking of a diet as a serious health endeavor that shouldn't be taken lightly.

Table 4-4 lists some popular diets. Bear in mind, these are just a fraction of the available diets out there. All have varying success rates and different pros and cons. Some can be dangerous, so be careful if you choose to go on one. Again, consult a doctor before doing anything drastic.

Table 4-4	Popular Diets
Diet Name	*Characteristics*
Atkins diet	Limits carbohydrates to control the amount of insulin in the blood. In this diet, proteins serve as the primary energy course, not carbohydrates, which are the recommended energy source.
Zone diet	Aims for a nutritional balance of 40% carbohydrates, 30% fats, and 30% protein at each meal.
South Beach diet	Aims to control insulin levels by having individuals eat unrefined "slow carbs" (complex carbs, like whole grains) instead of "fast carbs" (simple carbs, like enriched bleached flour).
Mediterranean diet	Includes principles of traditional Italian, Spanish, Portuguese, French, North African, and Greek diets, where olive oils, whole grains, fresh fruits and vegetables, lean meats, limited saturated fat, and wine are key.
3-Day diet	Keeps caloric intake at very low levels. The majority of weight lost in the three days is usually water weight.
Cabbage Soup diet	Restricts the majority of your diet to a concoction of cabbage, water, onions, celery, bell peppers, and V8 juice for seven days.
Paleo diet	Restricts diet to include only foods our cavemen ancestors were likely to have eaten and excludes processed sugar, salt, grains, legumes, dairy, coffee, or alcohol. Limits potatoes as well.

Be wary of products that claim to produce results that are almost too good to be true. Certain supplements and diets will have minimal, if any, effectiveness in helping you reduce body fat, build muscle, reverse the aging process, and so on, but they may actually be dangerous and perhaps even deadly. Only trust peer-reviewed research, a valid, trusted professional, or a government source on recommendations for dietary regimens. Before making any type of dietary change, consult your doctor first!

Accepting that the solution is long term

What if I told you that you that you can reverse some effects of aging, reduce chances of wrinkles, and yes, even lose weight by simply eating food? Hard to imagine that simple dietary regimens that are relatively cheap can outperform any of the expensive, invasive, unproven, or even dangerous therapies sold daily in the form of supplements or diets.

Although many health products being sold on today's market are very beneficial when taken in the correct dosage under the direct supervision of a physician consultation, most physicians will tell you that the best way to lose weight, reduce cholesterol, reduce your risk of heart disease, stroke, and cancer, and live a healthier life is to eat a nutritious diet full of vegetables and fruits that is balanced with whole grains and lean meats.

Clinical nutrition preaches that optimum wellness is achieved over time with healthy behavior choices (healthier diets and more exercise), not a mysterious wonder drug that claims to produce results in hours.

Although wanting immediate gratification is natural, healthiness is, for the most part, achieved over the long term. Part of a responsible life change when trying to achieve optimum health status — like changing the way you eat, increasing exercise, quitting smoking, or whatever — takes time. You won't get the results you desire immediately. It will take months and possibly years to achieve your desired goals. That's okay. It's normal and, most importantly, it's healthy. Don't expect immediate satisfaction.

Part II
You Are What You Eat

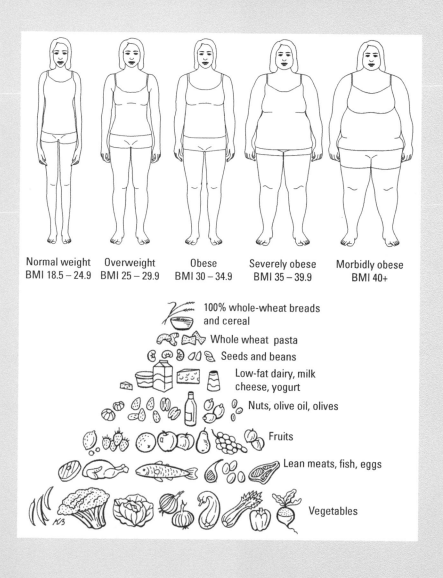

Normal weight
BMI 18.5 – 24.9

Overweight
BMI 25 – 29.9

Obese
BMI 30 – 34.9

Severely obese
BMI 35 – 39.9

Morbidly obese
BMI 40+

100% whole-wheat breads
and cereal

Whole wheat pasta

Seeds and beans

Low-fat dairy, milk
cheese, yogurt

Nuts, olive oil, olives

Fruits

Lean meats, fish, eggs

Vegetables

web extras

Find out why eating too many carrots can turn you orange and create other problems (beyond attracting wascally wabbits) at www.dummies.com/extras/clinicalnutrition.

In this part. . .

✔ Learn why obesity is rapidly spreading around the world — even into nations that have traditionally avoided this health problem — and the ramification this phenomenon is having on health outcomes around the world

✔ Identify the foods that can help prevent cancer and cardiovascular disease

✔ Understand how diet is linked with diabetes and kidney disease and what key changes you can make or suggest to fend off this danger

✔ Get familiar with the food alterations, food contaminants, and foodborne illnesses and find out how to protect yourself from these threats

Chapter 5

Observing Obesity

· ·

· ·

*O*ne almost impossible-to-ignore trend is that societies are becoming larger. Yes, they're growing in population numbers, but they are, quite literally, growing in body weight as well, and they're growing fast. Alarmingly, populations around the world are doubling their obesity rates in only a few decades. Researchers now project that some regions around the world will have an adult overweight rate of over 90 percent! In those countries, nine out of ten adults will be overweight, and many of those will be obese.

Although body fat is essential for life, you must be very careful that you maintain a healthy amount and not gain or lose too much. An equilibrium must be met to produce the best health outcomes. As you discover in this chapter, nations around the world are losing that battle. Populations are losing the momentum to maintain a healthy body weight and are becoming sicker and dying younger because of that fact.

Gaining Basic Info about Obesity and Being Overweight

Obesity is essentially an accumulation of excess body fat as a result of overconsumption of calories and a lack of exercise to burn the extra energy off. Very simply, when your body has an excess of energy — either through fat, protein, or carbohydrate sources — it usually converts those extra calories into fatty-acid chains (triglycerides) that are stored in adipose tissue. *Adipose tissue* is another name for body fat.

All humans need a certain amount of body fat to maintain, or gain, optimum health status. Fat is essential for life. As I discuss in Chapter 2, you need fat to digest and utilize fat-soluble vitamins. Without fat, your body wouldn't be able process those vitamins, and the result would be a deficiency disease and possibly even death.

Fat is so essential for a healthy body that not having enough body fat can increase your risk of death. During periods of famine or if an individual develops or contracts a *wasting disease* (a disease where muscle and organ tissues degenerate due to poor intakes of nutrition or nutrient losses due to infection), having too little body fat can actually increase the likelihood of death. However, by far, the highest risk of death and disease from body mass/fat stems from having too much. Ranging from obesity to diabetes to heart disease to some cancers, having too much body fat can be very deadly.

The key is to have the right amount of body fat — not too much and not too little. Table 5-1 lists body fat ratings for both men and women. Although being too heavy and too thin both increase your risk of death and disease, being obese greatly increases that risk.

Table 5-1	Body Fat Rating for Men and Women	
	Amount of Fat as a Percentage of Body Weight	
Body Fat Rating	**Men**	**Women**
At risk due to high body fat	>30%	>40%
Excess fat	21–30%	31–40%
Moderately lean	13–20%	23–30%
Lean	9–12%	19–22%
Very lean	5–8%	15–18%
At risk due to low body fat	<5%	<15%

Your mortality risk increases as your body fat rating falls or rises to dangerous levels.

Balancing energy intake and output

To gain weight, you simply consume more energy than you burn/use (check out Chapter 2 for a detailed explanation of the energy-in/energy-out equation for body weight changes):

Energy In (calories consumed) – Energy Out (calories expended)
= Change in energy stores (excess/loss/equilibrium)

However, just eating a few extra calories here and there doesn't mean you'll become obese. Gaining weight is a slow process of chronic intake of excess calories. In addition, if you exercise, you'll burn off many of those extra calories, thus preventing body weight increases.

As I explain in Chapter 3, a healthy diet makes room for *discretionary calories* each day. These calories are ones that can come from any food source you like — even from items you're normally instructed to stay away from, like those that are high in sugar or fat. The problem is that people often abuse their discretionary allotment, and that's what gets them into trouble. If you are trying to lose weight or maintain your weight, you need to be mindful of the discretionary calories you eat in a given day. Remember, every 3,500 calories you consume in excess of what you need causes you to gain one pound of body fat.

Determining how much energy intake you need

To determine the appropriate level of energy requires you to factor in gender, age, height, and activity level. Consider these examples:

- ✔ **A very active, taller than average (say 6' 2" tall), 25-year-old professional male football player who weighs 210 pounds:** This person needs somewhere between 3,000 to 4,000 or more calories a day to fuel his active lifestyle — quite a bit more than the normal 2,000-calorie-per-day allotment. If he ate only enough calories to sustain an average activity level, he would burn more than he consumes.

- ✔ **A 130-pound, 5' tall, 85-year-old woman who leads a relatively sedentary lifestyle:** She needs to consume markedly fewer calories per day than the football player and even fewer than the 2,000-calorie-a-day average. She would probably need, on average, around 1,700 calories per day of nutrient-dense food to maintain her health.

To set a limit on the calories consumed per day, you must reflect on your lifestyle. Proper energy balance is directly related to your demographic information (age, weight, and so on) and activity level. Head to Chapter 3 to find a numerical breakdown on healthy energy levels for people over the age of 30 with different activity levels.

Monitoring your daily caloric intake and amount of exercise is essential for maintaining healthy body weight. Use the energy-in/energy-out equation for body weight changes to estimate how many calories you should be consuming in a given day. Remember, if you need to lose weight, the calculation needs to produce a negative value. To gain weight, the calculation must produce a positive value.

Measuring Weight and Body Fat

Measuring body weight is pretty straightforward: Step on a scale and note the number displayed. Weight is measured with standard units of pounds, kilograms, stones, and so on, depending on where you live. More challenging is figuring out whether your body weight is healthy or unhealthy.

Determining a healthy body weight requires that you factor in gender, age, height, and activity level. As I note earlier, a healthy body weight for a 25-year-old professional male football player is quite a bit different from the healthy body weight of an 85-year-old sedentary woman.

You can measure how much body weight is considered normal, overweight, underweight, and/or obese by using a number of tools, which I explain in this section. No tool is 100 percent error-free, however, and all have their strengths and weaknesses. However, some of these tools are more popular than others. A tool's popularity may be due to how easy or simple it is to use, not necessarily because it is better than another.

Calculating Body Mass Index (BMI)

The body mass index does not actually measure body fat; it measures body compositional characteristics (height and weight). These characteristics *correlate,* or relate, with varying types of body fatness. Comparing BMI to body fatness yields the six general categories of BMI, outlined in Table 5-2. Notice how having too low a BMI and too high a BMI are both bad for you. Figure 5-1 represents these classifications graphically.

Table 5-2	Body Mass Index Classifications
Classification	*BMI*
Underweight	<18.5
Normal weight	18.5–24.99
Overweight	25–29.99
Obese (Obese I)	30–34.99
Severely obese (Obese II)	35–39.99
Morbidly obese (Extreme Obese)	>40

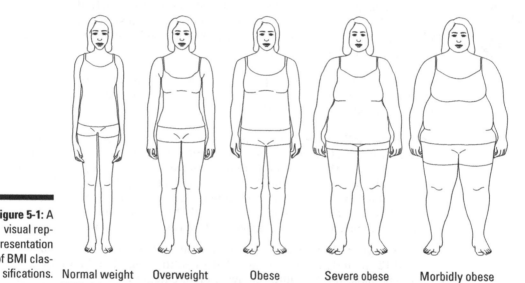

Figure 5-1: A visual representation of BMI classifications.

| Normal weight BMI 18.5 – 24.9 | Overweight BMI 25 – 29.9 | Obese BMI 30 – 34.9 | Severe obese BMI 35 – 39.9 | Morbidly obese BMI 40+ |

Illustration by Wiley, Composition Services Graphics

BMI is calculated by the following equations:

The English equation:

$$BMI = \frac{\text{weight (lbs)}}{\text{height (in)} \times \text{height (in)}} \times 703$$

The metric equation:

$$BMI = \frac{weight\ (kg)}{height\ (m) \times height\ (m)}$$

The primary problem with BMI is that it doesn't differentiate between body fat and muscle/bone mass. As a result, it may misclassify some individuals into higher or lower categories of BMI. Professional athletes, for example, are probably in the prime of their lives in terms of fitness and health but are often classified as overweight or obese, according to the BMI. The issue is that many athletes of have high muscle mass — not fat.

It's not uncommon for elite athletes to be labeled obese by a BMI chart yet to have only 8 percent body fat, which is nowhere near obese status. Incorrect BMI categorization and mislabeling can stop some individuals from getting the help they need to gain or lose weight.

Revisiting the 25-year-old male professional football player and the 85-year-old sedentary woman (refer to the earlier section "Balancing energy intake and output"), consider what their BMI levels are.

- ✔ **The football player:** According to the BMI chart, he needs to be somewhere between 145 and 195 pounds to fall in the normal weight and normal BMI range. If this football player is like other professional football players, he's probably bordering on the upper end of the body weight interval and is probably considered overweight according to the BMI. But, as I note earlier, the fact that the BMI does not take into account muscle and bone mass, the BMI results are skewed.

- ✔ **The 85-year-old woman:** She needs to be somewhere between 95 and 125 pounds to be considered at a healthy weight and BMI. At 130 pounds, she falls into the overweight category.

BMI may not be the most accurate method to assess whether an individual is overweight or obese. Because it does not account for muscle and bone mass, it can produce an inflated calculation and thus misrepresent your true body weight category. Therefore, athletes should not rely on the BMI. Nevertheless, for those who do not fall into those groups, the BMI classifications can accurately indicate whether someone is truly overweight, obese, and so on.

A case in point — my own

I am currently 6 feet tall (on a good day!) and weigh 183 pounds. I have an athletic build and exercise regularly. Even though I'm not thin, I wouldn't consider myself overweight. Rather, I'm a healthy weight — at least I think so. While writing this chapter, I asked my family, friends, and colleagues to give me an honest answer when I asked whether I was overweight. The overwhelming responses? "Huh? You're not overweight. What are you talking about?"

But according to the BMI calculation, my body mass index is 24.8, just a hair below overweight status. Hence, the problem: In reality, I'm not overweight. Yet, the BMI is essentially telling me that, if I eat one more double cheeseburger, I will graduate into the overweight category.

Using anthropometric body fat tests

Anthropometric (the measurement of the human body) analyses use various measurements to assess body mass. These tests predict total body weight composition — the percentage of bone, muscle, and fat in an individual — by measuring weight, height, and *girth* (your waist measurement) and performing a fat-fold test.

The primary goal of body fat tests is to determine what percentage of your body is composed of fat, not whether the relationship between how tall you are and how much you weigh is a good one.

Because these tests use multiple body measurements, they yield better assessments of healthiness related to body weight than does a simple BMI. However, they aren't good for everyone. Some people, including those who are obese, may find these measurements less accurate than others for assessing bone density and overall health.

Assessing total body fat is the most accurate way to measure an individual's overall state of healthiness. As a rule, the more body fat you have, the more at risk you are to be overweight or obese. As with BMI and energy intake, how much body fat a person should have varies with age and gender. Women tend to have more body fat than men, primarily because of the needs of childbearing. Older individuals have more body fat than younger, due primarily to the muscle mass degeneration that occurs as people age. Figure 5-2 shows the total body fat ranges for different ages.

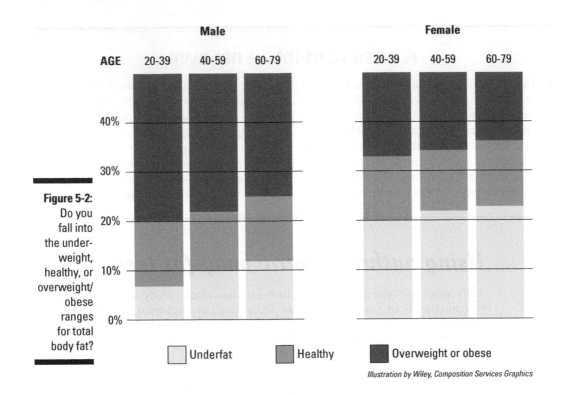

Figure 5-2:
Do you
fall into
the under-
weight,
healthy, or
overweight/
obese
ranges
for total
body fat?

Performing a fat-fold test

To conduct a body fat analysis, you perform a fat-fold test, which involves pinching different parts of the body (don't worry, it doesn't hurt) with a pair of calipers to measure in millimeters how much skin (and fat) is folded when the tool clamps down. Typical areas tested for fat fold are hips, triceps, biceps, stomach, and pectoral regions of the body. Generally, you add together the measurements to get a final value.

Table 5-3 shows a chart similar to one you may use to determine the percentage of body fat of individuals of different ages, based on the results of a fat-fold test. (Different charts will tell you what measurements are used for the calculations.) As you can see here, a 32-year-old male with a 35 millimeter measurement would have approximately 17.7 percent body fat. A 48-year-old woman with a 75 millimeter measurement would have almost 36 percent body fat (35.9).

Table 5-3	Equivalent Fat Content, as a Percentage of Body Weight						
	Men				**Women**		
Skinfolds (mm)	*17-29*	*30-39*	*40-49*	*50+*	*16-29*	*30-39*	*40-49*	*50+*
20	8.1	12.2	12.2	12.6	14.1	17.0	19.8	21.4
25	10.5	14.2	15.0	15.6	16.8	19.4	22.2	24.0
30	12.9	16.2	17.7	18.6	19.5	21.8	24.5	26.6
35	14.7	17.7	19.6	20.8	21.5	23.7	26.4	28.5
40	16.4	19.2	21.4	22.9	23.4	25.5	28.2	30.3
45	17.7	20.2	23.0	24.7	25.0	26.9	29.6	31.9
50	19.0	21.5	24.6	26.5	26.5	28.2	31.0	33.4
55	21.0	22.5	25.9	27.9	27.8	29.4	32.1	34.6
60	21.2	23.5	27.1	29.2	29.1	30.6	33.2	35.7
65	22.2	24.3	28.2	30.4	30.2	31.6	34.1	36.7
70	23.1	25.1	29.3	31.6	31.2	32.5	35.0	37.7
75	24.0	25.9	30.3	32.7	32.2	33.4	35.9	38.7
80	24.8	26.6	31.2	33.8	33.1	34.3	36.7	39.6
85	25.5	27.2	32.1	34.8	34.0	35.1	37.5	40.4
90	26.2	27.8	33.0	35.8	34.8	35.8	38.3	41.2
95	26.9	28.4	33.7	36.6	35.6	36.5	39.0	41.9
100	27.6	29.0	34.4	37.7	36.4	37.2	39.7	42.6
105	28.2	29.6	35.1	38.2	37.1	37.9	40.7	43.3
And so on . . .							

Just as with BMI, anthropometric measurements aren't 100 percent accurate. The fat-fold test measures only subcutaneous fat, not *visceral fat* (fat that lies deep underneath the skin around major organ systems). Visceral fat can be an important factor in measuring true body mass, fatness, and your overall state of healthiness.

Where you carry fat can affect your risk of death and disease. Although the fat-fold test tries to account for this by including measurements of different parts of the body, it doesn't truly capture the phenomenon of fat accumulation or make correlations regarding higher risk.

Calculating your waist-to-hip ratio

Another way to measure body mass as it relates to overall health is to use the waist-to-hip ratio test. In this method, you take a measurement of your waist at the narrowest point and your hips at the widest point (see Figure 5-3). Then simply divide the waist measurement by the hip measurement to get your ratio. Depending on the size of that number, you can approximate how much body mass you have and where that body mass is located.

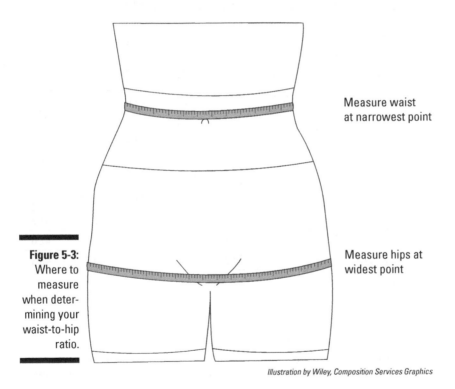

Measure waist at narrowest point

Measure hips at widest point

Figure 5-3: Where to measure when determining your waist-to-hip ratio.

Illustration by Wiley, Composition Services Graphics

Table 5-4 shows waist-to-hip ratio standards for both men and women.

Based on the preceding information, take a look at Figure 5-4 and see whether you can tell which man has a larger waist-to-hip ratio: Figure A or Figure B? If you guessed the man on the right (Figure B), you're correct. He's the unhealthier of the two because he carries more fat around his stomach and belly than around his hips, giving him a larger waist-to-hip ratio and putting him at greater health risks due to too much body fat.

Table 5-4	Waist-to-Hip Circumference Ratios and Disease Risk				
Men					
Age (yrs)	**_20–29_**	**_30–39_**	**_40–49_**	**_50–59_**	**_60–69_**
Low	<0.83	<0.84	<0.88	<0.90	<0.91
Moderate	0.83–0.88	0.84–0.91	0.88–0.95	0.90–0.96	0.91–0.98
High	0.89–0.94	0.92–0.96	0.96–1.00	0.97–1.02	0.99–1.03
Very high	>0.94	>0.96	>1.00	>1.02	>1.03
Women					
Age (yrs)	**_20–29_**	**_30–39_**	**_40–49_**	**_50–59_**	**_60–69_**
Low	<0.71	<0.72	<0.73	<0.74	<0.76
Moderate	0.71–0.77	0.72–0.78	0.73–0.79	0.74–0.81	0.76–0.83
High	0.78–0.82	0.79–0.84	0.80–0.87	0.82–0.88	0.84–0.90
Very high	>0.82	>0.84	>0.87	>0.88	>0.90

Source: Heyward VH, Stolarcyzk LM: Applied Body Composition Assessment. Champaign IL, Human Kinetics, 1996

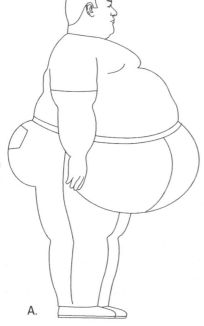

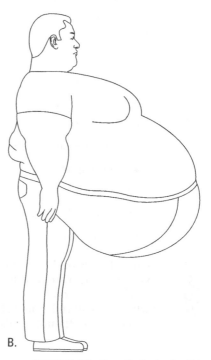

Figure 5-4:
Which has the unhealthier waist-to-hip ratio? Answer: The man on the right (B).

A.

B.

Illustration by Wiley, Composition Services Graphics

Comorbidities: Encountering Obesity and the Diseases That Go with It

Millions of Americans and people worldwide are overweight or obese and at risk for serious diseases like heart disease, diabetes, some cancers, gallbladder disease, and even respiratory problems. This phenomenon — having multiple diseases at the same time, usually stemming from one central disease — is called *comorbidity*.

The number of diseases that can be linked with excess body fat is mind-boggling. Did you know, for example, that the risk of developing diabetes is tripled for obese people? Simply put, being obese puts you at risk for a multitude of adverse health outcomes, as I explain in this section.

Introducing obesity-related diseases

The more body fat you have — or the more obese you are — the more likely you are to develop potentially deadly illnesses, like the following. These diseases can stem from complications related to being obese (you can read about several of these health concerns in the remaining chapters of this part):

- Cardiovascular disease (Chapter 7)
- Some cancers, like colorectal and pancreatic (Chapter 6)
- Type 2 diabetes (Chapter 8)
- Respiratory problems
- Kidney disease (Chapter 9)
- Sleep apnea
- Arthritis
- Gallbladder disease
- Mental and social health concerns

Other things besides your diet affect how much you weigh. Elements such as your genetic history, your physical environment, and your personal behavioral choices contribute to how much body fat you accumulate (or not) and where it is stored. Some of these are modifiable, or changeable, risk factors; you can alter them to make yourself healthier. However, some risk factors, like genetics, are non-modifiable. They may predispose you to having more body fat accumulated in certain areas of your body, and you can't really do too much about that.

Bellying up to bar: Central adiposity

Central adiposity, or *visceral fatness,* refers to the amount of fat accumulated in and around your abdomen (see Figure 5-5). Some people are shaped like pears, carrying their fat in and around their hips and buttocks. Others are shaped like apples; their fat tends to accumulate around their midsections. Whether you are apple- or pear-shaped can be determined by the waist-to-hip ratio, which I discuss earlier in "Calculating your waist-to-hip ratio."

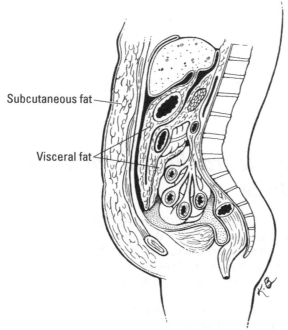

Subcutaneous fat

Visceral fat

Figure 5-5:
Subcuta-
neous
versus
visceral fat.

Illustration by Kathryn Born, MA

"Apples" have a higher risk of death from all causes than "pears" do. In fact, central obesity is one of the most concerning issues for health professionals. Being centrally obese is as much of a risk for poor health as is using tobacco regularly.

Being centrally obese causes more problems than being less centrally obese for two major reasons:

- ✔ **More adipokines:** *Adipokines* are hormones that regulate inflammatory processes in tissue. Centrally obese people have more adipokines, increasing inflammation and the risk of heart disease. In addition, increases in adipokines increase the risk of insulin resistance, which raises the risk of developing type 2 diabetes (head to Chapter 8 for more on diabetes).

- ✔ **More fatty acids:** Visceral fatness increases production of fatty acids and inflammatory proteins that are transferred into your blood. Higher *blood lipids* (fat in your blood) increase your risk for coronary heart disease (CAD) and stroke. In addition, excess lipids build up in your fat tissues and liver, and they become inflamed. The proteins stemming from this state of inflammation also increase your risk of death and disease.

People most at risk for central obesity are men of all ages and post-menopausal women. Women of childbearing ages (approximately 14 to 40 years old) tend to be more pear-shaped and have less central obesity. In addition, excessive alcohol consumption and lack of exercise can also increase your risks of visceral fatness. Although you can't change your age or gender, you can control the behaviors that put you at greater risk: Moderate your drinking and stay active.

Underlying mental health complications of being obese

The physical risks stemming from obesity are a major reason to prevent and/or treat the disease, yet the potential mental health issues associated with being overweight are sometimes overlooked, even though they can be just as problematic. Usually when someone is being treated for obesity, a common procedure is to assess whether an underlying mental health issue exists.

A key question in the discussion about obesity and mental health is whether the obesity causes the mental health issue, or whether an underlying mental health issue causes the obesity. Research suggests that, if an individual is obese, the social pressure to be thin can cause depression, anxiety, and a range of other emotional problems. However, many cases of obesity are the *result* of depression, anxiety, and even post-traumatic stress disorder (PTSD). Therefore, understanding the time sequence of the weight gain that led to

Inheriting obesity: Fact or fiction?

Is obesity a genetically predisposed condition? Some recent studies have tried to answer that very question. Here's the quick version of the complicated findings: Yes, genetic inheritance can play a role in the development of obesity in a child. Some research suggests that if one of the two parents is obese at the time of the child's birth, that child has a 30 percent increased risk of becoming obese him- or herself. If both parents are obese, the risk of the child becoming obese increases to 70 percent.

You may be thinking that the question is answered, but not so fast. Here's the complicated part: The evidence isn't totally conclusive.

Ask yourself this question: Does the study conclusively show whether genetics or childrearing leads to the increased risk? If the child is reared by obese parents who overconsume calories daily, is the child also learning to overconsume? Or is the child's weight really a result of something genetic?

The fact is that the answer to the question is largely unknown. What is known, however, is that obese women who plan to have children should lose weight before becoming pregnant to minimize the risk of complications, such as gestational diabetes and hypertension, while pregnant.

obesity and identifying any mood disorders that occurred prior to, during, or as a result of the weight gain is important. This information can help healthcare providers identify underlying mental health issues.

Any physical assessment of an individual who is overweight or obese needs to have a mental health assessment as well. Many times, a latent mental health concern is a causal factor in the development of obesity, not the other way around.

Achieving and Maintaining a Healthy Body Weight

The primary way to treat and/or prevent obesity is to make a total life change that revolves around the following:

- Eating healthy (a diet that is rich in fiber, fruits, and vegetables and low in fats, sugars, and salts; incorporates plenty of water; and refrains from excess caloric consumption)
- Exercising regularly

✔ Maintaining a positive mental health status

✔ Having the willpower to continue with the changes

A lifestyle that includes these components guarantees the best possible results as it pertains to healthy weight loss. In this section, I outline two kinds of therapy that can help people combat obesity.

Consulting a dietary health professional about losing weight

Every individual is different: different metabolic rates, genetics, and demographic information. These differences may make an individual more or less prone to becoming obese. As a result, each treatment, therapy, or prevention plan is different for each person.

Although diet plans may be similar between people or groups, each person responds to a diet plan differently. Each has his or her own needs, own goals, own resources, and own capabilities — or challenges — when taking the actions necessary to attain a healthy weight. One thing is common, though, across all groups: Lifestyle changes *must* incorporate responsible, healthy eating; regular exercise; and the willpower to refrain from eating too many calories.

The best solution when attempting to begin dietary and exercise regimens is to consult a physician. You can discuss options and decide together the best possible solution for your own specific lifestyle needs. Another person to consult is a nutritionist (your physician may give you a referral to a recommended source). Because of their special training in understanding the relationship between diet and bodily function, nutritionists can help you understand this connection, plan a healthy diet, and choose appropriate lifestyle behaviors that can promote the best possible health outcomes.

Do not fully commit to radical diets or supplements to achieve weight loss without consulting a physician first. Many of these dietary remedies have not been evaluated by qualified professionals, make suspect claims at best, and may be dangerous. Be careful with adopting any regimen not endorsed by verified, qualified personnel.

Losing weight is hard, and having to lose a lot of weight can be overwhelming. But there is good news: Across all groups, smaller victories in the war of the waistline can boost self-esteem enough to continue. Consider these points:

- ✔ **Losing even a little weight can yield positive results.** Recent literature suggests that your risk of developing type 2 diabetes can drop by nearly 30 percent if you lose between 8 and 12 pounds. In addition, when you lose weight, insulin sensitivity is improved, which helps you limit the deleterious effects that diabetes has on the body.

- ✔ **Physical effects from changing eating and exercising habits are almost immediate for obese people.** For example, hypertensive people (those with high blood pressure) who significantly limit total fat and salt content of their foods can produce positive results in less than a month.

- ✔ **Weight loss is easier in the beginning for obese people.** And these immediate effects are crucial for the long-term sustainment of the individual's lifestyle change.

Implementing medical therapy

For the severely obese for whom nutritional guidance and lifestyle changes are not successful, surgical solutions may be an option. The goal of these procedures is to make the stomach smaller (about the size of a chicken egg) in order to induce feelings of fullness more quickly and to prevent overeating and reduce obesity.

One such procedure is gastric bypass surgery. In this procedure, a surgeon essentially creates a new, smaller stomach and attaches your intestines to this new stomach, thus bypassing your original one. People who undergo these surgeries are prohibited from eating too much food and from eating greasy foods and foods that are high in fat. Not following the required eating instructions — eating too much, for example, or having certain types of food — can result in vomiting.

Strict guidelines must be met to qualify for these surgical procedures:

- ✔ You must be severely obese. The specific requirements vary, but double your normal weight is common.

- ✔ You must have repeatedly failed to lose weight using the traditional methods of diet and exercise.

- ✔ You must have developed a disease associated with your obesity.

- ✔ You must undergo and pass mental health assessments. Patients must be cleared of certain mental health diagnoses that could undermine their chances of success; they must also learn how to cope with the possibility of a new body. Sometimes the shock of transformation from obesity to normal weight can create mental issues itself.

The reason for the strict standards is that surgeons want to ensure that patients fully understand the invasiveness and cost of the surgery and that they are prepared for the changes that are to come post-surgery. These surgeries require that patients make a lifelong commitment to change adverse health behaviors in order to prevent the issue from resurfacing. If the patient becomes obese again, which is not that uncommon, the resources expended by both the patient and surgeon on the procedure were to no avail.

Rising Global Morbidity Rates

A common misconception is that only populations in the developed world (the United States, Western Europe, Australia, Canada, Japan, and so on) gain excessive (unhealthy) amounts of body fat. The truth is that, as Chapter 4 suggests, chronic diseases, including obesity, are now a global issue. Countries in the developing world that have traditionally been viewed as being at risk for deficient caloric intake now have some of the largest issues with overconsumption and, therefore, a rising overweight and obese population.

There are approximately 1.5 billion overweight and 650 million obese people around the globe. You read that correctly: Over 2 billion people around the world are overweight or obese. That's about one in three people. If this trend continues into the middle of the 21st century, the world will quite possibly have 2.5 billion overweight and 1.5 billion obese individuals — numbers that are mindboggling to most people.

Doing a survey of the people and regions affected

So who is most affected and where do they live? Southeast and East Asian nations, along with countries in Sub-Saharan Africa have the lowest rates of obesity (less than 5 percent of the adult populations in these places is obese), whereas the Polynesian islands and other island nations in the South Pacific have the highest number of obese people in the world (over 60 percent of their adult populations is obese). Western nations like the United States, nations of Western Europe, some Middle Eastern nations, Australia, and Argentina also have some of the higher rates in comparison to the rest of the world.

Table 5-5 lists the world's most obese countries. Notice that eight of them are Pacific Island nations. Kuwait and the United States are the only non-Polynesian nations that make the top ten.

Table 5-5	The World's Most Obese Countries
Country	*Percentage of Overweight Adults Ages 15 and Over*
Nauru	94.5
Micronesia	91.1
Cook Islands	90.9
Tonga	90.8
Niue	81.7
Samoa	80.4
Palau	78.4
Kuwait	74.2
U.S.	74.1
Kiribati	73.6

Source: World Health Organization

Understanding the spread of obesity around the world

Two key factors have contributed to the development of obesity worldwide:

✔ **The drastic increase in available food energy:** In nations that suffered under cycles of famine and starvation in the early parts of the 20th century, the majority of their populations are now overweight or obese. This is due to a number of factors, two of which are

- **Food becoming more readily accessible:** In countries that have traditionally experienced food insecurity, the availability of food is certainly not a bad thing. The problems arise, however, when those foods are unhealthy ones.

- **The Westernization of cultures and, ultimately, diets:** Fast-food establishments are sprouting up all over the developing world and making food cheaper to obtain. These foods aren't nutrient-dense, but energy-dense. Coupled with more sedentary lifestyles, this drastic increase in caloric intake is contributing to an obesity outbreak.

✔ **A rising trend of sedentary lifestyles:** The advent of cellphones, personal computers, and other technological advancements makes physical exertion sometimes unnecessary. For example, would you choose to climb six flights of stairs or take the elevator? Exactly. Most of us would choose the elevator.

The global obesity trends are increasing yearly with little hope for a turn-around any time soon. As global rates continue to climb, public health professionals and policymakers have their work cut out for them since changing the behavior of individuals, let alone entire nations, is a very difficult task. In the meantime, the best we can do is encourage individuals to choose healthy behaviors: to eat healthy and not overeat, to exercise regularly, and to refrain from alcohol abuse and tobacco use.

Chapter 6

Concerning Yourself and Cancer

For the past 50 to 60 years, few events have been as devastating to society's overall health and wellness status as the dramatic rise in the incidence of cancer. Although you can argue that obesity-related heart disease and diabetes — even the HIV/AIDS epidemic — rival the threat cancer poses to human longevity, cancer is still, in my opinion, the number one threat to human health.

Cancer deserves its place at the top of the "big threats to human health" list because of the sheer number of people affected and the fact that more and more causal factors of cancer are being discovered daily, from the relatively obvious (tobacco use, for example) to the most seemingly innocuous, like the grill markings on a hamburger (yes, that black char has been shown to be a *carcinogen,* a cancer-causer) or the use of a mobile phone (evidence is beginning to mount that cellular phone waves cause brain tumors).

Fortunately, medical treatment has come a long way in the past half-century, and researchers, health professionals, and regular people like you and me are doing plenty to fight back. A lot of new research has been done on prevention measures, including the role diet plays in both developing and preventing cancer. In this chapter, I examine these issues, provide an overview of cancer fundamentals, and explain how cancer affects your body.

Grasping Cancer Basics

Cancer is the leading cause of death worldwide. According to projections, an estimated 13.5 million cancer deaths occur each year. Ask yourself this question: How many of those 13.5 million cancers are related, even loosely, to the digestion process (that is, the gastrointestinal tract)? The answer? Approximately 40 percent of reported cancers involve your intestinal tract, suggesting that diet may be a contributing factor.

Take a look at the pie chart in Figure 6-1. This chart is divided into three sections: cancers of the gastrointestinal tract, lung cancers, and a collection of other cancers. Although 40 percent of all cancers occur in the gastrointestinal tract and, therefore, presumably have a connection to diet, the other cancers, particularly those in the "Other Cancers" slice, also have links to diet. For some of these cancers, like bladder cancer, the link is fairly strong between the cancer and what you eat and drink over the course of a lifetime. For others, the link is less clear but still likely a factor.

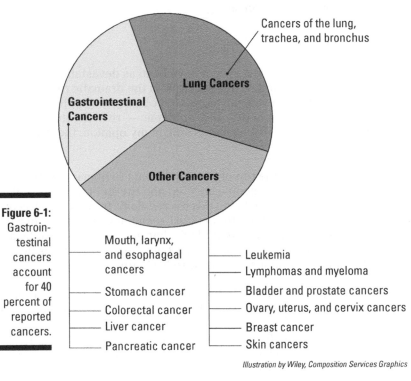

Figure 6-1:
Gastrointestinal cancers account for 40 percent of reported cancers.

Illustration by Wiley, Composition Services Graphics

So does your diet *definitely* cause cancer? No. It *probably* does. Researchers agree that diet plays a larger role than once thought in the development of cancer; however, as you discover in this chapter, very little with research — and especially cancer research — is definite. Because so many factors and exposures to so many different things can cause cancer, stating definitively that a particular item is *the* cause of cancer is rare among health professionals. However, what researchers do state definitively is that between 20 percent and 50 percent of all cancers stem from some aspect of your diet.

If you want to understand cancer, you first need to understand the basic science and physiology behind the disease. In this section, I give you a very brief overview of what happens upon exposure to a *mutagen* (an agent that causes mutations at the cellular level) and explain who is getting cancer, what kinds of cancers they're getting, and the risk factors — particularly those related to poor nutrition and exercise habits — that put certain groups at greater risk for a cancer diagnosis.

Mutations (changes at the genetic level) may cause a cell to act abnormally, which can lead to irregular functions of those cells. This irregularity can eventually lead to a cancer diagnosis.

Understanding global cancer epidemiology

Previously thought to be a problem mainly for the developed world, cancer now affects all countries. In fact, some of the highest incidence rates of cancer in the world occur in populations from developing countries in Latin America, Sub-Saharan Africa, and parts of Asia. (An *incidence rate* refers to the number of new cases of a disease in a population over a given period of time.)

In addition, researchers predict that cancers, like lung and prostate cancer, that currently have higher incidence rates in the developed world (most of Europe, Japan, Australia, the United States, and Canada), will, within a few decades, have a higher incidence rate in the developing world.

What's the deal with all this uncertainty stuff?

With cancer research, although reports may indicate increased risks of cancer from certain exposures, rarely, if ever, do you read that those exposures definitely cause it. That's because, when discussing statistics or research results, scientists never say that anything is proven with 100 percent certainty.

This protocol, however, doesn't mean that the research is uncertain. Scientists, for example, still will not say with 100 percent certainty that gravity causes things to drop. Why? Because in order for experiments to be valid, they must be disprovable. And the chance, no matter how small, that something can be disproven keeps scientists from making definitive claims. And who knows? In some galaxy somewhere — one that scientists just haven't found yet — gravity may cause objects to spin counterclockwise on their heads.

Identifying general reasons for the change

As I note, researchers predict that in the future, the incidence rate of cancers will be higher in developing countries than in developed ones. Why the change? For two reasons:

- ✔ **Globalization:** Today foods, lifestyles, cultures, and technologies spread globally, not regionally or nationally. Whereas in decades past, it would take years, perhaps decades or centuries, for cultures to adopt the mainstays of other cultures, today those things traverse the world in nanoseconds.

- ✔ **Resources:** The developed world has more resources than the developing world does to invest in research and to promote healthy behaviors and cancer prevention measures.

Here's an example: In the 1950s, approximately 45 percent of the U.S. adult population smoked cigarettes. Today, that rate is about 17 percent, which over time will result in lowering incidence rates of lung cancer. Present-day China, on the other hand, is the largest consumer and producer of tobacco. In fact, China has more smokers than the entire *total* population of the United States and about 60 percent of Europe's population. Although China doesn't have the highest lung cancer rates in the world today, within 20 to 30 years, that country will probably rank in the top five worldwide — a scenario that is also true for other developmentally similar countries, like Turkey and Vietnam.

The primary forces driving each society through the epidemiologic transition are technological, scientific, and industrial advancements. (The *epidemiologic transition* refers to the changes and progression a society goes through in the context of disease, which you can read about in Chapter 4.) Although the advancements that come as a society makes the transition produce overwhelmingly positive outcomes, like medical and public health discoveries, they have some negative effects as well. For example, one of the most serious negative consequences from the transition is an increased sedentary lifestyle; increasingly technological societies foster physically inactive populations.

This trend is repeated across most other adverse health behaviors: poorer dietary patterns, increasing alcohol abuse, increasing energy intake, lack of exercise, and so on. And the result, if these populations don't commit to taking a healthy approach, will be more chronic disease, including much more cancer.

Noting the connection to calorie consumption

Table 6-1 shows the change in approximate calories consumed per day in different parts of the world. Take particular note of the rise in calories per day in the developing world compared with those consumed in the developed world; then look at the projections into 2015 and 2030. From 1965 to 2030, the largest increase in calories consumed per day occurs in the developing world, with some regions experiencing over a 40 percent increase in energy consumption. Compare that to the developed world that has approximately a 15 percent increase.

Table 6-1	Real and Projected Daily Calorie Consumption, 1965–2030					
Region	*1965*	*1975*	*1985*	*2000*	*2015*	*2030*
Developing countries	**2,050**	**2,150**	**2,500**	**2,700**	**2,900**	**3,000**
Near East and North Africa	2,250	2,600	3,000	3,006	3,100	3,200
Sub-Saharan Africa	2,000	2,050	2,100	2,200	2,350	2,550
Latin America and the Caribbean	2,400	2,500	2,700	2,800	3,000	3,200
East Asia	1,950	2,100	2,500	3,000	3,100	3,200
South Asia	2,000	2,000	2,200	2,400	2,700	2,900
Developed countries	**3,000**	**3,100**	**3,200**	**3,400**	**3,450**	**3,500**
World	**2,400**	**2,450**	**2,700**	**2,800**	**3,000**	**3,050**

Source: Adapted from the WHO and FAO report, "Diet, nutrition, and the prevention of chronic diseases"

Health professionals suggest that this rise in energy consumed per day is a good thing because large swaths of these regions are prone to famine. Although in the short term, this rise in energy is beneficial, it will be a detriment to these regions over time. As I explain in later sections of this chapter, an increasing trend of energy consumed per day is correlated positively with cancer development. In other words, higher calorie intake over long periods of time is directly linked to increased incidence of cancer.

Whenever you discuss cancer, keep in mind that risk is not distributed equally between different demographic groups. For example, 60-year-old men, and women who are between 40 and 80 years old die of cancer more than any other disease. Scandinavian men have the highest risk for testicular cancer. Black American males are at a higher risk for prostate cancer than other male populations in the U.S. Women in Sub-Saharan African are at greater risk of developing cervical cancer than women from any other country in the world. Bottom line: Age, gender, ethnicity, and other demographic information play a part.

Discovering how cancer develops: Free radicals and carcinogens

Cancer manifests in your genes. Cells, when exposed to a cancer-causing material, may become mutated. The question is, what causes, or initiates, cellular mutation?

Two terms you're likely to hear in any conversation revolving around causal factors of cancer are *carcinogens* and *free radicals:*

✔ **Carcinogens:** A *carcinogen* is simply any agent — types of food (for example, high-fat foods), foreign substances (like pesticides), and radiation, among many others — that can cause cancer.

✔ **Free radicals:** A *free radical* is an atom or molecule that is highly reactive due to unpaired electrons. Electrons like to travel in pairs. An unpaired electron will seek out another electron, and it'll capture the needed electron from the nearest stable molecule. When the stable molecule loses its electron, it becomes a free radical itself. This unstable free radical then seeks an electron to make a pair, and the cycle continues. Eventually, this stealing of electrons can disrupt cellular function. Researchers theorize that this chain reaction of electron stealing can mutate cells' genetic components, thus resulting, over time, into cancer.

Both carcinogens and free radicals can mutate cellular DNA and thus initiate the process of a healthy cell becoming a cancerous cell. You can find these substances almost anywhere and in most anything, particularly in the food you eat.

Consider, for example, liver cancer, which can result from a diet chronically very high in fat. Figure 6-2 shows how free radicals can mutate liver cells; they eventually disrupt normal cell function and can affect the DNA in the cell's nucleus. Notice that poor nutrition is one of the causes.

In Figure 6-3, you see the same process as it pertains to the entire organ itself. A high-fat diet leads to fat accumulation in the liver. This fat is seen as a foreign substance, and macrophages and neutrophils (types of white blood cells that fight infection) are dispatched to fight the "infection." If the inflammation persists over long periods of time, tissue damage — and possibly cancer — can result.

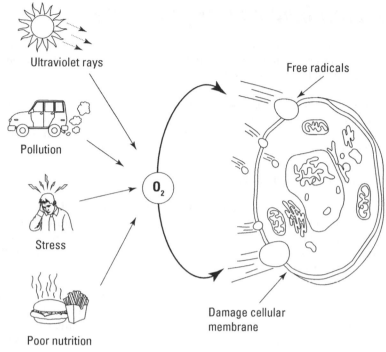

Figure 6-2:
How free radicals damage a cell.

Illustration by Wiley, Composition Services Graphics

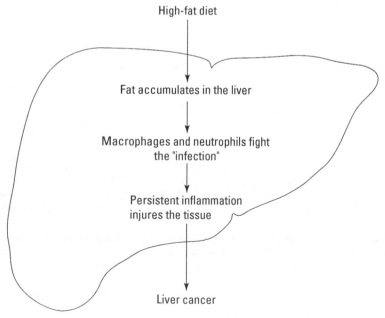

Figure 6-3:
How a high-fat diet can lead to liver cancer.

Illustration by Wiley, Composition Services Graphics

Seeing how cancer progresses

Cancer manifests in your genes. If one of your cells is exposed to a cancer-causing material, the DNA in the cell may become mutated. One bad cell doesn't spoil the whole batch, does it?

To answer that question you have to know a couple of things about cells: First, they reproduce by splitting, which means 1 cell produces 2 cells that, barring any mutations that make the daughter cells different, are exactly identical to it. These 2 cells split into 4 cells, which split into 8 cells, and then into 16 cells, and, well, you get the picture. Second, if something goes wrong in a cell, it has a self-destruct mechanism.

Here's the problem: Once damaged, a cell may lose the ability to self-destruct or stop reproducing. Therefore, if your cellular DNA is mutated from carcinogens, like tobacco use, alcohol abuse, high-energy diet, cellular phone waves, and so on, your mutated cells may continue to replicate and divide uncontrollably.

Cells that endlessly divide begin to grow into a tumor. When these mutated cells grow numerous enough, and if no intervention occurs to stop them, they take over the functions of healthy tissue surrounding the cancer site, then take over the entire organ, and then spread *(metastasize)* to other locations in the body and often cause death.

Four major steps occur in *carcinogenesis,* the process of cancer development (see Figure 6-4):

1. Initiation.

The cells are exposed to cancer-causing agents, and their DNA mutates.

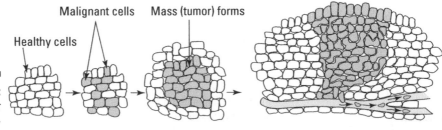

Malignant cells   Mass (tumor) forms

Healthy cells

Figure 6-4:
Cancer progression from exposure to metastasis.

Initiation: Cells are exposed to carcinogens and mutate

Promotion: Mutated cells divide.

Latency / transformation / progression: Malignant cell masses form.

Tumor/metastasis: Mass of malignant cells take over tissue functions and major organs and spread to other regions in the body.

Illustration by Wiley, Composition Services Graphics

Why cell death is better than cell injury

Which is better, a dead cell or an injured cell? If the cell has become mutated because of repeated exposure to a carcinogen or free radical, without doubt, you want a cell death. Think about it: A tumor is essentially a large mass of mutated (injured) cells that take over the functions of healthy tissue and organs, causing them to fail and, in the end, causing you to die. Better for the mutated cell to die than for it to live only to cause problems.

Your body is a resilient machine. It has failsafe mechanisms that help prevent cancer development. When cellular DNA mutates during initiation phase (refer to the section "Seeing how cancer progresses,") your body can activate (or *express*) a self-destruct gene that causes the cell to die to prevent it from replicating its mutated DNA.

---

2. **Promotion.**

   The mutated cells begin to undergo the process of *mitosis* (cell division) and propagate uncontrollably.

3. **Latency Period/Transformation/Progression.**

   The mutated cells transform into malignant cell masses. Essentially. this is the period between initiation and the clinical discovery of the disease, which can range in length, depending on the type of cancer.

4. **Tumor/Metastasis.**

   A mass of malignant cells takes over functions of tissue and major organs while spreading to other regions of the body. This stage leads to disability and usually death.

Noting Nutritional Risks

Some diets encourage cancer: A primary risk factor for cancer development is a diet that includes any one or more of the following characteristics, especially when combined with a physically inactive lifestyle:

- ✔ Is high in fat and low in fiber
- ✔ Includes lots of processed foods
- ✔ Includes excessive amounts of alcohol
- ✔ Relies primarily on red meat as the main protein source

Unfortunately, this list describes the diets of many, if not most, people, who may not truly understand the link between what they eat and their increased risk of developing cancer.

Eating a high-energy diet with a side of sedentary lifestyle

Fat appears to be a cancer promoter in animals. When calorie intake rises and energy expenditure through exercise decreases, cancer rates tend to rise in response. In addition, the type of dietary fat may be important, with some fats promoting cancer and others protecting against it:

- Omega-6 polyunsaturated fatty acids may promote cancer; omega-3 fatty acids from fish, walnuts, or flaxseeds, on the other hand, may protect against some cancers and may support recovery during cancer treatment.

- Saturated fats and trans-fats increase cancer risk among people who chronically consume high amounts.

In addition, the buildup of adipose tissue in and around your major organs (which often occurs from lack of exercise and eating too much) may cause inflammation, which could lead to certain cellular mutations. Table 6-2 lists some cancers related to significant rises in body fat, total energy intake, and source of fat.

Table 6-2	Cancers Linked to Excess Body Fat	
Type of Cancer	*Percentage of Cases Linked to Obesity*	*Number of Cases per Year*
Breast	17%	33,000
Colorectal	9%	13,200
Endometrial	49%	20,700
Esophageal	35%	5,800
Gallbladder	21%	2,000
Kidney	24%	13,900
Pancreatic	28%	11,900

Source: American Institute for Cancer Research, 2012

As I explain in Chapter 5, most populations around the world are experiencing a rise in daily energy consumption. This increase in energy (that is, glucose) is contributing to *insulin-like growth factors (IGF),* adipokine-related inflammation, and other complications.

Insulin-like growth factors

IGF stems from the body's saturation of excess glucose. Your pancreas responds by manufacturing insulin to move the glucose from the blood into the cell. Essentially, if the cell is chronically saturated with insulin, the insulin signaling system (how the cell utilizes and receives insulin) is at risk for mutation. If the insulin receptors become mutated, the risk of cancer increases exponentially.

Research has shown that tumor cells thrive on high levels of glucose and really cannot survive without it. A few of your cells, like neurons, do not need insulin to absorb glucose from the blood flowing by them, but most of your healthy cells need appropriate levels of both insulin and glucose.

Adipokines

Adipokines are hormones that regulate inflammatory processes and energy metabolism in tissues. When you are more obese, particularly more centrally obese due to physical inactivity and overeating, the overabundance of adipokines promotes inflammation and insulin resistance (you can read more about insulin resistance in Chapter 8), which raises your risk of developing diabetes, coronary heart disease, and even cancer.

If you are obese or diabetic, you should not drastically change your diet without consulting your healthcare provider. People with these conditions have distinct dietary needs. Altering your diet without understanding fully the disease and its connection with food can be dangerous and possibly deadly.

Consuming a lot of red meat

Evidence links diets high in red meat with a moderately elevated risk of breast cancer, prostate cancer, and cancers of the digestive tract. Processed meats seem to be of special concern. The problems with red meat are multifold:

- ✔ **The presence of nitrites and nitrates in the meat:** These compounds kill bacteria (they're particularly useful in preventing botulism), enhance flavor, and give color to meats. They are great for curing bacon, hams, and deli meat. However, there is some controversy around using nitrates because they can lead to the formation of *nitrosamines,* a cancer-causing compound.

- ✔ **Animal-based saturated fats:** A study by the National Cancer Institute suggests that saturated fat may be a cause of intestinal cancer. Besides possibly causing cancer, saturated fats are a known factor in heart disease.

- ✔ **The way the meat is cooked:** Research links broiled, fried, grilled, and/or smoked meats to cancer. These cooking methods can generate carcinogens. Particularly risky is charring the meat. Blackened flesh demonstrates carcinogenic qualities in research studies.

As Table 6-3 indicates, global meat consumption is rising dramatically. From the early 1960s to the amount projected for 2035, people around the world will eat eight times more meat. As I note earlier in the chapter, much of this increase will occur in the developing world, particularly in regions where meat was once rare but is becoming more available as meat production becomes more efficient and costs decrease. As meat consumption rises, expect even more cases of cancer resulting from the foods people eat.

Table 6-3	Increases in Global Meat Consumption, in Metric Tons
Year	*Total Global Meat Consumption*
1961	~50 million
1971	~100 million
1981	~125 million
1991	~175 million
2001	~225 million
2011	~260 million
2025	~350 million

Drinking too much alcohol

Alcohol alone is associated with cancers of the mouth, throat, and breast. Although liver cancer is more commonly associated with alcohol abuse, parts of the body more at risk are the esophagus, oral cavity, pharynx, and larynx. In addition, cancers of the head and neck are strongly correlated with the combination of alcohol and tobacco use and low intakes of green and yellow fruits and vegetables. Table 6-4 lists cancers related to alcohol.

Table 6-4	Percentage of Fatal Cancers Related to Alcohol
Cancer	*Percentage Related to Alcohol*
Esophageal cancers	75%
Mouth cancers	50%
Larynx cancers	50%
Liver cancers	30%

Taking Charge of Your Nutrition to Ward Off a Cancer Diagnosis

Dietary patterns can put you at risk for developing cancer. Carcinogens and free radicals in your food and from pesticides and other toxins, eaten consistently over time, can increase your risk of cellular mutation and cancer. Fortunately, you can take control of these risk factors.

Promoting a healthier lifestyle that includes making responsible food choices and exercising is the remedy for cancer prevention. Unfortunately, making the changes necessary to achieve this goal isn't always so easy. In this section, I outline things that can make a positive difference.

Promoting healthy lifestyles through a multifaceted approach

Promoting healthy diets and lifestyles to reduce cancer requires a multifaceted approach. Any type of promotion campaign must do the following:

- ✔ **Include different styles of messaging.** Not everyone listens to a message the same way or responds to the same type of message. Some people, for example, may respond to fear or threat in a message; others don't. As a nutritionist, you need to develop different methods of communicating to reach and motivate as many people as possible.

- ✔ **Involve different sectors of society in decision-making and support services.** At the family level, for example, a diet plan would involve all family members in meal planning and cooking activities.

- ✔ **Provide viable, easy-to-access options for food and exercise opportunities.** Efforts to promote healthy eating should include easy-to-make recipes, tips on how to shop cheaply and healthily, and other suggestions to make meal prep easy. Similarly, exercise options must include strategies that people can adopt. A cash-strapped mother who works two jobs to make ends meet, for example, has neither the time nor the financial resources to make use of a gym membership.

In Chapters 19 and 20, I discuss health communication and behavioral intervention strategies. This information can help you understand what drives decisions and how you can develop persuasive ways to communicate with your patients.

Adapting behaviors to reduce cancer risk

Eating a high-calorie, high-fat diet, coupled with a sedentary lifestyle, tobacco use, alcohol abuse, and other adverse health behaviors puts you at exponentially higher risk of developing cancer than does eating a healthy diet and maintaining a healthy lifestyle.

In short, scientists know that to reduce your risk of cancer you must begin to eat healthy and exercise. Table 6-5 summarizes healthy behavior choices and notes which cancers they protect against. Pay particular attention to the diet, exercise, alcohol, and body weight–related columns.

Table 6-5	Recommendations to Decrease Your Cancer Risk					
	Avoid Tobacco	*Be Physically Active*	*Maintain Healthy Weight*	*Eat Healthy Diet*	*Limit Alcohol*	*Avoid Excess Sun Exposure*
Bladder	X			X		
Breast		X	X	X	X	
Cervix	X					
Colorectal	X	X	X	X	X	
Esophagus	X		X	X	X	
Kidney	X		X			
Larynx	X			X	X	
Lung	X			X		
Oral	X			X	X	X
Pancreas	X			X		
Prostate	X	X	X	X	X	
Skin						X
Stomach	X			X		
Uterus			X			

Source: World Cancer Research Fund/American Cancer Institute for Cancer Research

Making healthy changes to your diet

To counter the dangers outlined in the preceding sections, dietary strategies must promote eating adequate quantities of healthy, nutritious food. The current American diet tends to have these characteristics:

- ✔ Higher overall energy intakes

- ✔ Increased saturated fat consumption (mostly from animal sources)

- ✔ Lower than recommended consumption of complex carbohydrates, fiber, fruits, and vegetables

In this section, I outline some of the dietary changes you can make to reduce your cancer risk. Table 6-6 highlights the dietary factors that either increase or decrease your risk of developing certain cancers.

Table 6-6	Dietary Factors and Their Relationship to Cancer Risk	
Type of Cancer	*Factors Increasing Risk*	*Possible Protective Effect From*
Bladder[1]	High alcohol intake; weak association with coffee consumption	Fruits and vegetables, adequate fluid intake
Breast[2]	High intakes of calories, saturated fats, red meat, and alcohol, and low intakes in vitamin A; obesity	Monounsaturated fats, vegetables and fruits, calcium, vitamin D
Cervical[1]	Folate deficiency (**Note:** Viral infection is also a risk factor)	Adequate folate intake, possibly fruits and vegetables
Colorectal[1,2]	High intakes of fat (particularly saturated fat), red meat, alcohol, and supplemental iron; low intakes of fiber, folate, vitamin D, calcium, and vegetables; obesity	Vegetables (especially cruciferous [cabbage-type]), fruits, calcium, vitamin D, and dairy; possibly whole wheat and wheat bran
Kidney[1]	Possibly high intakes of red meat (especially fried, sautéed, charred, or cooked well done); obesity	Fruits and vegetables (especially orange and dark green ones)

(continued)

Table 6-6 (continued)

Type of Cancer	Factors Increasing Risk	Possible Protective Effect From
Mouth, throat, and esophagus[1]	High intakes of alcohol (especially in combination with tobacco use) and preserved foods; low intake of vitamins and minerals; obesity	Fruits and vegetables
Liver	High intakes of alcohol; iron overload (**Note:** Hepatitis infection is also a risk factor)	Vegetables (especially yellow and green ones)
Lung[1]	Low vitamin A intake; beta-carotene supplements (in smokers) (**Note:** Air pollution is also a risk factor)	Fruits and vegetables
Ovarian	High lactase intake	Vegetables, especially green, leafy ones
Pancreatic[1]	High intakes of red meat	Fruits and vegetables (especially green and yellow ones)

[1]Tobacco use is also a risk factor.
[2]Physical inactivity is a risk factor.

Beware of diets that claim to cure cancer. Coffee consumption, for example, has been linked to preventing basal cell carcinoma, but interestingly, it's not been shown to provide protection against the deadlier melanoma. Still, some individuals are being counseled to drink as much as five times the daily recommendation of coffee to not only prevent cancer growth but to cure it. Be skeptical of any such claims or recommendations. The hypothetical benefits that are supposed to come from drinking excessive amounts of coffee after a cancer diagnosis don't come anywhere close to the increased risks of raising your blood pressure, reducing beneficial sleep, and developing kidney stones. If you are thinking about altering your diet, make a doctor's appointment and talk it out.

Increasing fiber and drinking water

Significant evidence shows that eating a diet rich in high-fiber, low-fat foods and drinking plenty of water are good for you. Specifically, these actions can decrease your risk of developing colon and bladder cancers. Although it's unclear whether the fiber itself or some other characteristic of a high-fiber diet lowers the risk of colon cancer, researchers know that a colon full of fiber can perform miracles. As my wife tells me, "A healthy colon equals a healthy you." Words to live by.

In addition, staying adequately hydrated is essential in promoting the best possible health outcomes. Here's why:

- ✔ People who drink adequate fluids each day may be less prone to developing colon or bladder cancer because they are flushing out their bodily waste more frequently than those who don't drink as much.

- ✔ To digest, fiber requires bacterial fermentation. The rise in this fermentation increases the likelihood that the carcinogenic nitrogen compounds found in red meats and other animal products will bind to the fiber, helping to neutralize the effects of these potential cancer-causers and excrete them out of the body quickly.

- ✔ Fiber acts as a *chelating agent,* a substance that removes select compounds, in the colon. Water, certain vitamins, minerals, and even bile (a detergent-like digestive product made by the liver, stored in the gallbladder, and used to break fats into smaller pieces so enzymes can complete digestion) are in a sense attracted to fiber, leading to more rapid excretion. Because the potential exists for cancer-causing products to enter your guts, the faster it moves through, the lower your risk of developing cancer, especially colorectal or anal cancer.

 Folate is found in high-fiber foods. Research shows that folate deficiency seems to increase the risk of cancers of the cervix, colon, skin, and other sites. Researchers don't understand yet why this is so, but you can help protect yourself from these cancers by making sure you get enough folate in your diet.

Getting enough vitamin E: The antioxidant

Antioxidants are the entities, like vitamin E, that protect cellular integrity from the damaging effects of free radicals (refer to the earlier section "Discovering how cancer develops: Free radicals and carcinogens" for details on what free radicals are). Vitamin E is generally viewed as the element best suited to counteract the effects of free radicals in the body. Table 6-7 lists foods that are high in vitamin E.

Table 6-7	Foods High in Vitamin E	
Food	*Serving Size*	*Percentage of RDA*
Sunflower seeds	1 ounce	76
Sunflower oil	1 tablespoon	66
Almonds	1 ounce	50
Peanut butter	2 tablespoons	21
Avocados	1 cup, sliced	13
Olive oil	1 tablespoon	11
Spinach	1 cup, cooked	11
Pumpkin seeds	1 ounce	2

The percentage of adults worldwide who consume five or more servings of fruits and vegetables each day is staggeringly low, particularly in the more developed world. Approximately only 20 percent to 30 percent of adults eat adequate amounts of vitamins and minerals per day from fruit- and vegetable-based foods. The point? People are at risk for not getting enough vitamin E.

Although an excess of vitamin E can actually encourage negative effects of free radicals, a consensus exists among nutritionists and dietary health professionals that healthy amounts of vitamin E discourage cancer growth in the body. However, this may not be true for esophageal and prostate cancers.

Vitamin D may protect against skin cancer. So make sure to get your recommended daily dose of this vitamin. Great sources of vitamin D include fatty fish (salmon, tuna, and sardines), dairy (lower fat forms fortified with vitamin D), and egg yolk. But avoid cod liver oil. Although it is a great source of vitamin D, it's also way too high in preformed vitamin A, which is the only form that can cause toxicity.

Eating a rainbow: Phytochemicals and you

What elements make hot peppers hot, make the aloe plant great for sunburns, make ginger tangy, make fennel taste licorice-y, and make eggplants purple? The answer: phytochemicals.

Phytochemicals are chemicals that confer taste, color, and other qualities to plant matter. Although the exact nature and function of these elements are still largely unknown, many of them are greatly beneficial to the body. Some phytochemicals in fruits and vegetables are thought to reduce the risk of heart disease, cancer, and the effects of stress, and to increase immune system response.

The vast majority of people worldwide are not benefitting from potentially fantastic sources of cancer prevention due simply to a poor diet. To avoid this problem, eat fruits and vegetables of all colors. Doing so is an easy way to ensure you're getting all the health benefits phytochemicals have to offer. Table 6-8 lists some common phytochemicals that you can find at your local grocer.

Table 6-8	Foods and Their Phytochemicals
Food	**Phytochemical**
Aloe	Emodin
Artichoke	Silymarin
Basil	Ursolic acid
Carrots	Beta-carotene

Food	Phytochemical
Cloves	Eugenol, isoeugenol
Cruciferous vegetables (cabbage, cauliflower, green, leafy vegetables)	Sulforaphane
Fennel	Anethole
Garlic	Diethyl sulfate, ajoene, s-allyl cysteine, allicin
Ginger	6-gingerol
Pomegranate	Ellagic acid
Red chili	Capsaicin
Red grapes	Resveratrol
Soybean	Genistein
Tea	Catechin
Tomato	Lycopene
Turmeric	Curcumin

Eat more cruciferous vegetables and tomatoes. They're two of the best foods for cancer prevention:

✔ **Cruciferous vegetables:** Research shows that individuals with very low intakes of these vegetables are at significantly higher risks to developing colon cancer than those who eat healthy amounts.

✔ **Tomatoes:** The phytochemical lycopene in tomatoes makes this food one of the best to eat to help fight against cancer. So next time you're wondering what to order at a restaurant, try the pasta and get the marinara sauce. Not only will it taste delicious, but you'll also be preventing cancer at the same time!

Chapter 7

Cracking the Cardiovascular Case

- -

In This Chapter

▶ Understanding the different forms of cardiovascular disease

▶ Outlining the risk factors for cardiovascular disease

▶ Identifying which foods promote heart health

▶ Assessing your cardiovascular disease risk

- -

*I*f you take a look at the leading causes of death in the Western world, heart disease reigns supreme, even surpassing cancer as the number one killer in our society. Globally, cardiovascular disease (CVD) kills millions of people per year. Consider these numbers:

✔ In 2011, the Centers for Disease Control and Prevention (CDC) noted that approximately 27 million U.S. adults were diagnosed with heart disease. Further, around 600,000 died of the disease, making it the number-one cause of death.

✔ In Canada, yearly deaths attributed to CVD hover around 30 percent.

✔ In the United Kingdom, nearly 35 percent of all deaths are attributed to the disease.

✔ In Europe, over 4 million people per year die as a result of CVD complications.

✔ One Australian dies every 12 minutes from CVD.

Despite the bleak morbidity and mortality rates, there is some good news: Through proper diet and exercise, CVD can be treated and prevented. By incorporating some very easy, practical wellness activities into your everyday routine, you can live your life with very low risk of developing heart disease.

In this chapter, I tell you what you need to know about heart disease, discuss the physiology behind the disease, and explain how diet and nutrition are key components of any strategy designed to lower your risk factors and any treatment plan designed to minimize the disease's effects.

Clarifying Confusing Terminology about Cardiovascular Disease

The job of the cardiovascular system is to oxygenate and transport blood throughout your body. It consists of your blood vessels and your heart, as shown in Figure 7-1, as well as your lungs. This system feeds your body oxygen and assists in removing carbon dioxide from the body.

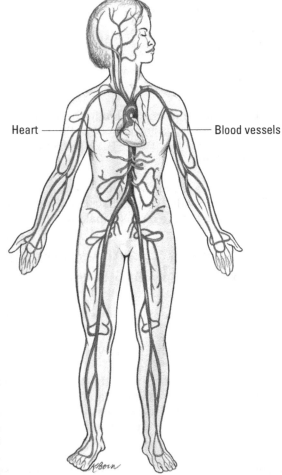

Heart ————————————————— Blood vessels

Figure 7-1:
The cardiovascular system includes your heart and blood vessels, as shown here, as well as your lungs.

Illustration by Kathryn Born, MA

I am sure you have heard of heart disease, cardiovascular disease, coronary heart disease, stroke, hypertension, heart attack, and so on. In fact, an endless list of diseases seems to stem from cardiovascular issues. Before you can understand how proper diet and exercise programs can assist in lessening your risk of experiencing one or more of these adverse health outcomes, you need to know what these terms actually mean.

For the most part, *cardiovascular disease (CVD)* is an umbrella term that includes diseases of the heart and circulatory system. This term includes many different health issues, like actual heart disease or some other circulatory issue. CVD is the number-one killer worldwide and includes a number of diseases of the cardiovascular system, which swells its ranks.

Following are some of the diseases that are all lumped under the CVD umbrella:

- ✔ **Atherosclerosis:** Atherosclerosis is a fatty hardening of the arteries. In atherosclerosis, plaque builds up on the arterial walls and impedes the flow of blood. Because it is the most common way to develop heart disease and because you can significantly reduce your risk of developing other cardiovascular problems by addressing the risk factors that lead to atherosclerosis, I devote the entire next section to this topic.

- ✔ **Coronary heart disease (CHD):** In CHD, your heart suffers damage from atherosclerosis (see the preceding item in this list).

- ✔ **Heart attack:** In a heart attack, heart tissue dies when oxygenated blood cannot be delivered to the heart muscle because of coronary arterial blockage. A heart attack causes permanent damage to the heart muscle.

   The phrase *myocardial infarction* is another name for heart attack. Myocardial infarction is the result of a *thrombosis* or an *embolism,* both of which are basically fatty deposits that form in the arteries and block the flow of blood. Myocardial infarction causes very rapid heart tissue death. You can read more about thrombosis and embolism in the later section "Clotting up a storm.")

- ✔ **Stroke:** In a stroke, a cerebral arterial blockage prevents oxygen from reaching the brain, resulting in the death of brain tissue.

- ✔ **Hypertension:** With hypertension (also called *high blood pressure*), the pressure within the arteries increases to a unhealthy level. When this happens, more strain is placed on the heart, which has to pump the blood through the body via blood vessels.

Attacking Atherosclerosis

As I explain in the preceding section, atherosclerosis is the technical term for a condition that many people simply call a hardening of the arteries. Most, if not all, of us have at least some form of the disease already. Although having atherosclerosis isn't normal, it is very common.

Atherosclerosis presents myriad dangers to your health, and it develops slowly over time, putting undue strain on your heart and leading to possible clotting, which, in all too many people, results in heart attacks and strokes. In this section, I examine the heart strain and clotting more closely.

Watching how atherosclerosis develops

Here's how atherosclerosis usually progresses (see Figure 7-2):

1. **Filmy streaks of fat line the arterial walls.**

2. **These streaks begin to accumulate into a mass, which can begin to block the blood vessel.**

   The material that actually hardens is called *plaque.* Plaque is a buildup of fatty acids in the arteries that has hardened over time. Where an artery branches into two or more vessels, the plaque can easily get lodged at the branch and block the artery.

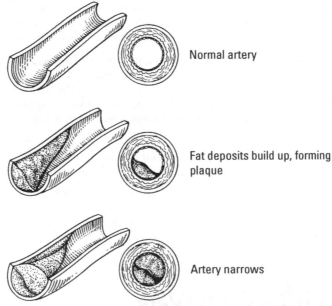

Normal artery

Fat deposits build up, forming plaque

Artery narrows

Figure 7-2: The development of plaque impedes blood flow.

Illustration by Kathryn Born, MA

3. **As the artery becomes more and more blocked, blood flow is more and more restricted.**

   Restricting blood flow reduces the amount of oxygenated blood available to nourish the body. As it becomes more and more difficult for the blood to flow through the artery, the heart must pump that much harder. This process is one way to develop hypertension: The narrower the artery, the more pressure that must be used to pump the blood.

4. **If left untreated, eventually a complete blockage can result, causing massive heart failure and/or stroke, and possibly death.**

   When blood can't pass through due to a blockage, your heart goes into distress, culminating in a heart attack, which can cause death because your heart stops beating or becomes so damaged that it cannot be revived. For stroke victims, the cerebral infarction can cut the blood supply off to the brain, causing massive brain damage.

Unfortunately, rarely do symptoms warn you that you're developing atherosclerosis. And for the most part, you really don't know how much of any particular vessel is blocked and hardened by plaque.

Your best bet is to eat a high-fiber, low-fat diet and exercise to prevent the disease outright or to limit its buildup. A diet low in saturated fats and cholesterol, coupled with a regular exercise regimen, can reduce your risk of plaque buildup and arterial hardening. Head to the later section "Eating Your Way to a Healthy Heart" for details on how dietary and exercise habits can help reduce your risk of developing atherosclerosis and other cardiovascular-related diseases.

Plucking away at your heart strains

Your body's organs and tissues need a certain amount of oxygen to function properly. Your heart's job is to make sure that all the parts get the oxygen they need. When narrowed or blocked blood vessels reduce blood flow, your heart has to repeatedly exert itself above and beyond normal to ensure that your tissues and organs still get the oxygen they need. Putting your heart under this added pressure can lead to significant adverse health outcomes.

Think about it: Your heart is a muscle, just like any other muscle, and it can get tired. Could you walk up 50 flights of stairs without the muscles in your thighs getting tired? Probably not, unless you're Superman or extraordinarily fit. For us normal folk, walking up 50 flights of stairs would definitely wear out our legs. The point: Muscles get tired and worn out after repeated use above and beyond their normal strain. And in this context, "normal" is the strain the muscle is accustomed to. For very unfit people, normal may be no farther than a few steps; for firefighters in peak condition or world-class athletes, normal would take them significantly farther.

Your heart is no different. If your heart has to repeatedly pump blood with more and more force just to get the appropriate amount of blood through clogged arteries, the muscle will flat out get strained, eventually tire, and then, unfortunately, stop working.

Clotting up a storm

The fact that your blood can clot is a good thing. Blood clotting is part of the body's internal healing mechanism. When a blood vessel has been injured, *platelets* (a certain kind of blood cell) and *plasma* (the fluid part of your blood) form a clot to cover the injury site and prevent excessive bleeding. When healing is complete, the clot naturally dissolves. However, atherosclerosis and related issues can cause abnormal clotting, which poses a direct threat to your health and your life.

One key difference between regular clots and abnormal clots is that abnormal clots do not dissolve back into the blood as normal clots do. If these clots do not dissolve, they become obstructions in the vessel that can cause some major health problems, such as the following:

- **Aneurysm:** In an aneurysm, a blood-filled bulge in the wall of a blood vessel forms. This bulge is the result of a weakening of the arterial wall and built-up pressure within a blood vessel.

- **Thrombosis:** In thrombosis, shown in Figure 7-3, a blood clot forms within a blood vessel and remains attached to its place of origin. The technical term for this type of clot is a *thrombus*.

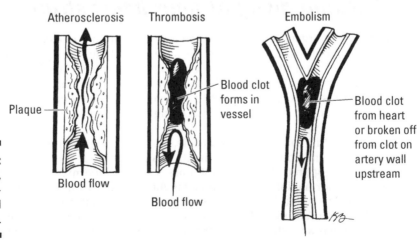

Figure 7-3: Aneurysm, thrombosis, and embolism.

Illustration by Kathryn Born, MA

> ✔ **Embolism:** With an embolism, also shown in Figure 7-3, a blood clot or an air bubble is transported by the blood stream and becomes lodged in a blood vessel and impedes the circulation. The technical term for the material that gets stuck is *embolus*.

Another difference between regular and abnormal clots is that, whereas regular clots form as a result of injury, abnormal clots can form even without an obvious injury, primarily as a result of built-up plaque in your arteries. If the plaque ruptures suddenly, a clot develops because your body believes the ruptured plaque is an injury.

Scientists hypothesize that abnormal clots don't dissolve as readily due to the continued presence of the plaque and, thus, the continued perceived injury by the body.

Figuring Out the Risk Factors of CVD

Diseases of the cardiovascular system manifest themselves slowly throughout your life. They aren't typically sudden onset events, even though the outcomes may be sudden — an unexpected massive heart attack, for example. In most cases, decades-long buildup of risk factors lead to these "sudden" events. For many, if not most, people, the buildup begins early in life and continues throughout their lifetimes. In fact, most people have no idea they are developing these conditions unless they are carefully screened by their physicians.

So the question remains: What can put you at an increased risk for CVD? Many things, actually. Look at this list for some of the primary risk factors for CVD:

✔ **Family history:** You're more likely to have CVD if a history of the disease exists in your family.

✔ **Aging:** Your risks for developing CVD increase as you get older.

✔ **Sex:** Scientists hypothesize that men get the disease more than women due to their genetic differences, as well as social and environmental differences (differing average workplace exposures, for example).

✔ **Race/ethnicity:** Different racial/ethnic groups, as well as other demographic subgroups, can be at an increased risk of developing CVD than others.

Figure 7-4 shows the stats from California. These rates would be at least mildly mirrored in other modern societies. Table 7-1 outlines the data for this chart.

If you are more at risk due to your demographic, you need to take extra special precaution to help ward off CVD. Definitely consult your physician before implementing any new diet or lifestyle regimen.

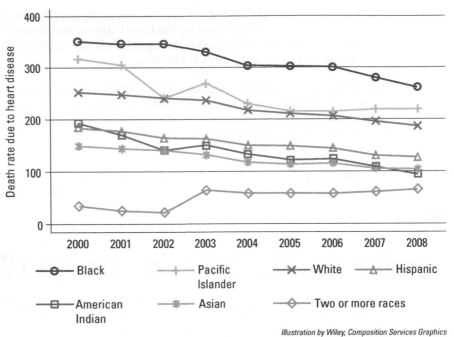

Figure 7-4: Age-adjusted death rates for heart disease in California, 2000–2008 (Source: California Department of Public Health).

Table 7-1			Heart Disease Age-Adjusted Death Rates by Race/Ethnicity (California, 2000–2008)						
	2000	*2001*	*2002*	*2003*	*2004*	*2005*	*2006*	*2007*	*2008*
Black	351.2	347.3	347.1	333.3	304.5	302.1	301.8	280.4	262.2
Pacific Islander	317.3	306.0	241.2	269.4	230.1	216.4	215.0	220.1	219.0
White	251.8	248.2	240.2	236.4	218.1	211.1	206.6	196.2	187.3
Hispanic	184.8	177.0	165.4	163.3	150.3	148.5	143.8	130.1	127.4
American Indian	192.6	170.3	142.0	150.1	133.7	123.0	123.8	110.1	93.8
Asian	150.2	144.7	142.0	132.1	117.0	114.5	115.6	106.5	103.9
Two or more races	34.1	25.5	22.7	64.7	58.7	58.0	58.2	60.9	65.8

Source: California Department of Public Health http://www.cdph.ca.gov/programs/ohir/Pages/Heart2008PrinterVersion.aspx

✔ **Eating a high-fat, low-fiber diet:** This kind of diet is such a risk factor that it's known as the *atherogenic diet* due to its strong links to atherosclerosis.

✔ **Inactive lifestyle:** Lack of exercise is a leading contributor to developing CVD.

✔ **Being obese:** Obesity alone increases your risk, but the fact that most cases of obesity also involve high-fat, low-fiber diets and inactive lifestyles compounds the risk.

✔ **Tobacco use:** People who use tobacco are 70 percent more likely to develop heart disease than nonsmokers. If you are a nonsmoker who lives with a smoker, you are 30 percent more likely to get heart disease.

✔ **High cholesterol:** Cholesterol contributes to the buildup of plaque on arterial walls, thus increasing your risk of developing thrombosis and, eventually, embolism (refer to the earlier section "Clotting up a storm" for more on these conditions).

✔ **Hypertension:** High blood pressure causes your blood vessels to clog or weaken. When you are hypertensive, your heart is overworked, thus raising your risk of heart disease.

✔ **Having diabetes:** Diabetes is a risk factor because people with type 2 diabetes also often have other risk factors, such as obesity, high-fat, low-fiber diets, hypertension, and so on.

The good news is that the vast majority of these risk factors are modifiable. That is, these behaviors can be changed; they are not permanent. Obviously, increasing your level of activity and eating a healthy diet can mitigate the lifestyle and diet risk factors. But doing so can also mitigate other risk factors as well, such as obesity, cholesterol, hypertension, and diabetes. Bottom line: Your diet is one of the leading contributors, if not *the* leading contributor, to developing heart disease.

Most of the risk factors for heart disease are modifiable, meaning that you can change them. Table 7-2 outlines actions you can take to prevent and/or treat CVD.

Table 7-2	Ways to Decrease Risks of Heart Disease
To Combat This Risk Factor	**Take This Action**
Obesity	Lose weight
Having diabetes	Control carbohydrate intake (sugars)
Tobacco use	Refrain from or quit smoking

(continued)

Table 7-2 *(continued)*	
To Combat This Risk Factor	**Take This Action**
Inactive lifestyle	Continue or begin to exercise
High cholesterol	Monitor you blood cholesterol
Hypertension	Control salt intake and stress
Eating a high-fat, low fiber diet	Eat a high-fiber, low-fat diet (what I call the anti-atherogenic diet)

Eating Your Way to a Healthy Heart

Lifestyle changes are your best bet for achieving heart healthiness. You can adopt a number of behaviors to promote a higher quality and increased quantity of life. And believe it or not, these behaviors are not that difficult to fully incorporate into your life. As a bonus, eating a healthier diet, getting more exercise, refraining from smoking, and keeping stress low work not only to prevent CVD, but also to help prevent other diseases, like obesity, diabetes, and even some cancers.

To promote the best possible health for your cardiovascular system, you need to follow some specific guidelines, especially if you're over 40 years old. I outline these suggestions in this section.

Controlling cholesterol

Cholesterol is a wax-like material that is manufactured in your body (your liver produces it), and it's found in the animal-based foods you eat.

Cholesterol made by your liver is called *endogenous cholesterol,* and cholesterol obtained from your food is called *exogenous cholesterol.*

Although most people think only bad things when they hear the word *cholesterol,* cholesterol is actually necessary for good health. It's needed to make vitamin D and hormones, it assists in digestion (cholesterol helps with the manufacture of bile), and it helps maintain cell integrity. Remember, cholesterol is an essential part of a long and healthy life. Without it, you wouldn't survive.

Read on to discover the different types of cholesterol, how much cholesterol you should get in a day, and how a high-fiber diet can help you control your cholesterol levels.

Good guys versus bad guys: HDL and LDL cholesterol

There are two main types of cholesterol: *high-density lipoproteins (HDL)* and *low-density lipoproteins (LDL)*. Together, HDL and LDL transport needed fats and other nutrients to and from the cells.

Still, HDL cholesterol is considered good cholesterol, and LDL is considered bad cholesterol. Why? The quick answer is that LDL is packed with more fat, and HDL is packed with more protein.

Physicians suggest that people raise their HDL cholesterol level and lower their LDL level. The idea is that having more lean than fatty cholesterol (HDL has more protein and less fat than LDL) discourages an excess of fat and cholesterol being delivered *to* cells. The goal is to have excess fat and cholesterol carried *away* from cells, and HDL is just the substance for these tasks.

Controlling your cholesterol intake

As I mention earlier, in addition to your body making cholesterol, you can also get cholesterol from the foods you eat. For that reason, you need to control how much cholesterol you ingest because a diet high in cholesterol can contribute to high blood cholesterol levels, which can promote CVD.

Here are the guidelines:

- **For healthy adults:** A healthy adult should limit dietary cholesterol to less than 300 mg/day (your liver makes about 1,000 mg/day).

- **Adults with health issues:** If you were diagnosed with CVD, if you have diabetes, or if you have high LDL/low HDL, you should limit your dietary cholesterol to less than 200 mg a day.

Most animal-based foods contain some amount of cholesterol, and foods high in fat tend to have more cholesterol in them. You want to monitor how much of these foods you consume to avoid excess cholesterol, which can contribute to the development of CVD.

As important as watching how much cholesterol you get from food is, don't think that that alone protects you from high cholesterol. Even though food cholesterol raises your blood cholesterol, it isn't the main culprit in raising cholesterol to dangerously high levels. Sure, food cholesterol has an impact, but not as much as trans-fats and saturated fats do. Trans-fat and saturated fat have more influence over the levels of your endogenous cholesterol than exogenous cholesterol sources do. Crazy, right? To read more about those kinds of fats, head to the later section "Taking care of fats."

Being a good egg

I've always found it kind of a shame that most people hear the word *cholesterol* and automatically have a negative reaction. Years and years of bad press on this substance have made people believe that it's one they ultimately must avoid. To that, I say hogwash.

Do me a favor: Ask the next adult or two you see whether they like to eat eggs. If the answer is yes, ask whether they eat eggs every day, to which they'll probably reply, "No." If you ask them why, they'll probably respond in one of two ways:

✔ Eggs are too high in fat.

✔ Eggs are too high in cholesterol.

Granted, eggs do have both fat and cholesterol, but not to the extent that they have to be avoided completely.

Contrary to what most people believe, eggs are not a taboo food. They are good for you. You should eat eggs. They are full of vitamins (particularly the vitamin A precursor, beta-carotene, and vitamin D), good fats, protein, and yes, cholesterol — all essentials for a healthy diet. Just don't eat an omelet made from eight extra-large eggs for breakfast every day. One or two small eggs a day is fine.

Here's what the science says: Although eating too many eggs can increase your cholesterol, eating four egg yolks or fewer a week hasn't been found to increase your risk of heart disease. It's all about moderation. Refer to the Chapters 2 and 3 for a refresher on those discussions.

Eating a high-fiber diet to control cholesterol levels

Eating a high-fiber, low-fat diet can do many wonderful things for your health. Ranging from keeping your colon strong to reducing the amount of excess fat in your diet, fiber is one of those food substances that is crucial if you want to live the healthiest life possible. Fiber is also a fantastic tool for controlling cholesterol levels in your body.

Here's how fiber in the diet can help control cholesterol:

✔ **Fiber moves things along.** In the small intestine, when bile (made by the liver from endogenous cholesterol) assists with fat digestion, fiber must be present to help speed along the process of getting the digested food through the intestines.

✔ **Fiber, especially soluble fiber, acts as a sponge.** This sponge soaks up excess water, some minerals, and vitamins. Most importantly, it soaks up excess bile — and the cholesterol in it — and transports it out of the body. Soluble fiber is the type of fiber that does the best job soaking up the cholesterol from bile.

Bile is made up of cholesterol components, and in a low-fiber environment, any bile left over after the digestion process is sent back into the bloodstream, slightly raising your total body cholesterol. In this scenario, the cholesterol isn't being excreted; it's being recycled, which is not necessarily a good thing. If this recycling continues, eventually your cholesterol levels will be so high that they'll begin to pose a threat to your cardiovascular system.

Here's a step-by-step explanation of how soluble fiber can lower cholesterol (see Figure 7-5):

1. **Soluble fiber and cholesterol from foods reach the stomach and travel from there to the small intestine.**

2. **Meanwhile, cholesterol from the liver goes to the intestines.**

3. **Soluble fiber forms a gel that binds some cholesterol to the small intestine and takes it out of the body.**

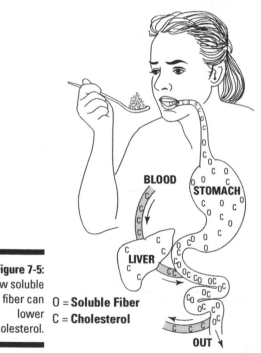

Figure 7-5:
How soluble
fiber can
lower
cholesterol.

O = **Soluble Fiber**
C = **Cholesterol**

Illustration by Wiley, Composition Services Graphics

Excess cholesterol in your body encourages the growth of plaque in the arteries. If left unchecked, this plaque begins to harden and clog the arteries, which can lead to very serious adverse health outcomes. Although you need to be careful not to eat too much fiber (because it could soak up too much water and other nutrients), you must ensure that you get enough to regulate any excess cholesterol in your diet.

Looking at good sources of fiber

Most food packages don't show soluble fiber separately. Instead, the total fiber content is listed simply as *dietary fiber.* So it pays to know some sources of soluble fiber. Table 7-3 lists foods that are high in soluble fiber and shows the fiber content in a serving. Try to incorporate these foods into your diet. Your heart will thank you for it.

Table 7-3	High-fiber Foods	
Food	*Serving Size*	*Total Fiber (grams)*
Artichoke	1 medium	10.3
Black beans, cooked	1 cup	15.0
Flaxseed	1 tablespoon	3.0
Green peas, cooked	1 cup	8.8
Kale, cooked	1 cup	2.6
Kidney beans	1 cup	13.1
Lentils, cooked	1 cup	15.6
Lima beans, cooked	1 cup	9.0
Navy beans, cooked	1 cup	19.1
Oats, dry	1 cup	16.5
Pinto beans, cooked	1 cup	11.0
Split peas, cooked	1 cup	16.3
Raspberries	1 cup	8.0
Soybeans, cooked	1 cup	7.6

Source: USDA, National Nutrient Database for Standard Reference

Taking care of fats

Back in the 1960s, research that highlighted the dangers that cholesterol and saturated fats posed to heart health led to an enormous push to eliminate foods containing those substances from people's diets. Advertising campaigns advised eliminating saturated fats and cholesterol from diets and promoted using trans-fats as a heart-healthy substitute. Boy, they were wrong.

As it turns out, the story on fat and how to incorporate it into a healthy diet is fairly complicated. Here's what you need to know:

- ✔ **Fat is essential for well-being.** It serves as a storage facility for some vitamins, it's a source of energy, and it protects major organs of the body.

- ✔ **There are two general categories of fat — saturated and unsaturated.** Saturated fats are found in animal products and processed foods. A saturated fat is fully saturated with hydrogen atoms and is solid at room temperature. Saturated fats are considered bad, because they can raise your LDL cholesterol.

  Unsaturated fats are considered heart-healthy because they help lower LDL cholesterol and raise HDL cholesterol. These kinds of fats are found in foods such as nuts and some fruits and vegetables, like avocados. They are liquid at room temperature and differ from saturated fats in their chemical structure; they are not fully saturated with hydrogen. They can be unsaturated at one spot in the fatty acid chain (monounsaturated fats, such as in olives) or more than one spot (polyunsaturated, such as in vegetable oil [omega-6 fats] and flaxseed oil [omega-3 fats]).

No fat is purely healthy. They all have percentages of saturated, polyunsaturated, and monounsaturated fats. What makes one fat healthier than another is the percentages of each of these. Obviously, healthier fats are those that have a higher percentage of unsaturated fats and a lower percentage of saturated fats. Table 7-4 lists the different kinds of oils and shows their breakdown into good and bad fats.

The less saturated fat, the better. Also, steer clear of overeating animal fats, coconut and palm oils, and butter. Monounsaturated fats (olive and safflower oils) and fatty fish oils are best for keeping your arteries clear and your cardiovascular system at its healthiest.

DASH-ing your diet for good health

The Dietary Approach to Stop Hypertension (DASH) diet is the number-one recommendation on how to reduce your risk of morbidity and mortality associated with CVD. This diet reduces blood pressure through the following actions:

- ✔ Reducing sodium
- ✔ Increasing magnesium, calcium, and potassium
- ✔ Increasing the amount of vigorous exercise
- ✔ Eating more whole grains, fruits, and vegetables
- ✔ Keeping calories and fat to lower levels
- ✔ Keeping stress levels low

Table 7-4	Comparing Dietary Fats			
Dietary Fat	*Saturated*	*Polyunsaturated*		*Monounsaturated*
		Omega-6	*Omega-3*	
Canola oil	7%	21%	11%	61%
Safflower oil	8%	14%	1%	77%
Flaxseed oil	9%	16%	57%	18%
Sunflower oil	12%	71%	1%	16%
Corn oil	13%	57%	1%	29%
Olive oil	15%	9%	1%	75%
Soybean oil	16%	54%	8%	23%
Peanut oil	19%	33%	>1%	48%
Cottonseed oil	27%	34%	>1%	19%
Lard	43%	9%	1%	47%
Palm oil	51%	10%	>1%	39%
Butter, melted	68%	3%	1%	28%
Coconut oil	91%	2%	0%	7%

Source: Sizer & Whitney, 2012

Were our ancestors healthier?

Humans have been eating saturated fats and cholesterol for millennia. From the ancient Egyptians to the World War II era, meat, dairy, and other natural sources of saturated fats and cholesterol were dietary staples. Given what earlier research was saying about these substances, you'd think that people who ate these diets were keeling over from CVD and other dietary-related chronic diseases at a much higher rate than people of the modern era. Well, you'd be wrong.

Interestingly, the incidence of CVD and diet-related chronic diseases such as diabetes in that earlier era were much lower than the rate of those health issues in populations from the 1960s to the present day.

Eliminating cholesterol and saturated fats from the diet and substituting trans-fats in their place didn't make society any healthier. In fact, I would go out on a limb and say people today are worse off. Consider that, if you look at CVD rates post-1960, you see no significant drops in morbidity or mortality related to this change.

As it turns out, trans-fats increase the risk for CVD just as much as saturated fats do. *Trans*-fats are created artificially, when humans *hydrogenate* (literally add hydrogen to) unsaturated fats. The hydrogenated unsaturated fats become straighter in shape and act in the body like saturated fats. You're better off eating naturally occurring unsaturated fats to reduce your CVD risk. Even naturally occurring saturated fats are better for you than trans-fats, but they still need to be limited.

By making these diet and lifestyle changes, the DASH diet sets in motion a chain reaction that leads to improved health and decreased risk of CVD:

1. By reducing sodium, increasing exercise, and promoting the intake of healthier foods, you reduce hypertension and reduce the amount of calories eaten.

2. Eating fewer calories reduces cholesterol and fat levels and helps regulate obesity.

3. A healthy body weight, in addition to the other changes, ultimately reduces your risk of developing CVD.

Putting Together Your Action Plan

Although CVD is the number-one killer around the world and even though it may seem that many of the risk factors are unavoidable, you can take action now that will significantly reduce your risk of developing cardiovascular disease in the future. Here are some things you can do:

✔ **Keep salt at low levels.** Salt (sodium) raises blood pressure in the body. People with high blood pressure are at a higher risk of heart disease. Be sure to limit your salt intake.

✔ **Exercise!** Physical activity offers so many benefits: It helps you maintain (or achieve) a healthy weight, it lowers cholesterol, it relieves stress . . . the list goes on and on.

✔ **Keep fat and calories at manageable levels.** You should get about 25 percent to 35 percent of your calories from fat. If you chronically get too much fat in your diet, you are at a higher risk of developing plaque in your arteries. Refer to the earlier section "Clotting up a storm" to read about the dangers that plaque poses.

✔ **Choose healthy fats.** These include monounsaturated and polyunsaturated fats. Keep your saturated fats, trans-fats, and food cholesterol at lower levels.

✔ **Chill out!** Keep stress low! Stress is linked with panic and anxiety, which is linked to higher risks of heart disease.

✔ **Eat more whole foods like whole grains, fruits, and vegetables.** Doing so not only ensures that you're eating low-fat foods that are chock-full of nutrients and fiber, which promote heart health, but it also means that you're getting fewer of your calories through foods that are high in saturated fats, trans-fats, and cholesterol.

✔ **Don't smoke.** And if you do smoke, quit now.

✔ **Keep alcohol to moderate intake levels.** High alcohol intake promotes high blood pressure, which is a risk factor for heart disease. Take it easy and drink responsibly.

Even though the solutions themselves are pretty straightforward, many people struggle to make these changes. The first thing you need to do is have confidence. The next is to understand that this process is easier than you think. You have to take baby steps at first to get used to the changes in your diet and lifestyle, but don't worry. It gets easier. I promise.

I will leave you with this list, courtesy of Skinny Mom (www.skinnymom.com), to help you plan your diet for a healthier heart and life! These foods contain one or more nutrients known to protect the heart, lower cholesterol levels, reduce high blood pressure, and protect blood cells and blood vessels.

Almonds	Oranges
Apples	Papaya
Asparagus	Popcorn
Banana	Raisins
Black or kidney beans	Red bell pepper
Blueberries	Red wine
100% whole-wheat bread	Salmon
Broccoli	Soy milk
Brown rice	Spinach
Cantaloupe	Sweet potatoes
Carrots	Tea
Dark chocolate	Tomatoes
Flaxseed	Tuna
Lentils	Walnuts
Oatmeal	Yogurt

Chapter 8

Discussing Diabetes

Diabetes mellitus, commonly referred to simply as *diabetes,* is a very serious disease that seems to be getting more prevalent, not only in the industrialized, developed world, but globally as well. Theories abound regarding why the incidence and prevalence of the disease are increasing and pinpoint everything from genetics as the culprit to high-fructose corn syrup.

In this chapter, I explore what diabetes is, explain the factors that put you at risk for the disease, and look at what dietary patterns you can adopt to help keep this disease at bay.

Outlining the Physiology of the Disease

To understand what diabetes actually is, you need to understand some basic human physiology first. Specifically, you need to be familiar with blood glucose and insulin and how these two substances interact in the body.

Gaining insight on blood glucose

The body desires carbohydrates for energy. Glucose is the foundational unit of carbohydrates and the principal sugar your body burns for energy. Glucose is an essential building block of your body and its processes. In other words, without glucose, your body wouldn't work; in fact, it wouldn't survive.

Your body gets glucose through a series of three chemical processes that occur when you eat:

- ✔ When your body digests carbohydrates

- ✔ When the liver uses amino acid *precursors* (the raw, unprocessed form of amino acid) to produce glucose in a process called *gluconeogenesis*

- ✔ When *glycogen,* the principal form of glucose in your body, is broken down in the liver, in a process called *glycogenolysis*

Your body, for all its hardiness, is a very finely tuned machine that needs only a certain amount of glucose, and it goes to extraordinary lengths to keep the glucose levels in line. With both types of diabetes (type 1 and type 2), that balance ends up out of whack, and you end up in trouble.

What does blood glucose do for you?

Glucose performs a number of important functions in the body:

- ✔ **It helps facilitate eating.** How so? When glucose levels decrease in the blood, usually after a period of not eating, your brain is alerted that you need food. Your brain then triggers a sensation of hunger, and in response, you find food and eat it. At that point, your blood glucose levels rise back to normal levels.

 Glucose levels are usually lowest in the morning before breakfast and fluctuate throughout the day as you eat lunch, dinner, and snacks. As a rule, they remain elevated for about an hour or two after meals.

- ✔ **It provides fuel and nutrients to keep cells alive and functioning.** Your cells require energy to perform all the functions needed to properly do their work (link amino acids together to form proteins, divide, and so on).

- ✔ **It provides the fuel needed to give you energy for activities and physical exertion.** Any type of activity you perform — even ones that take place without your conscious involvement (temperature regulation, digestion, and so on) — requires energy; glucose is the primary source of that energy.

Obtaining blood glucose and keeping it at healthy levels

Blood sugar levels vary among people, depending on their physiology, family history, and behaviors.

Normal fasting blood glucose levels differ, depending on whether you have diabetes (*Note:* Glucose levels are measured in milligrams per deciliter, or mg/dL):

Category	*Fasting Glucose Levels*
People without diabetes	70–99 mg/dL
People with prediabetes	100–126 mg/dL
People with diabetes	127–150 mg/dL

After eating, the glucose levels rise. For those without diabetes, the levels rise to about 140 to 150 mg/dL. For those with diabetes, levels can get to 180 mg/dL, but they shouldn't consistently stay above 180 mg/dL.

Understanding the purpose of insulin

Insulin is a protein that enables your body to use energy (that is, sugar and other carbs). Therefore as you eat, your blood becomes rich with energy. Insulin, secreted by the pancreas, allows that sugar/energy to be used by the cells.

The problem in people with diabetes is that their bodies don't secrete insulin (type 1 diabetes) or their bodies are resistant to its effects (type 2 diabetes). (Read about the different types of diabetes in the upcoming section "Distinguishing between type 1 and type 2 diabetes.") Many people with diabetes must take exogenous (artificial) insulin by injections in order to allow the blood sugar to enter the cells and be used.

When you eat increased amount of refined carbohydrates (white flour or rice, simple sugars, and so on), your insulin levels spike. This situation can lead to a rise in triglycerides in the blood. If you are already insulin resistant, this effect is worsened.

Defining Diabetes

Diabetes mellitus is a chronic metabolic disorder that is primarily defined by a high fasting blood glucose level (that is, your blood glucose is tested after a period during which you refrain from eating). The status of high blood glucose level, or *hyperglycemia,* usually results when insulin, a hormone you can read about in the preceding section, is no longer created by the body or no longer works as it's supposed to.

Because glucose can't get into the cells to do its work, people with diabetes end up with excess glucose molecules floating in the plasma of the blood. This is why people with diabetes are often said to have high blood sugar.

Diabetes is characterized by chronic hyperglycemia; however, the body can also become *hypoglycemic. Hypoglycemia* occurs when blood sugar levels drop too low. Someone with blood sugar levels that are too low may experience sluggishness, weakness, irritability, and excessive sweating. Alarmingly, this condition can cause you to pass out and, if it is chronic, can lead to brain damage. People with diabetes can become hypoglycemic if they take too much insulin.

Diabetes, if uncontrolled, can do some very serious damage to the human body, including the following:

✔ It causes blood vessel, nerve, and eye damage, which can lead to amputation, blindness, and even death.

✔ If it gets too concentrated, people with diabetes can go into a very hyperglycemic state and die.

The incidence of diabetes around the world is rapidly increasing — and not just among older people, a population that has traditionally experienced high rates of the disease. Now young adults, sometimes even children, are being diagnosed with type 2 diabetes.

Distinguishing between type 1 and type 2 diabetes

Diabetes comes in a variety of forms: two primary types (type 1 and type 2), gestational diabetes (seen among pregnant women; head to Chapter 15 for details), and a form of the disease — prediabetes — that is experienced before the full-blown version of the disease appears.

In this section, I cover the four different types and/or stages of the disease. Different risk factors lead to different classifications, so be sure to take note of which factors are distinct and which are shared among different varieties.

Prediabetes

Prediabetes is a health condition in which fasting blood glucose levels rise to slightly above normal levels, ranging approximately from 100 mg/dL to 125 mg/dL. Even slightly elevated blood glucose levels can cause problems: For starters, tissue damage can occur during this stage, paralleling the same kind of damage someone with full-blown diabetes would experience.

One of the most alarming concerns about prediabetes is that very few people who have it know they have it. Therefore, if you think you may be at risk for prediabetes, be sure to have yourself tested, and if you are overweight or obese (with a BMI above 25) — a primary risk factor for developing prediabetes — have your blood glucose levels checked regularly. Delayed discovery and/or treatment of the condition can make the situation worse. If you want to check out your risk, take the Diabetes Risk Test at `http://www.diabetes.org/diabetes-basics/prevention/diabetes-risk-test/?loc=DropDownDB-RiskTest`.

Diabetes insipidus

Another disorder, called *diabetes insipidus,* is unrelated to *diabetes mellitus.* People with diabetes insipidus experience excessive thirst and excrete very large quantities of urine, just as people with diabetes mellitus do. But diabetes insipidus differs from diabetes mellitus in some specific ways; one primary difference is the lack of glucose in the urine, one of the hallmarks of diabetes mellitus.

Interestingly, when the ancients first discovered disease mellitus, they named it for these two characteristics: the excessive amount of urine and the sweetness of the urine. *Diabetes* is the Latin word meaning "siphon" (sufferers urinated frequently), and *mellitus* is the Latin word meaning "honey" (some intrepid early physician tasted the urine and found it to be sweet).

Type 1 diabetes

Type 1 diabetes is a genetic, autoimmune disorder. It usually arises when the person's own immune system misidentifies insulin as an enemy and attacks the cells of the pancreas that produce it. Eventually, the pancreas cannot produce insulin.

Approximately 5 percent to 10 percent of all cases of diabetes are type 1. Because it is typically diagnosed during childhood and adolescence, it was once called *juvenile diabetes,* but the fact is that it can occur at any age, even later in life (but diagnosis usually occurs prior to age 35). Incidence rates of type 1 diabetes are on the rise. In fact, it is the leading chronic disease among children and adolescents.

The International Diabetes Foundation indicates that the ten countries that have the highest incidence of type 1 diabetes in children are the following (listed in order from highest to lowest): Finland, Sweden, Norway, the U.K., Canada, Australia, Denmark, Germany, New Zealand, and Puerto Rico (a U.S. territory). This list is partly the result of more vigorous diagnostic practices in these countries versus the rest of the world and possibly because of a combination of genetic predispositions and dietary habits.

As I explain earlier, the fuel that cells use to live and function is glucose, and insulin is the gatekeeper that lets glucose into the cells. In type 1 diabetes, after you eat, glucose concentration builds up in the blood while body tissues are simultaneously starving for glucose. The treatment for type 1 diabetes is insulin injections. Once insulin is present, the cells can take up and use the glucose from the bloodstream.

In the research world, there's been some chatter that a vaccine for type 1 diabetes is under development, as is an insulin-producing pancreatic cell transplant procedure. It will probably be years before either of these treatments is actually available, but the mere idea that they're being considered demonstrates fantastic advancements in the field!

Type 2 diabetes

In type 2 diabetes, body tissues lose their sensitivity to insulin. The problem is that insulin is no longer effective at getting into the cells. Unlike type 1 diabetes, which is characterized by a lack of insulin, in type 2 diabetes, plenty of insulin is available; it's just not doing its job.

Type 2 diabetes represents about 90 percent to 95 percent of all diabetes cases. Just like type 1 diabetes, the incidence of type 2 diabetes is rising in an alarming way around the globe. Nations whose populations 30 years ago experienced nowhere near epidemic levels of diabetes (the developing nations) are now among the most at risk. The Middle East, for example, is on track to have the largest percentage increase, with an almost 200 percent increase in existing cases!

The main risk factors for type 2 diabetes include being overweight or obese, age, and physical inactivity. As a rule, people who are apple-shaped (that is, their fat accumulates in the abdomen) are more likely to develop type 2 diabetes than those whose bodies are pear-shaped (the fat accumulates on the hips and buttocks).

Type 2 diabetes is many times called *adult-onset diabetes* because it occurs mostly in adults, after long-term, chronic, excessive calorie intake. Alarmingly, however, type 2 diabetes is now being diagnosed in children, who are succumbing in growing numbers to the same ills (being overweight and physically inactive and eating an unhealthy diet) that previously characterized the lifestyles of older sufferers.

Gestational diabetes

Gestational diabetes occurs in pregnant women. What makes this type of diabetes so interesting is that the women who are diagnosed with the disease did not have diabetes prior to their pregnancies, and the diabetes resolves itself after the women give birth. Experts estimate that approximately 20 percent of all pregnancies result in a diagnosis of gestational diabetes.

No one is really sure what causes gestational diabetes, but health professionals hypothesize that the cause is one of the following:

✔ **Very high intake of calories by the mother:** High energy consumption leads to significant and rapid weight gain, which puts the mother temporarily in a state of insulin resistance.

Losing sensitivity to insulin, step by step

How does the body lose its sensitivity to insulin? These steps explain what happens:

1. A person chronically overconsumes calories, including sugar, resulting in higher amounts of sugar in the blood and probable weight gain.

2. As glucose rises in the bloodstream, the pancreas compensates by producing larger and larger amounts of insulin.

3. Eventually the pancreas is so overworked that it begins to slow down insulin production,

and blood sugar spins even further out of control.

4. The muscles and *adipose tissues* (fat deposits) no longer respond to increased glucose in the blood and don't absorb it.

5. The person now has a condition called *insulin resistance*, which produces the major health problems associated with type 2 diabetes.

✔ **A hormonal condition related to the placenta:** Health professionals suggest that hormones from the placenta affect the ability of the mother's insulin to move sugars from the blood into the cell. In this way, gestational diabetes is essentially a form of insulin resistance.

For more information on gestational diabetes, head to Chapter 15.

Toxic effects of diabetes

When your body has too much glucose in the blood, some serious adverse health outcomes can occur. This section outlines the major physiological problems stemming from diabetes.

Altering cell metabolism and function

Being hyperglycemic can literally alter the metabolism of virtually every cell in the body — a pretty powerful effect, if you ask me. Cell metabolism refers to the cycle of chemical transformations in the cells that enable them to sustain proper function. One primary end product of cell metabolism is the formation of energy. Too much glucose can overwhelm this system.

Here are some of the effects of excess sugar in the blood:

✓ **Toxic alcohols are created from too much fructose.** You consume fructose when you eat fruit, honey, or high-fructose corn syrup, which your liver metabolizes much in the same way it metabolizes alcohol; therefore, processing fructose produces much the same effect on your liver as excessive alcohol does.

✓ **Certain cells may swell.** When blood sugar levels are chronically high, water collects in the cells, causing them to swell. If this occurs in the cells that make up the lenses of the eyes, for example, vision can be distorted.

✓ **Proteins may lose the ability to function properly.** Some cells attach excess glucose to proteins in abnormal ways. When this happens, the proteins cannot function properly or, in some cases, cannot function at all. The end result can cause some major problems, like nerve and blood vessel damage.

Affecting blood flow and nerve sensation

In people who have diabetes, the structure of blood vessels and nerves become damaged. This damage can lead to a loss of circulation and nerve function, which has these deleterious effects:

✓ **Kidney damage:** The loss of blood flow to the kidneys damages them, thus limiting their ability to cleanse the blood. For details on kidney function and disease, head to Chapter 9.

✓ **Increased risks from infection:** When you have an infection, you need blood flow to help carry wastes away from and needed antibodies to the infected area. When you have diabetes, not only are you more likely to suffer from infection, but the loss of both circulation and proper nerve functioning can lead to situations in which you are unaware of problems because you don't feel the discomfort that someone with proper circulation and nerve function would feel.

This loss of sensation is one of the reasons why people with diabetes must have their feet regularly checked — to ensure that no undetected injury or infection is present. Alarmingly, if left untreated, such injuries can lead to amputation (mostly of legs and feet) or even death.

Paying attention to warning signs

The following list outlines some warning signs of diabetes. Keep in mind that having just one or two of these does not necessarily mean that you have diabetes. However, if you have three, four, or more — or if you experience any of these symptoms chronically — go to your physician and get your blood glucose levels checked:

- Excessive urination and thirst
- Urine that smells sweet and fruity (may be a sign of glucose in the urine)
- Unexplained weight loss with nausea, fatigue, weakness, and irritability
- Cravings for sweets
- Frequent infections of the skin, gums, vagina, or urinary tract
- Blurred vision
- Slow healing of cuts and bruises
- Pain in legs, feet, and hands

Clarifying the risk factors

The risk factors for diabetes are pretty straightforward and, if you think about them, not very surprising. In the following list, I outline some major risk factors of the disease; although other factors exist, these are the most prominent:

- **Obesity:** If you are obese, your risk of developing diabetes is tripled, mainly because people who are obese tend to exhibit several other risk factors as well: low physical activity, unhealthy diets, and a family history of diabetes.

- **Stress:** Stress can make you eat more and exercise less, thus increasing your risk of developing diabetes.

- **Little or no physical activity:** The less you exercise, the less likely you are to burn off unneeded energy. The less energy you burn and the more weight you gain, the more at risk you are for developing diabetes.

- **Increasing age:** As you age, your risk of diabetes increases because you are apt to eat more refined sugars and exercise less, impeding your body's ability to process these sugars effectively.

- **Eating an unhealthy diet:** Your risk is higher if your diet consists of processed, refined foods with very high levels of simple carbohydrates (simple sugars/glucose) and low levels of complex carbohydrates, fiber, and water.

- **Family history:** You are more at risk of developing diabetes if you have a history of the disease in your family, especially if an immediate member (parents, grandparents, or any siblings) had the disease.

These risk factors may seem particularly alarming if they describe your life right now: Maybe you are obese and don't eat a good diet and don't exercise. Maybe you're getting past middle age and have a lot of stress at your job as you near retirement. Maybe both your parents had diabetes, and several of the other risk factors hit a little too close to home. What do you do? First, don't panic. It's going to be okay. The good thing is that four of these six risk factors are *modifiable;* they can be changed. In the next sections, I tell you how you can use diet and lifestyle to prevent — or treat — diabetes.

Preventing and Treating Diabetes through Diet and Lifestyle

Believe it or not, you can treat, prevent, and even reverse the damage done by diabetes through diet. If you are trying to lower your risk factors, you must follow a healthy diet and engage in regular exercise. If you already have diabetes and you're using diet to treat or reverse the disease, your diet will be even further specialized and more strict. This section outlines dietary guidelines that can help with treatment and prevention.

As I explain in the preceding section, four of the six risk factors for diabetes are preventable. Sure, you can't do anything about getting older or being part of a family with a history of diabetes, but you can focus on the factors you can do something about. Here are some simple suggestions that you can undertake immediately:

- ✔ **Change your diet and get moving.** One of the most impactful steps you can take is to stop eating poorly and begin exercising. These changes don't have to be drastic to be effective. Start small and try increasing your dietary restrictions and exercise sessions every week as you grow more fit. This approach will lead to weight loss if you burn more calories than you consume (refer to Chapter 5 for specific suggestions on combating obesity).

  You don't necessarily have to give up your favorite foods. However, you do need to modify how you eat. You can continue to eat some of your favorite foods, but you absolutely must moderate how much you eat. In other words, it's not so much quality, but quantity, that matters.

- ✔ **Reduce stress.** Look for ways, even little ways, to reduce the amount of stress you experience in a given day. Breathing exercises work, as does meditation. Taking a leisurely walk around a park where I can do some people-watching with my wife is my favorite way to relax!

These changes aren't complex, but they can be hard, especially mentally. I get that, but don't let that be an obstacle or excuse that stops you from making changes that can help you ward off this terrible disease. Remember, you have the power to be successful. Consult your doctor for guidance and then take the steps you need to to get your life on track to prevent (or treat) diabetes. Read on for more detailed information that will help you as you get you started.

Controlling blood glucose levels

To control diabetes, you must control your insulin levels. The biggest challenge in this battle for control? Simple carbohydrates, or sugars (glucose), in foods. Most people consume a moderate- to high-carb diet.

Most health professionals agree that the best way to control blood sugar is to avoid or limit the foods that cause an increase in unhealthy blood glucose levels in the first place. Those foods are ones that include carbohydrates, especially simple carbs. Therefore, the key is to reduce the amount of carbs you eat.

Although cutting back on carbs may seem like an easy task, it's actually a bit more difficult than most people initially suppose. Why? Because carbs are in almost all the foods that people love to eat. In the next section, I shed some light on how you can reduce your carbohydrate intake yet still enjoy your food.

Reducing your carbs

Eating a reduced-carb diet has been a craze now for two decades. Most of this interest stemmed from the popularity of a quick weight-loss method. However, in this section, I explore this diet from the perspective of diabetes maintenance.

Before you get into the nitty-gritty details of reduced-carb diets, I want to take a few lines to cheerlead for getting healthy and staying healthy. You have a unique opportunity. Unlike many diseases, diabetes is a disease that you can, to a large extent, treat and possibly reverse simply by adopting certain behaviors. By following a strict diet, exercising, and taking any medications prescribed by your doctor, you can not only take care of this disease but also become the healthiest you possible.

Looking at key features of reduced-carb diets

In a reduced-carb diet, you simply cut back on foods that contain large amounts of carbohydrates. Doing so enables you to control your body's blood sugar levels. Not too complicated, right?

Cutting back on carbs can be difficult, especially for people who are used to eating a lot of bread, drinking coffee with sugar, and eating pizza, chips, and what seems to be almost every tasty food imaginable. Fortunately, you can still eat tasty foods and also control your glucose levels.

Some diet plans offer advice on how to eat when you have diabetes. For the most part, they preach limited carbohydrates, particularly from grain products, but also from fruit and vegetable sources, to help control blood sugar levels.

Figure 8-1 shows the low-carbohydrate diabetes food pyramid. In this plan, usually given to people who are first diagnosed with the disease, vegetables are the primary staple in your diet. This plan shows people how to get the majority of their carbohydrates from complex carbohydrate sources, which is recommended over the grain-based carbs, many of which tend to be simple carbs (from refined breads and rice, for example).

Following this food plan helps you keep blood sugar under control. The key, of course, is to limit your portions and be aware of natural sugars found in the foods — even those that you may assume don't contain sugars (fruits and potatoes, for example).

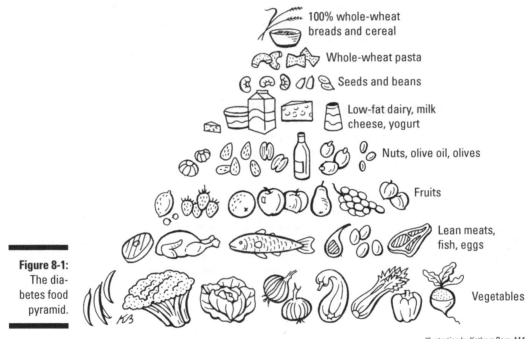

Figure 8-1:
The dia-
betes food
pyramid.

100% whole-wheat breads and cereal

Whole-wheat pasta

Seeds and beans

Low-fat dairy, milk cheese, yogurt

Nuts, olive oil, olives

Fruits

Lean meats, fish, eggs

Vegetables

Illustration by Kathryn Born, MA

Other tips and advice to successfully manage diabetes

As you create a meal plan to control your blood sugar, keep these guidelines in mind:

✔ **Eat more from the foods at the bottom of the pyramid and less from the foods at the top.** As you can see in Figure 8-1, the carbs from grain sources are at the top of the pyramid, which means that these food items are the ones you should eat the least of each day.

✔ **Be careful of how much fruit you eat.** Fruits appear in the middle of the pyramid because they contain high levels of natural sugars (called *fructose*).

✔ **Choose your protein carefully.** Protein-rich foods (besides beans, which contain a lot of carbs) are an important part of a reduced-carb diet. However, you need to be careful. Protein-rich foods tend to be higher in calories and saturated fat. So as you incorporate different proteins into your diet, be sure to keep your red meat intake in check and be wary of eating too many saturated fats.

Following are some options you can choose from when you're preparing a meal ideal for someone with diabetes. These foods help keep blood sugar down:

Apples	Lean protein
Asparagus	Melon
Beans	Nuts
Berries	Omega-3–rich fish
Broccoli	Red onion
Carrots	Soy
Citrus	Sweet potatoes
Dark, leafy greens	Tea
Fat-free milk and yogurt	Tomatoes
Flaxseed	Whole grains

Determining how stringent your diet must be

You can still eat carbs when you have diabetes, but you have to control them. How stringent this control must be depends on the severity of your diabetes: If your diabetes isn't severe, you have a bit more flexibility with the kinds of carbs and how much of them you can eat. If your diabetes is more severe, certain carbs may be off-limits, and other carbohydrates may need to be strictly controlled. Your physician can determine the severity of the disease and provide guidance.

The amount of carbs you need to incorporate in your diet depends on how severe your diabetes is. Perhaps somewhere in the range of 45 to 60 grams of carbs per meal is a good place to start, but be sure to consult your physician for specific guidelines.

Timing your meals

Controlling blood glucose through what you eat is only part of the equation when it comes to living healthily with diabetes. You also must pay attention to the timing of your meals. Basically, when you eat, your blood glucose levels rise as the food you eat is broken down during the digestion process. Between meals, your blood glucose levels fall as your cells slowly use the glucose up.

To keep your glucose levels from spiking (rising too high or too quickly) or falling to dangerous levels, do the following:

✔ Space out your meals and snacks evenly throughout the day.

✔ Eat roughly the same amount of carbohydrates at each meal.

Evenly spacing your meals can help you keep blood glucose levels from rising too high or falling too low.

You are in control of your disease; your disease is not in control of you. The best thing you can do is have a plan that incorporates these action items:

✔ Get informed. Read up on diabetes, talk with your physician, or go to any of a variety of websites that have helpful information, like http://www.diabetes.org/.

✔ Decide on a plan to incorporate a healthy lifestyle and start making some preliminary changes.

Experiment with what works and what doesn't and adapt as you need to to maximize your chances of success.

✔ Adjust your meal schedule to be sure you're keeping your blood sugar levels as even as possible throughout the day.

✔ Commit to the changes. Diabetes is a lifelong disease. The healthy changes you make need to last for a lifetime, too.

✔ Find a support system for help. You can usually find these groups in your local newspaper in the community events section. Or do a simple search on the web, using key terms like "local diabetes support groups" and your area.

Chapter 9

Caring about Kidney Disease

. . . .

In This Chapter

▶ Finding out what kidney disease is

▶ Identifying foods to avoid or treat kidney disease

▶ Discovering foods that are good for your kidneys

. . . .

*Y*our kidneys, along with the rest of your excretory system (see Chapter 14 for a more in-depth discussion on the entire system), are vital to keeping your body healthy and functioning. Your kidneys have two basic jobs:

✔ To assist with removing metabolic wastes from your body

✔ To maintain proper amounts of water and sodium (along with other nutrients) in your blood

When your kidneys don't work properly, impurities and contaminants remain in your blood and can wreak havoc on your health. Kidney disease is a very serious condition that can result in adverse health outcomes ranging from discomfort and inconvenience to severe disability and even death.

Because your kidneys are so important, you want to do all that you can to ensure that they're well taken care of. In this chapter, I familiarize you with the kidney, examine what kidney disease is and does, and explain how a well-balanced diet can help you prevent and even treat kidney disease.

Getting Comfortable with Your Kidneys

You can't understand kidney disease without understanding the kidney and its role.

Kidneys are essential for life. They are your body's filtering system, removing *metabolic wastes* (leftover elements of the excretory system process that your body can't use) and maintaining appropriate levels of water, salt, and other key nutrients in your blood. When the kidneys are damaged, wastes accumulate in your blood and create a toxicity that can lead to an early death.

Here are the basics (many of these things you probably already know):

✔ You have two kidneys, and they look like large beans (which is why kidney beans are called, well, kidney beans).

✔ Your kidneys are in your mid- to lower abdomen, toward the back (anterior) portion of your body (see Figure 9-1).

✔ If you make a fist with your hand, you can get an idea of the approximate size of one of your kidneys. (Use both hands, and you can "see" both of your kidneys.)

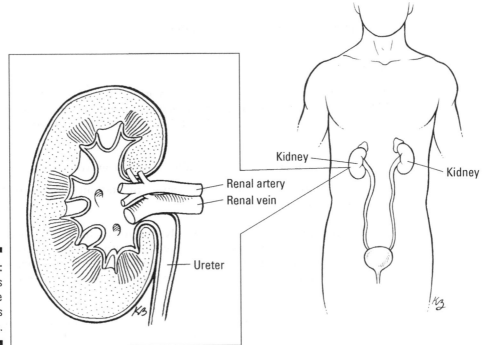

Kidney

Renal artery

Renal vein

Kidney

Ureter

Figure 9-1:
The kidneys and the kidney's parts.

Illustration by Kathryn Born, MA

In addition to illustrating the location of the kidneys, Figure 9-1 also shows key parts of the kidney:

✔ **Ureter:** The ureters are the muscular tubes that connect the kidneys with the bladder.

✔ **Renal vein:** These blood vessels drain the kidneys of wastes.

✔ **Renal artery:** These blood vessels supply the kidneys with oxygen and other nutrients.

Kidney disease is a serious health condition. In the remaining sections of this chapter, I explain how it develops, what the treatment options are, and how you can use diet to prevent it or help control its symptoms.

Understanding Kidney Disease

Kidney disease is the inability of your kidneys to remove wastes and regulate waste and sodium levels from the blood. Most cases of kidney disease stem from hypertension (high blood pressure), diabetes, family history, and/or cardiovascular disease (CVD). In addition, the ability of the kidneys to function at 100 percent efficiency lessens as you age. Thus, as you get older, your kidneys' cleansing mechanism decreases, contributing to the higher rate of kidney disease diagnoses in the elderly.

If you have diabetes, chronic hypertension, or cardiovascular disease, you are at very high risk of developing a medical condition called *vascular disease,* in which your blood vessels become weak and damaged. Vascular disease is a big problem for your kidneys because kidneys are very sensitive to a decrease in blood flow. Plaque that builds up in the renal artery can restrict blood flow to the kidney, causing the kidney to shrink and leading to impaired kidney function.

One way to prevent kidney disease is to watch what you eat. In addition to eating a healthy diet, pay particular attention to the amount of sugar and salt you eat:

- **Regulate your sugar intake.** An increasingly high amount of refined sugars in the blood increases your risk of developing diabetes.

- **Regulate how much salt is in your diet.** An increasing amount of salt in your blood strains the kidneys and also raises your risk of developing hypertension.

Also, get plenty of exercise. A well-balanced diet coupled with regular physical activity can assist in preventing the development of kidney disease. Head to the later section "Dieting to prevent kidney disease" for more ways to use diet to prevent kidney disease.

Moving through the stages

Kidney disease is a *chronic disease,* meaning that it usually takes years to develop, you live with it the rest of your life, it's incurable, and having the disease results in disability.

Kidney disease usually occurs in five stages, progressing from Stage 1 (normal kidney function but urine tests show some abnormalities) to Stage 5 (end-stage kidney failure). Depending on the presence of cardiovascular disease (CVD) or diabetes, the progression through these stages may be hastened. In this section, I give you the highlights.

Developing kidney disease

Each kidney has upwards of 1 million glomeruli. *Glomeruli* are tiny blood vessels that perform the actual filtering function in the kidneys. With kidney disease, the damage occurs over a long period of time, and it typically begins when the glomeruli deteriorate, weaken, or become damaged.

When an individual's blood vessels become compromised (weakened or damaged as they do in people with diabetes, chronic hypertension, and CVD), the glomeruli in the kidneys are at a very high risk of becoming compromised themselves. This, in turn, affects the ability of the kidneys to efficiently filter wastes from the blood. The result? The beginning of kidney disease.

Usually, no symptoms present themselves with early-stage kidney disease. There is relatively little pain or other physical indicators of its presence. How do you know you have it then? Scary, right? Don't worry. Blood or urine tests can help spot the presence of abnormally functioning kidneys.

If you have diabetes, hypertension, cardiovascular disease, or a family history of kidney disease, consult with your physician on how best to screen for kidney disease.

Figure 9-2 shows a healthy kidney and a kidney with kidney disease. Compared to a healthy kidney, a diseased kidney has a granular surface and is smaller in size. It also has decreased function. A urine test will reveal high levels of protein.

Healthy kidney

Diseased kidney

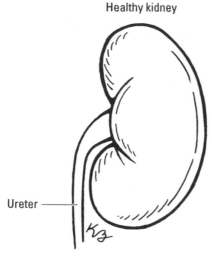
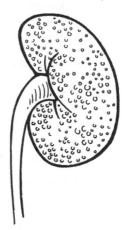

Ureter

Figure 9-2:
A healthy
kidney com-
pared to a
diseased
kidney.

• Healthy function

• Normal size

• Low urine protein

• Smooth surface

• Decreased function

• Smaller size

• High urine protein

• Granular surface

Illustration by Kathryn Born, MA

At this stage, the best way to treat kidney disease is to treat the disease that is causing the kidney damage in the first place. For example, people with high blood pressure and/or diabetes tend to have a higher risk of developing kidney damage. If these people also develop early-stage kidney disease, they can treat their kidney disease by controlling their high blood pressure and diabetes.

In addition to prescribing medications, physicians almost always promote a healthier lifestyle to control the underlying conditions to help treat kidney disease.

Progressing to kidney failure

As the glomeruli become more and more damaged, the kidneys lose more and more of their ability to filter the blood and regulate water and salt levels in the body. If this deficiency persists, outright kidney failure occurs.

Kidney failure is defined as the loss of more than 80 percent to 85 percent of your kidneys' efficiency. In other words, if your kidneys are working at only 15 percent to 20 percent of their capacity, you have kidney failure, or *end-stage renal disease (ESRD)*.

Symptoms of ESRD include the following:

- ✔ Significant fatigue
- ✔ Weight loss
- ✔ Headaches
- ✔ Nausea
- ✔ Excessive thirst
- ✔ Foul breath
- ✔ Loss of appetite

People with advanced kidney disease or kidney failure often undergo one of the following medical treatments:

- ✔ **Dialysis:** In dialysis, a machine filters your blood for you. Dialysis must be completed every day or every few days, and each session takes a few hours to complete.
- ✔ **Transplantation:** In this procedure, a healthy kidney replaces a diseased kidney (you can live with just one functioning kidney).

Calculating the global rate of chronic kidney disease

Kidney disease is a global issue. Most Western, or industrialized, nations have increasing morbidity and mortality rates associated with the disease. The growing prevalence of the disease is primarily due to the poor lifestyle choices made in regards to diet, exercise, stress, and other variables that have a great influence over health outcomes, either good or bad. Consider these numbers:

- ✔ In the United States today, nearly 15 percent of the adult population (approximately 30 million people) has chronic kidney disease. In the year 2000–2001, around 20 million people had the disease, indicating an increase of approximately 10 percent between then and now. Figure 9-3 shows where kidney disease is most prevalent in the U.S. — the South.

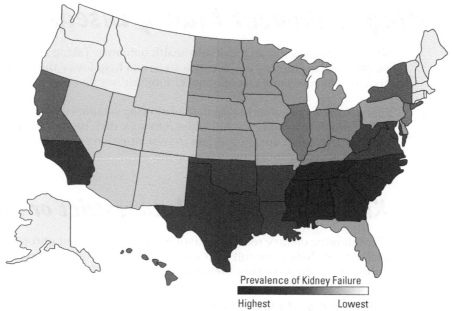

Prevalence of Kidney Failure

Highest   Lowest

Illustration by Wiley, Composition Services Graphics

> ✔ In Australia, one in three people is at risk of developing chronic kidney disease. Approximately 2 million Australian adults (nearly one in ten) are well on their way to developing the disease. Aboriginal populations have an increased risk compared to Australians of European descent.

> ✔ In England, nearly 40,000 hospital episodes per year are attributable to chronic kidney disease. Further, approximately 150,000 hospital bed-days are designated for chronic kidney disease treatment.

Kidney disease doesn't just affect countries in the Western world, however. Developing nations, like India and China, also have high rates of the disease. The question is, why?

China and India have very large populations and are quickly becoming Westernized. These nations exhibit behaviors typical of the Western world, but are adopting these habits much faster and to a much greater degree than any other nation on earth. Making the situation worse, people in these countries have less access to proper healthcare that can help limit the effects of kidney disease.

Dieting to Prevent Kidney Disease

Kidney disease is not an inevitable health outcome. Taking some small, easy-to-manage dietary and lifestyle steps can help lower the risk of you or someone in your family developing chronic kidney disease.

Discuss the suggestions I make in the following sections with your physician to see which you can or should adopt into your diet. He or she can help you make changes that are appropriate to your situation and that can lessen your risk of developing this disease later in life.

Knowing which foods to restrict or avoid

The following dietary recommendations can help prevent chronic kidney disease. As always, consult your physician before implementing any substantial change to your diet and/or lifestyle habits.

Controlling your protein intake

Kidneys have to work extra hard to filter the blood in individuals who eat very high protein diets. So limit your protein intake to about 80 to 100 grams per day. And make sure you select the right kinds and smaller amounts of proteins: lean means and skinless chicken, for example.

Usual protein intakes do not damage a healthy kidney. But when hypertension or diabetes starts to damage the kidney, protein restriction helps slow the damage and treat the disease. Lower protein levels reduce the burden placed on your kidneys during the digestion and filtration process.

As a general rule, five ounces of lean meat, coupled with one to three servings of dairy per day is sufficient. Of course, your specific recommendations depend on your age, your activity level, your gender, and any preexisting medical issues you may have, including family history of chronic kidney disease.

Limiting salt (sodium)

A low-salt diet helps prevent and manage chronic kidney disease. Keep sodium intake to no more than 2,000 mg per day. Don't overdo it with the salt shaker and be careful of condiments, sauces, dressings, and processed foods, which are often very high in sodium. Avoid fast food, which is also very high in sodium.

When cooking or shopping, be sure to do the following:

✔ Choose and prepare foods with less salt (sodium). Use less salt at the table.

✔ Read the nutrition labels on foods, especially for sodium, to help you pick the right foods and drinks. Refer to Chapter 3 for help on reading nutrition labels.

Watching out for foods high in phosphorus

Phosphorus is the second most abundant mineral in the body, but high amounts in your diet can be detrimental to your kidneys. Avoid or limit foods like whole-grain breads, wheat products, beans, and peas if you have an increased risk for chronic kidney disease. This admonition is especially important if you are in a more advanced stage (Stage 3 or 4) of chronic kidney disease.

Deciding which foods to eat

Certain foods can help prevent kidney disease. One of the most important things you can remember when choosing "kidney-friendly" foods is to select and eat foods that are high in antioxidants. (*Antioxidants* are molecules that prevent damage to other molecules and cells. Essentially, they help protect you from cancer and other diseases, like cardiovascular disease, possibly even Parkinson's disease, among many others.)

So which foods do you want to eat? The foods on this list are just some that encourage proper kidney function:

✔ Fresh seafood

✔ Olive oils and other monounsaturated fats

✔ Most fruits (apples, berries, and so on)

✔ Cucumbers

✔ Cruciferous vegetables (cauliflower, carrots, and cabbage, for example)

✔ Parsley

✔ Eggs (but mind the protein — eat one, not three!)

As a general rule, choose foods that are healthy for your heart, like lean cuts of meat, skinless chicken, fish, fruits, vegetables, and beans. They're often good for your kidneys, too, if for no other reason than because they can help you avoid health issues, like obesity or diabetes, that can increase your risk of kidney disease. Also be sure to drink plenty of water to ensure proper hydration.

Dieting to Treat Kidney Disease

The most important thing for those diagnosed with kidney disease is to slow its progression. Your diet can be an invaluable tool as you try to stop the progression of the disease or reduce the degree of disability you may suffer.

Focusing on food and fluid restrictions

Whether you were just diagnosed with kidney disease or you find yourself at the later stages of kidney disease, like ESRD, your objective is to reduce the burden your kidneys must endure to cleanse and regulate nutrient levels in your blood. Your diet is the primary factor impacting how great a burden your kidneys bear.

- ✔ **If you have kidney disease, steer clear of consuming significant amounts of the following foods: beef, poultry, pork, nuts, eggs, dairy, beans, and peas.** As I explain in the earlier section "Knowing which foods to restrict or avoid," the possible negative effects of protein, sodium, and phosphorus on the kidneys can be substantial. Therefore, if you have kidney disease, you need to limit the amount of foods you eat that are high in each of these nutrients.

- ✔ **Monitor your water intake.** If you have early-stage kidney disease, you must keep hydrated. Drinking lots of water helps flush your system of toxins. However, if the disease progresses to severe kidney disease, like ESRD, you actually need to limit the amount of fluids you get and adhere to a very strict diet. For this reason, if you have kidney disease, your fluid intake needs to be monitored so that you can identify the point at which restricting the amount of fluids becomes necessary. Your physician can be the gatekeeper who lets you know when fluid restrictions should begin.

Leaving the diet planning to professionals

If you have been diagnosed with kidney disease, your diet must be planned by a trained health professional, a dietician, your primary care physician, or any combination of these three.

There is no "one size fits all" diet for people suffering from kidney disease. Your diet plan will address all your dietary needs and will be specifically tailored to the stage of the disease you are in and your specific situation. In addition, as the disease progresses, your diet will be amended accordingly.

Casting No Kidney Stones

A *kidney stone* is a solid entity (literally, a stone made up of mineral deposits) that forms in the kidneys (see Figure 9-4). The stone, once formed, will travel down the ureter into the bladder, eventually into the urethra, and then out of the body.

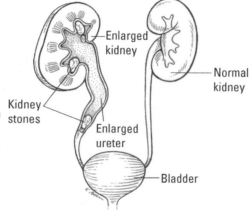

Enlarged kidney

Normal kidney

Kidney stones

Enlarged ureter

Bladder

Figure 9-4: Kidney stones form in the kidney.

Illustration by Kathryn Born, MA

Painful? Many times, yes. Sometimes, no.

Survivable? Of course.

The thing you have to be careful about with kidney stones is the stone becoming stuck. A stuck kidney stone can cause internal bleeding and extreme pain. Many times, the stone has to be treated via ultrasound (the sound wave breaks up the stone into pieces small enough to be passed through) or removed via surgery by a health professional.

Read on for more fun details on kidney stones.

Materials that make up kidney stones

The materials needed to create kidney stones are always present in the blood; it's only when those minerals and other materials are in high concentrations that they actually form into a solid piece.

Different foods in your diet can make you more prone to developing kidney stones: coffee, tea, and foods that are high in protein, phosphorus, and sodium. Specifically, watch out for the foods that contain high amounts of oxalate and purine.

The most important factor for reducing risk of any kind of kidney stone is drinking enough water every day.

Limiting oxalates

Oxalate is the most common stone-forming compound. Too much oxalate in the urine *(hyperoxaluria)* is responsible for up to 60 percent of calcium stones and is a more common cause of stones than too much calcium in the urine. Hyperoxaluria is usually caused by ingesting too many foods that are high in dietary oxalates, such as the following:

- ✔ Beer
- ✔ Vegetables like beets, spinach, swiss chard, and rhubarb
- ✔ Soy products
- ✔ Excessive quantities (like more than one cup a day) of nuts

Avoiding foods high in purines

Purine is a crystalline compound that, when broken down in the digestion process, forms uric acid. The more purine in your diet, the more uric acid is produced. If enough uric acid is present, uric acid crystals form, and these crystals can lead to kidneys stones (and gout — but that's a topic for Chapter 13). This type of stone is less common than calcium oxalate stones.

Purine is found in very high quantities in meat (particularly organ meat) and fatty fishes (mackerel and sardines). It is also found in lima beans, lentils, mushrooms, lobster, spinach, and oatmeal, among other foods that are higher in protein and among some other vegetables.

Chapter 10

All about Food Safety

*A*t any given time, billions of bacteria and other microbes hang out all over you, your belongings, and your food. Even as you read these words, your mouth, fingertips, pencils, and everything else in front of you are riddled with these creepy-crawly things. So should you panic and run for the nearest hazmat suit? No, because, for the most part, these invisible denizens of your world are okay. Most of them don't impact you at all; some are even good for you, performing needed functions like helping with digestion and inhibiting the growth of the bad bacteria.

Still, many microbes and contaminants can pose a threat to your health. Fortunately, your body has protective layers (your skin, the little hairs in your ears and nose, and so on) that create barriers between you and them. But when you eat, these nasty microbes can get into your system by hitching a ride on your food or on your fingers. That's why you need to know what steps to take to prevent harmful microbes from contaminating your food and making you sick.

In this chapter, I discuss microbial contamination, as well as the elements — like adulterants and non-microbial contaminants — that get added to food and can pose health risks. I also tell you how you can keep your food sources safe from contamination and prevent foodborne illness.

Assessing Food Adulteration

Adulteration is the deliberate addition of cheaper and/or potentially lower quality substances in food. "Well, why would anyone do that?" you ask. For plenty of reasons, but perhaps the primary motivation for adulterating food is economics.

Adding in a cheaper substance allows an individual or a business to stretch its supplies farther. In a way, any person who's ever made a little bit of hamburger into an entire meatloaf by adding extra bread crumbs and eggs is using the same principle. The difference is that Mom isn't pulling a fast one on the family to maximize her profit margins, and the ingredients she's adding aren't lowering the quality of the food.

Adulterants can be harmless for human consumption, like adding powdered beans in bread flour to make the flour go farther. But often, adulteration can be dangerous, even deadly. Unscrupulous people can put dangerous chemical compounds or other items not meant for human consumption into the food supply, thus resulting in serious health issues.

Understanding the motivation behind adulteration

Think of a bakery. The baker has his primary ingredients: flour, water, yeast, and salt. Now suppose that the first couple of Saturdays in the month have been particularly busy, and the baker thinks he may run out of flour before the next shipment at month's end. What does he do?

Well, he could just simply run out of flour and close the last weekend of the month, or he can try to stretch his remaining flour supply far enough to make bread for the rest of the month. He chooses the second option because it keeps him open *and* it lets him make even more profit because he's making more bread with less flour. How does he bulk up his flour? By using some inferior material, like powdered beans or chalk. Yes, literally chalk — the kind you write on blackboards with.

Businesses aren't the only entities that adulterate their food, and most people don't adulterate for sinister purposes. Often, people adulterate their food supply simply to make the food last longer so that they can save some money (think of Mom's meatloaf again). But when the adulteration involves non-food or contaminated items, the end result can actually make people sick or worse.

Identifying common types of adulteration

In addition to the health issues, another key issue with adulteration is consumer rights. Adulterations are often hidden and are meant to deceive consumers through inaccurate and misleading labeling or through adding undeclared ingredients. As reported in the *Deccan Herald,* the Food Safety and Standards Authority of India (2011) did a study that showed these common adulterations:

In meat:

- Selling nonorganic meat as organic
- Adding excess water to meat without declaring it
- Mixing spoiled meat in with fresh to extend the supply
- Adding beef and other meat to 100 percent pork sausages
- Selling "lean" meat that contains as much fat as standard meat does

In fish:

- Selling farmed fish as wild
- Mislabeling the geographic origin of the fish

In fruits and vegetables:

- Selling conventional produce as organic
- Giving the wrong geographical origin for the produce
- Selling cheaper varieties as expensive varieties
- Adding genetically modified soybeans to conventional beans without declaring them

In eggs, cheese, and olive oil:

- Selling battery farm eggs as free-range eggs
- Using cow milk rather than buffalo milk to make mozzarella
- Dying non-virgin olive oil dark green to make it look like extra-virgin olive oil
- Diluting olive oil with cheaper hazelnut oil

In orange juice and coffee:

- ✔ Diluting juice with inferior-quality juice
- ✔ Adding beet sugar to sweeten "naturally" sweet orange juice
- ✔ Adulterating highly sought-after Arabica beans with cheaper varieties

In alcohol:

- ✔ Selling counterfeit versions of big brands.

  Counterfeit alcohols may include dangerously high levels of methanol, which can cause permanent blindness or even death.
- ✔ Watering down spirits
- ✔ Substituting cheap varieties for premium brands in jars
- ✔ Adding extra sugar during winemaking to increase alcohol content

All these practices are deceiving because consumers think they're getting one thing when they're actually getting another. Although this list is specific to the kinds of contaminants uncovered by the Food Safety and Standards Authority of India, adulterations can occur anywhere. (***Note:*** India is a leading state on the presence of adulterants because much of the food produced and manufactured in India is at risk for adulteration.)

Looking for signs of adulteration in food

People have become more and more reliant on others to grow, produce, and prepare their food. In the past 60 or so years, people have become almost entirely removed from the food harvesting process, especially in developed, industrialized nations. We're also, for the most part, disconnected from the transportation and storage of our food as well — situations that leave us more and more vulnerable to the possibility of adulteration.

You can fight adulteration, however, by doing your homework about where your food is coming from, paying attention to how it's prepared, and being observant of what you're eating. If you can't actually see the food being made, look for any signs of adulteration or foreign matter. Use Table 10-1 as a mini-guide on how to test for adulterants in some common food products.

If you make your own food, purchase high-quality ingredients. Lower-quality ingredients are more at risk for adulteration.

Table 10-1		Testing for Adulterants	
Food	*Common Adulterant*	*How to Detect*	*Effects*
Bananas	Calcium carbide (ripens the fruit)	Look for banana stems that are green instead shiny yellow.	Can cause digestive system and liver cancers
Apples	Wax coating	Look for a very glossy, shiny skin.	Can lead to ulcers and gastric problems
Mangoes	Calcium carbide (ripens the fruit)	Look for uniform skin color on fruit and dark green patches on the surfaces where the mangoes are kept.	Can cause headaches, dizziness, and neurological problems
Chili powder	Brick powder	Add a small amount of chili powder to water; brick powder will settle on the bottom while the chili powder floats.	Can cause loss of vision and respiratory and digestive problems
Table salt	White chalk	Stir a small amount in water. Solution will turn white, and insoluble impurities will settle.	May cause appendicitis
Tea leaves	Coal tar dye	Scatter leaves on a damp paper towel and look for color spots after five minutes.	Is carcinogen and extremely poisonous
Ice cream	Washing powder	Add drops of lime juice to small amount of ice cream. If washing powder is present, the ice cream will froth or bubble.	Affects the kidneys, lungs, and heart
Green vegetables	Malachite green	Place vegetable on damp paper towel and look for discoloration on towel.	Is carcinogenic if consumed over long periods of time

Source: The Apollo Clinic, `http://www.theapolloclinic.com/`

The Pure Food and Drug Act of 1906 was the first law in the United States passed by the federal government to help control adulteration of food. One of the main goals of this law was to help regulate and protect bread flour from being tainted with lesser quality materials. This law, coupled with a series of consumer protection legislative actions assisted in the development of the Food and Drug Administration.

Controlling Food Contamination

In food contamination, a foreign substance is accidentally incorporated into the food supply. The contaminant could be dirt, hair (both human and animal, particularly rodents), animal feces or other waste, fungi, pesticide residue, insects (whole or in fragments), and so on. The questions you're perhaps asking yourself are

> "Does food always have some type of contaminant in it?"

> "If it does include a contaminant, will I get sick from eating it?"

> "How can food contaminants be prevented?"

In this section, I answer those questions.

Discovering the prevalence of contamination

Does your food always have some contaminant in it? Short answer: absolutely. Never, ever, will your food be 100 percent free of natural food contaminants. From the farm to the tableside, your food travels hundreds, perhaps thousands of miles — probably in the back of an 18-wheel rig in a crate for about three or four days — and is touched by many hands, all of which increase the chance that your food product will contain food contamination. Even if you grow your food in your own backyard and personally wash and prepare it yourself for consumption, you still can't completely avoid contaminants.

You will never be 100 percent free of food contamination. Every day you eat hairs, skin flakes, animal waste, insects, or any combination of these things, but you need to remember that most of it isn't harmful. Actually, sometimes, eating some of these materials could actually boost immune system function by exposing your body to different organisms for which it can develop an immunity. Or these items may not even contain potentially dangerous microbial contaminants. The problem with eating these items is when they do contain microbes that can cause harm. Then you have a problem.

In fact, it's so accepted that some contamination will occur that the U.S. Food and Drug Administration (FDA) has established rules for acceptable levels of both natural or unavoidable contaminations in food, which it calls its *defect action levels (DAL)*. Table 10-2, for example, lists some of the FDA's insect DALs in a variety of foods. (For more information about DALs, head to the later section "Taking steps to prevent contamination.")

Table 10-2	Acceptable Levels of Insect Contaminants in Food, According to the FDA
Food	*Acceptable Defects*
Broccoli (frozen)	Average of 60 or more aphids and/or thrips and/or mites per 100 grams
Chocolate	Up to 60 insect parts per 3.5 ounces
Peanut butter	Up to 30 insect parts per 3.5 ounces
Peaches	Up to 3 percent wormy
Peas	Up to 5 larvae per 18-ounce can
Spinach	Up to 10 aphids, thrips, and/or mites; or 1.6 leaf miners; or 0.4 caterpillar parts per 18-ounce can
Tomatoes	Up to 10 fruit fly eggs, or 5 fruit fly eggs and 1 maggot, or 2 maggots per 18-ounce jar
Wheat flour	Average of 150 or more insect fragments per 100 grams

Source: U.S. Food and Drug Administration

Recognizing the risks contaminants pose to your health

Will you get sick from food contamination? Short answer: Mostly not. After all, you eat contaminants every day (refer to the preceding section). Slightly lengthier answer: Whether food contaminants make you sick depends on how much of the contaminant you ingest; whether that contaminant is a microbe (virus, bacterium, parasite, and so on); and whether that microbe has toxic qualities.

Getting sick from microbial contamination of food is common, but, generally speaking, even when you eat food that has microbial contamination, you don't get sick. Why? Because your body has defense mechanisms to help stop potential infections from microbial contaminants in your food sources. Your saliva, for example, has antimicrobial qualities. In addition, stomach acid can pretty much kill most of the contamination that reaches the gut.

Still, these defenses aren't foolproof. Consuming contaminated food can definitely make you sick. Whether you get sick, how sick you get, and your prognosis for recovery all depend on the specific microbe involved and how much of it you ingest.

Some foods are more contaminated with microbes than others, due to the following:

✔ **They just happen to attract more microbes.** To find out how to minimize this danger, head to the later section "Handling potentially hazardous foods with care."

✔ **They've been subject to cross-contamination.** Find out how to avoid cross-contamination in the section "Avoiding cross-contamination."

Taking steps to prevent contamination

Can you prevent contamination? Short answer: No. It's just too easy for contaminants to come into contact with your food. From harvest to table, a nearly infinite number of ways exist for hair, dirt, feces, or whatever to get on or in your food. Whether your food grows in a patch outside your backdoor or in a field in the middle of Iowa or Saskatchewan; travels from a local farmer's market or in the back of semi-tracker trailer going cross-country; is prepared by Grandma, a fry cook, or a renowned chef at a famous bistro; is delivered to your table by wait staff or your kids; or is exposed at any other point in this process, accidental contaminants can get into your food at any time.

So unless you can grow, transport, prepare, and deliver your food in an absolutely sterile environment, you can bet that you'll eat some contaminants each and every day of your life. Weird, right? So relax. You've been eating these things since you were an infant and will continue to for the rest of your life.

All of this doesn't mean that contaminants don't matter. And, as I note in the preceding section, you need to be extra vigilant about microbial contaminants. Whereas a little waste and a few insect parts aren't going to hurt you, microbial contaminants can be dangerous. In this section, I explain what steps the FDA has taken to protect the food supply and outline things you can do to minimize contamination in your own kitchen.

Delving into defect action levels (DAL)

Governments now monitor contaminants in order to control and possibly even prevent them from getting into the food supply. To this end, the FDA developed defect action levels (DAL). DALs specify the maximum limit of contamination; in other words, if the contamination level is at or above this maximum amount, the government will take legal action to stop the product from being sold.

The DALs for oregano and curry

Pretty much any Italian food you eat has a very high chance of having oregano in it. Here's the DAL for ground oregano:

✔ **Insect filth:** Average of 1,250 or more insect fragments per 10 grams

Defect source: Insect fragments — pre-harvest and/or post-harvest and/or processing insect infestation

✔ **Rodent filth:** Average of 5 or more rodent hairs per 10 grams

Defect source: Rodent hair — post-harvest and/or processing contamination with animal hair or excreta

Like Indian food? Here's the DAL for curry powder:

✔ **Insect filth:** Average of 100 or more insect fragments per 25 grams

Defect source: Insect fragments — pre-harvest and/or post-harvest and/or processing insect infestation

✔ **Rodent filth:** Average of 4 or more rodent hairs per 25 grams

Defect source: Rodent hair — post-harvest and/or processing contamination with animal hair or excreta

And you always thought the secret ingredient was love.

You can find these and other DALs at the following URL: `http://www.fda.gov/Food/ GuidanceRegulation/Guidance DocumentsRegulatoryInformation/ SanitationTransportation/ ucm056174.htm#CHPTO`

A DAL is an upper limit, not the average, and it indicates the point below which a contaminant poses no danger to heath. So, yes, the government knows you eat these contaminants (as do the folks who set these levels), and it acknowledges that it cannot mandate that foods be 100 percent free from contaminants. But it will monitor contaminants to ensure that they do not rise to a level at which they become actual risks to human health. If a food exceeds the DAL limit, the FDA removes that food from store shelves.

Avoiding cross-contamination

Cross-contamination occurs when food is exposed to microbes in the environment. It occurs when microbes and dirt from people, raw meat, and raw fruits and vegetables come in contact — via hands, utensils, poor storage practices, and so on — with ready-to-eat foods.

You can do the following to prevent cross-contamination:

✔ Minimize hand contact with food and wash your hands after touching any raw food.

✔ Separate raw and cooked foods.

✔ Use separate utensils to handle raw and cooked foods.

The basic idea is to keep raw meat, raw seafood and fish, raw eggs, and untreated water away from cooked vegetables, cooked meat, cooked fish, and ready-to-eat foods like sandwiches, salads, cookies, and so on.

Handling potentially hazardous foods with care

You also need to be mindful of potentially hazardous foods. These foods grow microbes more easily than other foods. Table 10-3 lists foods that are considered potentially hazardous. When you use these foods, make sure you clean, refrigerate, and handle them properly.

Table 10-3	Potentially Hazardous Foods
Food	*Example(s)*
Raw meats and cooked meats	Mince, steak, casseroles, curries, sausages, poultry
Plant foods that have been heat-treated	Cooked rice, beans
Foods that include synthetic ingredients	Textured soy protein hamburger supplement
Dairy products	Milk, cream, cheese, custard, dairy-based desserts
Seafood	Fish, prawns, crab, crayfish, mussels, oysters
Processed fruits and vegetables	Prepared salads, ready-to-use vegetable packs, sliced melons, baked or boiled potatoes, prepared pasta
Processed foods containing eggs, beans, nuts, soybeans	Quiche, tofu, omelets
Foods containing any of the items listed	Tacos, pizzas, sandwiches

Maintaining safe temperatures for cooked and stored food

Microbial contaminants — particularly bacteria — like things nice and warm. Environments that are either too hot or too cold impede bacterial growth. You can use this knowledge to keep your food safe. Table 10-4 lists the safe cooking and storage temperatures and shows the temperature range that is ideal for microbial growth.

Table 10-4	Key Temperatures for Food Safety
Temperature	**Notes**
165°F	Minimum safe internal temperature for poultry, stuffing, casseroles, and reheated leftovers
160°F	Minimum safe internal temperature for beef, lamb, veal (medium), pork, and egg dishes
145°F	Minimum safe internal temperature for beef, lamb, veal, steaks, and roasts (medium rare), seafood
140°F	Minimum internal temperature for ham (fully cooked) and holding temperature for cooked foods
41°–139°F	DANGER ZONE
38°–40°F	Refrigerator temperatures
0°F and below	Freezer temperatures

Keep your food out of the danger zone of 41 to 140 degrees Fahrenheit. At these temperatures, microbial growth explodes.

Discussing Foodborne Disease

Foodborne disease, commonly called *food poisoning,* can result from causes found in nature, as well as from exposure to microbes via poor food handling or storage (refer to the earlier section "Discovering the prevalence of contamination" for details). In this section, I identify foods that are naturally toxic, explore the causes of foodborne illness, and explain steps you can take to avoid any problems.

Passing on the poison: Foods that are naturally toxic

The fact is that some foods are naturally toxic. Consider water hemlock, for example. This plant looks a bit like a parsnip, but it's definitely not as innocent nor as tasty. In fact, it's quite the opposite. Water hemlock is one of the deadliest plants in North America.

Other foods also have toxic effects on humans. Certain mushrooms and shell-fish, for example, have severely toxic effects on many people. Depending on the food eaten, death is almost a certainty in many cases.

The effects from naturally existing toxins cause a variety of reactions — vomiting, diarrhea and other types of gastrointestinal distress, delirium, organ failure, and even death — depending on who eats them and how much is consumed. Children and the elderly are often most at risk.

Be smart and don't eat anything you can't clearly identify or that includes ingredients you're not sure of. And if you suspect that you — or someone you know — ate something that you shouldn't have, consult a physician immediately. Better safe than sorry, I always say.

Minding your microbes: Foodborne illness caused by contamination

Although foodborne disease can occur from inborn toxins (as discussed in the preceding section), the vast majority of foodborne illness stems from some type of microbial contamination involving bacteria, viruses, parasites, or some other microbe.

As I explain in the earlier section "Controlling Food Contamination," *food contamination* refers to the accidental addition of dirt, hairs, feces, and so on into a food. *Microbial contamination* refers to the accidental addition of microbes in food and, as you would suspect, is much more dangerous than plain ol' food contamination.

Differentiating between food allergies and foodborne illness

Some people have allergies to certain types of foods. These allergies may result in symptoms that are very similar to the symptoms caused by foodborne illness. However, a distinct difference exists between foodborne illness and food allergies. In foodborne illness, it's not the food that has made you ill; it's the pathogen — a disease causing microbe — or the toxin that was in your food. In food allergies, your body has an adverse response to food proteins. Some allergies can be fatal (for example, nut and shellfish allergies

can cause airway constriction and suffocation), and some can be more mild (lactose intolerance, for example, causes gastrointestinal concerns).

If you suspect that you are allergic to certain foods, visit an allergist or other trained medical professional to help you figure out what foods you may be allergic to. Doing so may actually save your life. Most common food allergens include tree nuts, soy, fish, peanuts, shellfish, eggs, wheat, and dairy.

Looking at the prevalence of the problem

Foodborne illness caused by microbes is a very widespread problem that is expensive in terms of both money and human health. The world has billions of people who eat every day. That's potentially trillions of meals eaten daily. Obviously, not every meal is free of microbes. Worse, not all food is free from the kinds of microbes that can make you sick or perhaps even kill you. In addition, governments around the globe spend billions, perhaps even trillions, of dollars every few years to help control, treat, and prevent such dietary incidents.

Considering the fact that millions and millions of meals per day are infected with dangerous microbes, how can health professionals keep track? To successfully monitor every meal served around the world is so impossible that even the suggestion borders on the ludicrous. For the most part, health officials take a two-pronged approach:

- They establish rules designed to minimize the chances of microbial contamination and then follow up with inspections at agricultural, manufacturing, and transportation sites to ensure compliance with the regulations.

- They investigate outbreaks, establish remedial cleanup solutions (order the destruction of contaminated crops, for example), and then put in place preventative measures to help forestall future outbreaks.

The problem is that the potential sources of outbreaks is practically endless, whereas budgetary constraints often limit the scope of oversight.

In truth, the prevalence of the problem is unclear. Many cases of microbial contamination are rarely reported. The illness often gets passed off as a "24 hour bug" or a "case of the runs," or it's dismissed as something that just didn't agree with you (of course it didn't agree with you — it's why you're vomiting or having diarrhea). As a result, the numbers reported by governmental food safety administrations around the world are usually low. Can you imagine what they would be if foodborne illnesses were reported accurately?

Blaming bacteria, the biggest culprit

Bacteria, more than any other microbial contaminant, including viruses and parasites, cause the greatest number of outbreaks of foodborne illness. The most common types of bacterial contamination include the following:

- **Salmonella:** You usually find salmonella in uncooked poultry products. It used to be the most common contaminant, but it's now dropped below campylobacter jejuni (see the third item in this list). The most common symptom of salmonella poisoning is gastrointestinal distress.

- **E. coli:** You usually find *Escherichia coli (E. coli)* on unwashed vegetables and improperly processed meat products, which are then served undercooked (anything below well-done). *E. coli* causes severe gastrointestinal distress, and it may lead to kidney failure and death.

- **Campylobacter jejuni:** The most common type of bacterial contaminant today is *Campylobacter jejuni.* As with salmonella, mild to severe stomach and intestinal issues result. Undercooked meat and unwashed vegetables are the usual culprits.

- **Listeria:** One of the things that makes listeria such a problem is that it grows at low temperatures, so keeping meat or other food products in a refrigerator has only a limited effect on stemming its growth. Listeria affects a limited number of people but has one of, if not *the,* highest mortality rates of all these listed diseases. It is usually found on meat products and tainted vegetable and fruit matter.

  In 2011, a listeria outbreak occurred in the U.S. due to tainted cantaloupes. The highest number of cases occurred in Colorado, where, according to the U.S. Centers for Disease Control and Prevention (CDC), the farm linked to the contaminated cantaloupes was located. Kansas, New Mexico, Oklahoma, and Texas were also hard hit, and a few cases occurred elsewhere around the United States, as Figure 10-1 shows.

- **Staphylococcus aureus:** *Staphylococcus aureus* is a very common bacteria found almost everywhere. If it infects your guts, you will probably experience diarrhea or vomiting.

- **Botulism:** Botulism, caused by the bacteria *Clostridium botulinum,* is a very serious disease with a higher mortality rate than most of the other diseases in this list. It's usually found in contaminated cans of food or in undercooked food. The botulism toxin attacks the nervous system, and symptoms include double or blurred vision, drooping eyelids, slurred speech, difficulty swallowing, dry mouth, and muscle weakness. In severe cases, respiratory failure and paralysis occur.

  The botulism bacteria thrives in low-acid, low-oxygen environments, making it a particular concern for home canning of vegetables and meat (due to their low acid content). Before consuming home-canned vegetables, be sure to heat them to at least 176 degrees Fahrenheit for ten minutes. If you're eating home-canned spinach, corn, or meat, heat it to that temperature for 20 minutes. And if you notice any bulges, leaking, or odors from canned vegetables or meat you buy at the store, discard the food without opening. (As the botulism bacteria grows, it produces a gas that can cause the can to expand.)

Bacteria like warm, moist environments, and they multiply rapidly, particularly on and within potentially hazardous foods (refer to "Handling potentially hazardous foods with care" earlier for a discussion on these foods). A key way to protect your food from bacterial contamination is to avoid cross-contamination and to store it at appropriate temperatures (see the earlier section "Maintaining safe temperatures for cooked and stored foods" for more on food storage).

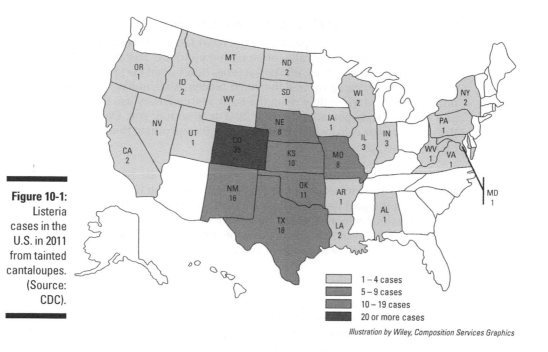

Figure 10-1:
Listeria
cases in the
U.S. in 2011
from tainted
cantaloupes.
(Source:
CDC).

1 – 4 cases
5 – 9 cases
10 – 19 cases
20 or more cases

Illustration by Wiley, Composition Services Graphics

Bacterial contamination is a global problem. Every day some region of the world seems to have to deal with cleaning up a botulism problem or attempting to control the spread of listeria. Table 10-5 illustrates the rate of growth of common bacterial contaminants in 2012.

Table 10-5	Food Safety Progress Report, 2012		
Disease Agents	**Percentage Change from 2006 to 2008**	**2012 rate per 100,000 population**	**Estimated Number of Undiagnosed Cases for Every Diagnosed Case**
Campylobacter	14% ↑	14.30	30
E. coli O157	No change	1.12	26
Listeria	No change	0.24	2
Salmonella	No change	16.42	29
Vibrio	43% ↑	0.41	142
Yersinia	No change	0.33	123

Source: U.S. Centers for Disease Control and Prevention

Viral contamination: Hepatitis A and norovirus

Although bacteria historically cause the most food outbreaks worldwide, an uptick in the number of viral contamination incidents has occurred in the past decade or so. Viruses, unlike bacteria, don't need certain types of food to grow on; they can grow and live most places. Also, unlike bacteria, they don't reproduce when they're on the food; instead, they use the food simply as a mode of transportation to their final destination: you. Once inside you, they hijack your cells, which they then use to reproduce their own genetic material and spread.

The two most common types of viral contamination are norovirus and hepatitis A. The incidence of norovirus contamination has seen a large increase in the past decade. These incidents are usually the result of cross-contamination by food workers who don't wash their hands after using the bathroom. Norovirus was responsible for nearly half of all foodborne illnesses in the U.S. between 2006 and 2010.

Parasites

Parasitic contamination is usually associated with sewage coming into contact with food, most commonly in water that you drink or that you use to wash your food. Like other microbial contaminants, parasitic contamination is also caused by food handlers who don't wash their hands and then touch your food.

Two foods that you need to be particularly careful of in terms of parasitic contamination are sushi and ceviche, dishes that feature raw fish or seafood. In fact, *any* type of raw fish or meat or, for that matter, any raw material that comes from an animal — like dairy products, for example — is particularly susceptible to parasites and other microbes.

Chances are you've seen this notice, or one very much like it, on restaurant menus:

> Consuming raw or undercooked meats, poultry, seafood, shellfish, or eggs may increase your risk of foodborne illness.

Restaurants include this warning for a reason: To alert you to the risk associated with eating raw foods. Be careful.

Being safe with food choice

Your risk of coming into contact with some type of food or microbial contaminant — dirt, hair, or something more serious like bacteria or a virus — is extremely high. That's why preventing foodborne illnesses is one key to a healthy life. Here are some ways you can reduce your chances of contracting a foodborne illness:

✔ **Eat foods that you make or cook yourself.** Although this doesn't elimi-nate the risk entirely, being in charge of the preparation practices — and following the suggestions I outline in the earlier section "Avoiding cross-contamination" — goes a long way toward keeping you safe from foodborne illness.

✔ **Know as much as you can about your food sources.** Contamination can occur at any point in the food-processing chain. Although contaminants don't always make you sick, they can. So be aware of what you eat, who makes your food, and where you buy it.

✔ **Minimize your exposure to contaminants.** The key to staying safe is to keep the amount of contaminants, particularly microbial contaminants, in your food low. Because high numbers of microbes usually need to be present in your body to make you sick, minimizing your exposure to bacteria, viruses, and so on is a good second step. The problem arises when billions of these microbes hang out in your soup or water or whatever you are eating and drinking. Refer to the earlier section "Taking steps to prevent contamination" for guidelines on how to safely handle food to protect yourself from contaminants.

Part III
Major Organ Systems and Nutrition

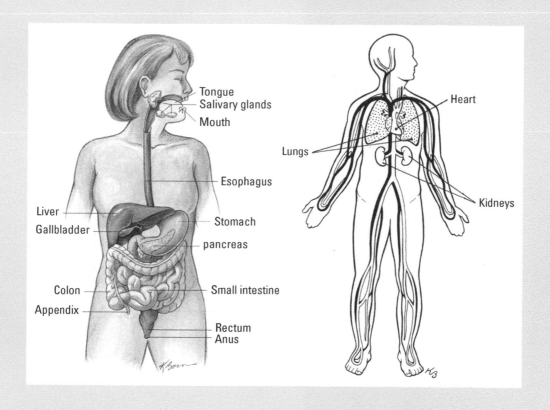

What you eat now definitely affects your life later. For an example of how the whole lifetime nutrition concept works, read about young female athletes and osteoporosis prevention at www.dummies.com/extras/clinicalnutrition.

Part III

Major Organ Systems
and Nutrition

In this part. . .

✔ Find out how proper nutrition can serve as an effective preventative and therapeutic tool for major organ systems

✔ Learn how nutrition can affect your gastrointestinal and cardiovascular systems and what foods can keep these systems in optimal health

✔ Understand the role of the pancreas in digestion and insulin regulation and how to modify your diet to prevent or avoid a diabetes diagnosis

✔ Determine how to keep your kidneys functioning properly through healthy diet and exercise

Chapter 11

Gaining Insight on the Gastrointestinal System

In This Chapter

▶ Outlining the major organs of the gastrointestinal (GI) system

▶ Discovering the major diseases affecting the GI system

▶ Adopting a diet that supports a healthy GI system

*B*ack at university, I knew an old man who was obsessed with his guts. He was always conscious of what he ate, specifically how the food he ingested made his stomach and intestines feel (either discomfort or not) and whether it made for a good bowel movement. (Looking back now, I realize these seem like odd topics for a conversation, but I did learn a lot!) In the end, I can condense all these conversations into one simple idea:

> Healthy guts = Healthy you

That's right. If your gastrointestinal system stays healthy and functions properly, for the most part, you'll probably be healthy, hopefully wealthy, and sometimes wise (my homage to my favorite 18th-century statesman, Ben Franklin). Although I'm treating this subject lightly, the lesson — that having a healthy, functioning GI system significantly increases your chances of having positive health outcomes — is worth learning early in life.

In this chapter, I introduce the parts of the GI system, explain some major diseases of the GI tract, and offer a few tips and tricks for what you can eat to bring about the best possible health outcomes for yourself.

Making Up the Gastrointestinal System

Your gastrointestinal (GI) system, also called the digestive system, is uniquely constructed to perform its specialized functions: turning food into the energy you need to survive and packaging the residue for waste disposal. To help you understand how the many parts of the digestive system work together, this section provides an overview of the structure and function of this complex system. As you read these sections, refer to the image in Figure 11-1.

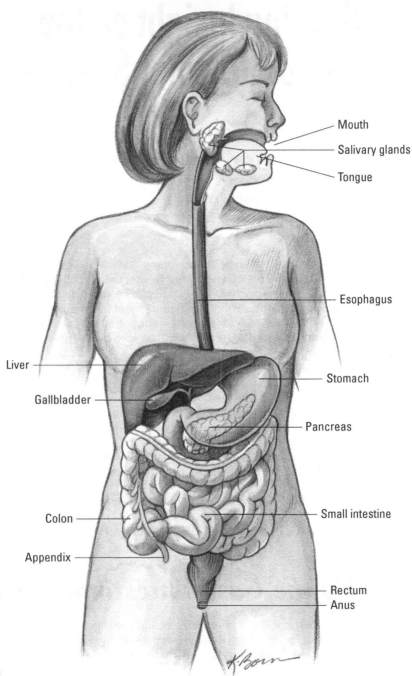

Mouth

Salivary glands

Tongue

Esophagus

Liver

Stomach

Gallbladder

Pancreas

Colon

Small intestine

Appendix

Rectum

Anus

Figure 11-1:
The gastro-
intestinal
system.

Illustration by Kathryn Born, MA

Mentioning your mouth

The GI system all begins here: your mouth. Digestion immediately starts the second you start to chew your food. When you chew, you're crushing, dicing, and slicing whole food into smaller pieces so that it can more easily be digested by the rest of your GI tract. Your teeth and tongue work together to get the initial job of digestion done. Also, saliva, when mixed with chewed food, has a digestive element that prepares your food for further digestion in your stomach and intestines.

Turns out your mother was right when she told you to chew your food thoroughly before swallowing. Carefully chewing your foods helps you avoid choking, swallowing too much air, and experiencing discomfort with digestion.

Moving the food around in your mouth is also essential for digestion. How would you be able to chew your food and swallow properly if you couldn't move it around? Exactly — and that's why your tongue is so important. It lets you move food around in your mouth as you chew. (Don't believe me? Try chewing *without* moving your tongue!)

Explaining your esophagus

The esophagus is an eight- to ten-inch tube (depending on your age and body size, of course) of muscles that connects your mouth and throat with your stomach. Through the process of *peristalsis* (contractions of your esophagus's muscles), your food is pushed down farther into your GI tract. The esophagus delivers food to your stomach.

Your esophagus isn't that wide, which is why you need to be careful of getting food stuck and possibly choking. For example, a large grape (unchewed) is just about the size of an adult esophagus opening. To avoid choking, be careful when you swallow, make sure your food is properly chewed, and don't laugh while you eat! (For a list of choking hazards for young children, head to Chapter 15.)

TECHNICAL STUFF

Tasty treats

In addition to moving food around your mouth as you chew, your tongue has one other important job: It allows you to taste your food (working alongside your sense of smell).

You have four primary tastes: bitter, sweet, salty, and sour. Some researchers indicate that a possible fifth taste, umami, may exist. Umami is the savory flavor, like that in broths, gravies, and meat-based dishes. Each taste has its own region on the tongue, as this image shows. The *papillae* (the taste buds, or the little bumps on your tongue) do the actual tasting.

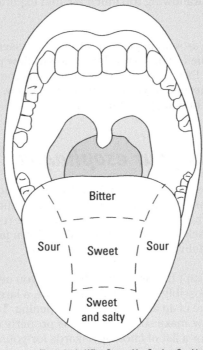

Illustration by Wiley, Composition Services Graphics

Understanding your stomach's role

Your stomach is a muscular container that receives food from your esophagus. The stomach walls secrete enzymes and acid that mix with the food and continue digestion. After a period of "marinating" in this acid bath, your food then moves into your small intestines for further digesting and nutrient absorption.

The acidity level of a food is indicated by its pH. The pH of gastric acid (stomach acid) is around 1.5, give or take. (Figure 11-2 shows acidity levels for several common substances.) Therefore, keeping acid from leaving the stomach is essential to prevent heartburn, ulcers, and other health concerns caused when stomach acid leaves the stomach and comes into contact with more sensitive organs. (The inside of your stomach is protected from this acid by a thick mucous lining.) Head to the later section "Discussing Some Functional Disorders of the GI Tract" for details on the problems that can result when stomach acid goes where it's not supposed to.

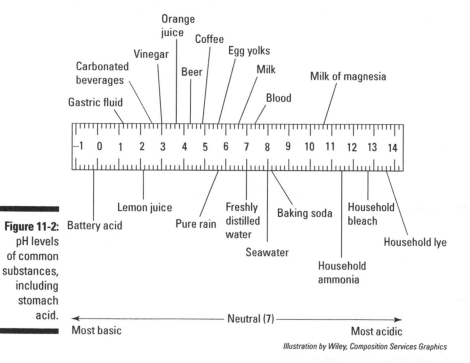

Figure 11-2: pH levels of common substances, including stomach acid.

Illustration by Wiley, Composition Services Graphics

Your wondrous small intestine

This amazing organ — your small intestine — is about 22 feet long. Think about that for a second. Look at your abdomen right now and imagine a 22-foot hose wrapped up and curled inside your gut. And that length doesn't even include the 5 or 6 feet that make up your large intestine.

The small intestine is responsible for digestion and nutrient absorption, tasks it performs with the help of the pancreas and liver. The food starts as a semi-solid state in the duodenum and ends as a semiliquid state as it empties into the large intestine. The process of peristalsis keeps the food moving through this organ.

Figure 11-3 illustrates the small intestine's three major sections: the duodenum, the jejunum, and the ileum. The *duodenum* primarily digests, and the *jejunum* and *ileum* primarily absorb nutrients and place them into your blood: The jejunum is where the secretion of digestive enzymes occurs. The ileum — the longest part of the small intestine — is the last part of the organ before the beginning of the large intestine. The absorption of B vitamins and bile salts take place in the ileum.

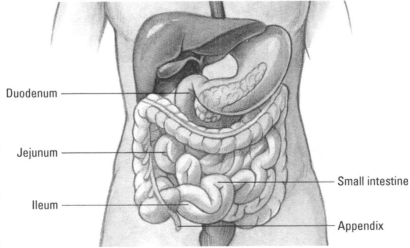

Figure 11-3:
The key areas of the small intestine.

Duodenum

Jejunum

Ileum

Small intestine

Appendix

Illustration by Kathryn Born, MA

Pertaining to the pancreas

The pancreas performs some very important jobs for the body:

✔ It secretes digestive enzymes into the duodenum, to help with the digestion process.

✔ It secretes sodium bicarbonate to help raise the pH of gastric acid to neutral (refer to Figure 11-2) so that the digested food from the stomach doesn't burn the sensitive small intestine.

✔ It manufactures insulin, the chief hormone for metabolizing blood glucose. You can read more about insulin and blood glucose (blood sugar) in Chapter 8.

The liver

The liver, in the context of digestion, performs two key functions:

✔ It processes nutrients absorbed from the small intestine.

✔ It manufactures bile, which is sent to the gallbladder for storage and then secreted into the small intestine to assist in digesting fat.

Concerning the colon (large intestine)

The colon (also called the large intestine) is about five feet long, and it connects the small intestine to the rectum. Figure 11-4 shows the major sections of the colon.

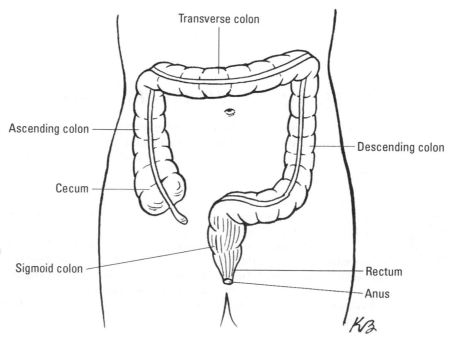

Figure 11-4: The parts of the large intestine.

Illustration by Kathryn Born, MA

- ✔ **The cecum:** The cecum is the pouch-like beginning section of the large intestine that receives undigested food from the small intestine.

- ✔ **The ascending colon (the right side):** Located on the right side of the body, the ascending colon's main function is to absorb water, nutrients, and vitamins from your food and return these things to the bloodstream.

- ✔ **The transverse colon:** The traverse colon travels across your body from right to left. This is where more water is absorbed from the food and where feces begins to form.

- ✔ **The descending colon (the left side):** This part of your colon absorbs the last remaining water from the digested matter and continues the food-to-feces process.

- ✔ **The sigmoid colon:** This portion of the colon connects to the rectum. The sigmoid colon stores feces until it is ready to be passed out of the body.

The job of the colon is to process waste (or *stool*) left over from the digestion process. Also, it absorbs water and other nutrients from the digested matter (mostly leftover food and a lot of bacteria). The digested food emptying into the colon from the small intestine begins as a semiliquid state and, due to the water removal, exits as a solid. Digested matter empties from the sigmoid colon into the rectum once or twice a day.

The bacteria in stool are very useful: They help process vitamins, help process leftover food, and even fight other, potentially harmful bacteria. They are pretty amazing little creatures!

Reviewing the rectum and anus

The rectum connects your large intestine with your anus. Its main purpose is to store stool and let you know when you have stool to pass. The anus is the final stop on the long digestive pathway. Together, the two help fecal waste leave your body.

Pay attention to your stool when you go to the bathroom. You can tell a lot about your health just by the consistency and color of your stool. Passed stool should be soft and a rich brown color. Stool that is hard, is in small pieces (like pellets), and is very dark brown means you're constipated (a possible indication that you're eating the wrong thing or have an underlying medical condition if the constipation is chronic). Further, if your stool is too loose (like diarrhea), your body is not absorbing enough water out of the digested food. This could lead to dehydration. Definitely go talk to your physician if you think there may be a larger issue.

What have you done for me lately?

So what's the appendix? Nothing much actually — it's just a small tube attached to the cecum that has no physiological purpose, at least none that's currently known. Although (as far as we know), the appendix has no real function, it can get infected, swell, burst, and possibly kill you if you don't get medical attention. For something that doesn't seem to have a purpose, it certainly can cause a lot of trouble. That's pretty much it.

Discussing Some Functional Disorders of the GI Tract

We all have times in our lives where our guts just don't work properly. Chances are you've clutched your stomach a time or two and grimaced in pain or discomfort. Maybe you had gas, a stomachache, nausea, constipation, bloating . . . the list goes on. Well, if misery loves company, you'll be happy to know that you're not alone: Up to one in four people have their digestive *motility* (the process of food moving through their GI tracts) affected due to one of these disorders. It can happen at any moment and for what seems to be no reason.

These *functional disorders* — conditions that impair the normal activity of the colon — are the most common health issues concerning the GI tract, but they particularly affect the colon and rectum. Often these disorders are the result of long-term behaviors or conditions, such as

✔ Having a sedentary lifestyle

✔ Eating a high-fat, low-fiber diet or consuming too much dairy in your diet

✔ Feeling chronic stress

✔ Being pregnant

✔ Taking too many antacids or laxatives

Non-functional disorders of the GI tract are health conditions — like chronic fatigue, stress, and even post-traumatic stress disorder (PTSD), for example — that aren't directly related to your digestive tract but can impact your colon and bowel habits.

In this section, I cover some major health concerns of the digestive system. This overview gives you an idea of some very common GI disorders and the possible dietary reasons why they exist. Keep in mind, however, that this discussion isn't meant to be a comprehensive review of all the diseases of the GI tract, nor is it a diagnostic tool.

Discussing constipation

When you can't pass stool — either you're unable to have a bowel movement or unable to have a satisfying bowel movement — you are *constipated*. A number of things can cause constipation, but many times the causes are

- ✔ A lack of fiber in the diet
- ✔ Inadequate water in the diet
- ✔ Stress and a disruption in your normal daily activity

Treating constipation isn't that difficult. In fact, it's quite easy. Eat a balanced diet, exercise regularly, and go to the toilet when you feel the urge.

If those things don't keep you regular, you can take a laxative to help stimulate your bowels. Keep in mind, however, that this solution cannot go on for a long period of time. Overusing laxatives can cause further functional disorders of the GI tract. Make sure you take laxatives sparingly and only when needed. Bulk laxatives, the kind that add fiber, are the safest.

Acid reflux

Acid reflux, or *gastroesophageal acid reflux (GERD),* occurs when gastric acid enters your esophagus. Gastric acid can damage the walls of the sensitive esophagus (or even the small intestine if it gets in there). These structures are not protected by a thick mucous membrane as the stomach is. The main symptom of acid reflux is a burning sensation in your esophagus, which gives this condition the name you probably know it by: *heartburn.*

Anyone can get GERD and often for unknown reasons. It occurs when the esophageal sphincter (a thin muscle acting as a gate between the esophagus and the stomach) weakens or isn't working properly and allows acid to leak upward. Other factors causing GERD include smoking cigarettes, being obese, having a genetic predisposition (possibly), and being pregnant.

The best way to avoid GERD is to live the healthiest way possible: eat a low-fat diet, don't smoke, limit your alcohol intake, get plenty of exercise, and reduce stress.

Left untreated, chronic GERD can lead to other, more serious health issues, such as Barrett's esophagus (which I discuss in the next section) and, potentially, esophageal cancer (covered in the section "Colon polyps and cancer").

Barrett's esophagus

Barrett's esophagus is a condition in which the cells of the esophageal walls have become mutated due to chronic exposure to gastric acid. The disorder is most often diagnosed in people with GERD, yet only a handful of people with GERD develop Barrett's esophagus.

Here's what happens: GERD causes your stomach's content, which is highly acidic, to push up into the esophagus, damaging the esophageal lining and changing the lining's cell structure. The change of the cell type is usually associated with Barrett's esophagus.

A major issue with Barrett's esophagus is that it increases your risk of getting esophageal cancer. Although only a small percentage of those with Barrett's gets cancer, that number is high enough to cause concern for those with chronic GERD.

If you have issues with GERD, lay off spicy foods, coffee, tomatoes, and other highly acidic foods. Consult a physician to determine which foods, exactly, you should avoid. The list can vary from person to person.

Peptic ulcers

Stomach acid doesn't present a problem only when it goes beyond the stomach. In some people, gastric acid literally eats through the mucous membrane of the stomach itself and begins to damage the stomach wall cells. When this happens, an ulcer develops.

People who have ulcers usually describe the feeling as a burning sensation in the middle part of the abdomen. Although these ulcers are pretty small, they can be big problems. Just ask anyone who has one. And don't think that you'll have trouble finding someone who has an ulcer. In the U.S. alone, ulcers affect 5 million people annually. In the Western world, the number of people suffering from peptic ulcers is also alarmingly high.

What causes peptic ulcers? *Helicobacter pylori (H. pylori)* bacteria. In years past, many people assumed that smoking and spicy food caused ulcers; they even suspected that stress may have caused them. No one imagined bacteria would be the culprit, but it is. Medications like aspirin have also been linked to causing ulcers. Still *H. pylori* bacteria are the culprits.

If you have a peptic ulcer, you may still want to avoid smoking, stress, and certain foods like tomatoes, coffee, and spicy foods, among others. Although research now suggests that these things don't *cause* the ulcers, they can trigger an ulcer episode.

Inflammatory bowel disease (IBD)

Inflammatory bowel disease (IBD), a condition in which the colon contracts more frequently than normal, has a number of aliases; two common ones include *irritable colon* and *spastic colon.* A number of things can trigger an IBD attack. The culprits include stress, specific foods, and certain medications.

People with IBD tend to suffer from stomach cramping, have frequent and urgent bowel movements, and experience other discomforts of their bowels, even including occasional bouts of constipation.

Two primary forms of IBD include the following (see Figure 11-5):

✔ **Ulcerative colitis:** With ulcerative colitis, usually only the large intestine (colon) is affected. In addition, ulcerative colitis typcially starts in one spot, almost exclusively in the colon.

✔ **Crohn's disease:** With Crohn's disease, the inflammation can happen anywhere along the digestive tract, ranging from oral to anal cavities. It can occur in patches along the digestive tract.

Ulcerative colitis   Crohn's disease

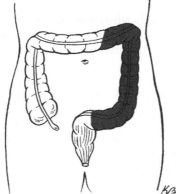
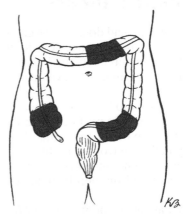

Figure 11-5:
Ulcerative colitis generally affects one area; Crohn's disease, multiple areas.

Illustration by Kathryn Born, MA

Because the conditions' symptoms are very similar, doctors sometimes have difficulty determining whether you have a case of ulcerative colitis or Crohn's. To make a proper diagnosis, your physicians will use a combination of X-rays, blood tests, and colonoscopies.

Just as those with ulcers or heartburn, people with IBD should avoid caffeine, acidic and/or spicy foods, and fried foods. Further, it also helps to control stress levels and increase fiber in the diet. These strategies won't cure the disease, but they can help lessen the symptoms and perhaps even help reduce the frequency or severity of flare-ups.

Despite the similarities of their symptoms and some general remedies to control flare-ups (as mentioned prior), the treatment for each is distinct:

- **With Crohn's disease:** The goal is to suppress the immune system that is causing the flare-ups in your GI tract. This suppression allows for the gut to heal itself. Surgically removing the affected part of the GI tract isn't really an option because flare-ups can occur — and recur — anywhere from the mouth to the anus.

- **With ulcerative colitis:** Surgery is an option because the affected areas are limited to the colon. Surgery is coupled with a series of treatments. However, because ulcerative colitis flare-ups can be infrequent, determining whether the treatment was effective can be difficult.

Discussing diverticular disease

Individuals with low-fiber diets tend to have weakened colon walls. When the walls bulge outward, diverticula result (see Figure 11-6). *Diverticula* are small pouches that form where the colon walls are weakest. Diverticula usually occur in the sigmoid colon (refer to Figure 11-1) because that section of the colon experiences higher pressure than the other sections.

In the Western world, approximately 15 percent of people over 40 and over 50 percent of those over 60 develop diverticular disease. Only a small portion of people with diverticular disease actually have complications, though. When they do occur, these complications include *diverticulitis* (inflammation of the diverticula resulting from fecal matter getting stuck in the small pouch), bleeding, and even colon blockage. Although these conditions are more rare than not, they can cause serious discomfort.

Eating a high-fiber diet with tons of fruits and vegetables can help keep diverticular disease at bay.

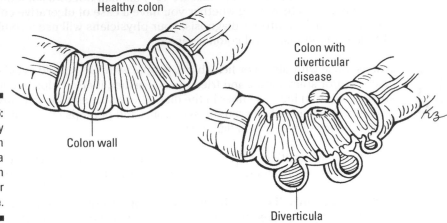

Healthy colon

Colon with
diverticular
disease

Figure 11-6:
Healthy
colon
versus a
colon with
diverticular
disease.

Colon wall

Diverticula

Illustration by Kathryn Born, MA

Colon polyps and cancer

Almost 1 million people globally are diagnosed with colorectal cancer. In the United States, this type of cancer is the second most common form, a scenario that is mimicked in other Western nations. One good thing: Colorectal cancer is highly treatable, and even more exciting, it's highly preventable.

Colonoscopies have saved many lives. In this procedure, a doctor uses a camera to look into your colon to see whether colon *polyps* (fleshy growths of abnormal cells) or, even worse, cancer is present.

Low-fiber, high-fat diets coupled with a sedentary lifestyle have been linked to the development of colorectal cancer. If you find yourself having irregular bowel habits, chronic constipation, pain in your abdomen, bloody stool, or sudden intolerances to food that you normally could eat, go to your physician to get checked. People over 50 years old should be regularly checked; how frequently you need to be checked depends on your risk factors, like family history of the disease and the presence of polyps.

Eating Your Way to Healthy Guts

In this section, I offer a series of dietary tips you can follow to help keep your GI system healthy and functioning properly. Again, as I state throughout this book, these are just suggestions. Before you adopt any of the following dietary recommendations, consult a physician to ensure these foods and diets are right for you.

As you go through these recommendations, think to yourself, "Can I do this?" "Is this in my best interest?" and "What can I do to incorporate these into my lifestyle?" Usually, people who read these tips with open minds and actively think about how to incorporate them tend to have more success than those who skim the list and pay no mind to the details.

Figuring out what foods to avoid

When you're targeting the health of your gastrointestinal tract, a good place to start is with a list of foods you should consider limiting, or even eliminating, from your diet. This one change is a key beginning to ensuring that your GI tract is working in tip-top shape.

Reducing the red meat you eat

People who frequently eat red meat are at an increased risk of GI diseases (they're also at increased risk for heart disease and several cancers) compared to those who eat it sparingly or not at all. Here are some guidelines:

- If you can avoid red meat entirely, fine, but you don't necessarily have to eliminate it completely from your diet. If you eat red meat, choose lean cuts, reduce your portion sizes, and eat it only occasionally.

- If you do eliminate red meat entirely, you must find alternatives that provide protein and iron; otherwise, you run the risk of becoming anemic or developing a protein malnutrition issue. Usually beans and legumes are good choices for protein. Eating cruciferous vegetables (vegetables from the cabbage family), among others, and fruit can help you cover all the vitamin and mineral needs.

Grilling eggplant or portobello mushrooms can give you a texture that is like red meat. If you put the right blend of spices on it, who knows? You may find your next favorite food!

Giving up or cutting back on gluten, if appropriate

Gluten is a protein that's usually found in wheat products, but it can also be found in other grains like rye and barley. Gluten can also be found in surprising places — in foods that you don't necessarily associate with wheat, such as ketchup, ice cream, cheese, and many other everyday foods.

Not everyone has an issue digesting gluten. These people don't need to cut back or eliminate gluten from their diets. But many people do have this health concern, and it's a very serious one.

Celiac disease, an allergic reaction to gluten, affects millions globally. This disorder can cause gas, bloating, and GERD, among other symptoms. It can also cause joint pain, muscle aches, memory loss, sluggishness, and even depression. The only way to control celiac disease is to eat a gluten-free diet.

A gluten-free diet is very restrictive, and although more and more gluten-free products are stocked on store shelves and offered in more restaurants, it is not a diet to adopt lightly. However, if you suspect that you may have a gluten allergy or celiac disease, you must get a proper diagnosis from a physician. And if you're experiencing unexplained GI symptoms, do *not* remove gluten from your diet until you've been tested; otherwise, the testing may be invalid.

If you do prove to have a gluten intolerance, you can substitute your gluten-filled diet with some gluten-free products, which, as I note earlier, are becoming more commonly available. Table 11-1 offers some suggested substitutions.

Table 11-1	Substitutes for Gluten-free Eating
Replace This	*With This*
Wheat tortilla	Corn, teff, or brown rice tortillas
White flour pasta	Quinoa, corn, or brown rice pasta
Wheat, rye, and barley bread	Brown and white rice-based bread
Oat-based granola	Puffed corn or rice-based granola
Wheat flour	Garbanzo bean, potato starch, or tapioca flour
Wheat-based breakfast cereals	Rice- or corn-based breakfast cereals

Cutting back on dairy

Lactose is a sugar found in dairy. If you are *lactose intolerant,* you cannot digest lactose. If you consume items that contain lactose, you'll experience mild to serious GI discomfort. Lactose intolerance affects hundreds of millions of people globally.

Nations whose populations have been farming and drinking dairy milk over generations tend to have fewer problems with lactose intolerance than nations that haven't had a large, cow dairy industry. Interesting, huh?

The good news is that you don't have to necessarily give up all dairy if you are lactose intolerant. Many times, those with lactose intolerance can enjoy certain types of dairy or can eat small amounts without feeling the effect. Avoiding milk will help, but you don't have to give up all dairy. Some lactose-intolerant people do fine with small amounts of milk.

If you're lactose intolerant, you may find these tips helpful:

- ✔ If you want to eat cheese, choose more aged cheeses, like cheddar, or cheeses that are drier in content, like Parmesan. These varieties are less harsh on the gut than softer, more milky cheeses. Why? Aged cheeses generally have less than a gram of lactose because the bacteria used in the cheese-making process eat the lactose. Fresh cheeses, like cottage, are coagulated by acid rather than bacteria and, therefore, retain more lactose.

✔ To calm your stomach, eat yogurt. Wondering why I am telling you to eat dairy when I just stated that people with lactose intolerance should be wary of dairy? It's because the millions, perhaps even billions, of bacteria in yogurt are actually very, very healthy for you; they help soothe your stomach. Head to the later section "Enjoying yogurt" for details.

Frowning on fried food

Thick, fatty foods, like pies, french fries, and greasy meat cause quite a few problems for your guts. First, these foods stay in the digestive system longer because they are usually low in fiber (fiber helps speed up transit through the GI tract). Second, they cause more acid reflux into the esophagus. So the next time you're craving buffalo wings or something like that, know that you can eat a few, but you don't want to eat an entire plateful.

Figuring out which foods to eat

Just as certain foods make the "do not eat (or eat very little)" list, other foods are actually good for the GI tract. In this section, you get a glimpse of the foods that can help you get (and keep) your GI tract in good health.

Foods high in dietary fiber

I call fiber the "snowplow" of the GI tract because it keeps food moving through your gastrointestinal system. This continual movement is important because it spurs regular bowel movements and helps you avoid constipation. When you are constipated, your very sensitive intestines absorb from your feces toxic waste products and other harmful elements, a situation that can cause health issues.

Fiber makes the walls of the colon strong by exercising them through contractions as your body moves your bowels. Table 11-2 lists foods that are high in fiber and absolutely delicious. As you can see, fruits, vegetables, and whole grains are the go-to foods for both fiber and taste!

Table 11-2	High-Fiber Foods	
Food	*Amount*	*Fiber (Grams)*
Baked potato	1 medium	5
Pear	1 average	4
Lentil soup	1 cup	14
Strawberries	1 cup	4
Orange	1 medium	3
Popcorn	3 cups	4

You should eat high-fiber foods regularly, but be careful not to eat too much fiber. An adult should get just above 30 grams of fiber a day. If you eat too much fiber, you can become constipated or lose precious nutrients from your body through your stool because fiber absorbs water and excess nutrients as it waits in the large intestine. If you eat too much fiber, the fiber will soak up too much of these nutrients and excrete them out of your body.

Enjoying yogurt

The number one probiotic food is yogurt. The active, or live, bacteria cultures in yogurt make it fantastic for soothing your guts. When you add yogurt to your diet as a way to help your GI tract, make sure to avoid yogurts that are high in sugar and artificial flavorings. Just get the plain, unsweetened one. You can add some nuts, honey, or fruit to make it more appealing.

As I state earlier, a major source of gut discomfort is dairy, but yogurt can save the day in many circumstances for many people who are lactose intolerant. However, make sure you speak with your doctor first to see how — and whether — you should introduce yogurt into your diet.

Approximately, four to five pounds of your body weight comes from the bacteria that live in your digestive tract! Amazing, huh?

Drinking water

Water is essential for healthy digestion. It not only keeps your guts flushed and hydrated, but it also prevents constipation. When you don't drink enough water, your colon extracts water from your digesting food (it's your body's way of protecting itself from dehydration). The result: constipation.

The more fiber you eat, the more water you need to drink. If you eat too much fiber and not enough water, you can become constipated.

Staying active to stay regular

Exercise can help support a healthy GI tract. Exercising allows food to move through the large intestine quickly. Intestinal muscles that contract during exercise also contribute to more efficient bowel movements.

Chapter 12

Caring for the Cardiovascular System

*E*veryone knows how important the cardiovascular system is to health, and we all know that taking care of the heart promotes the best possible health outcomes for ourselves and others. Yet heart disease reigns supreme as the number-one cause of death worldwide, particularly in the Western world. The American Heart Association suggests that up to one-third of Americans have cardiovascular disease — a number repeated in other Western countries. And, as I suggest in Chapter 4, cardiovascular disease is becoming the number-one cause of death in the developing world, as well.

Globally, heart disease and cardiovascular health concerns affect many people, and the numbers are increasing, even as you read this chapter. My goal is to spur you to think about what you can do to promote cardiovascular wellness. In this chapter, I give you an overview of the cardiovascular system and its major functions and outline some of the specific health concerns stemming from this system. I also share dietary recommendations that can help prevent cardiovascular disease and explain how some dietary regimens can be used to treat cardiovascular health issues after they occur.

Making Up the Cardiovascular System

The *cardiovascular system,* shown in Figure 12-1, is a complex system that includes your heart, arteries, veins, capillaries, and blood, as well as your lungs and kidneys. All these different components have their own jobs — and are even parts of different systems — but they all work as one to keep blood flowing through your body.

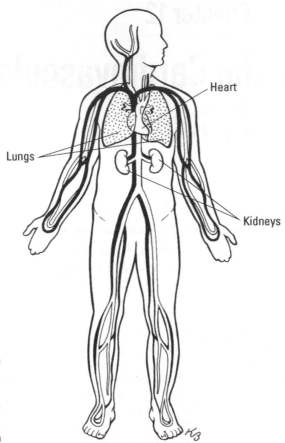

Heart

Lungs

Kidneys

Figure 12-1:
The cardio-
vascular
system.

Your heart is in control of this entire process. Its pumping action keeps blood circulating in the body through a network of blood vessels (veins, arteries, capillaries, and so on). Of course, blood doesn't just move through your body for the fun of it. Among other things, it carries oxygen and nutrients to all organs and tissues and helps remove the waste that your cells produce. The lungs and kidneys help in those functions:

- ✔ The *cardiopulmonary system* refers to the heart and lung system of respiration (breathing), which helps replenish and cleanse the blood.

- ✔ The excretory system (the kidneys, bladder, ureters, and urethra) filters out wastes from the blood.

The cardiovascular system is often called the *circulatory system*. However, to make a distinction, the circulatory system includes both the cardiovascular system and the endocrine system. Think of it this way: The cardiovascular system *circulates* blood, and the endocrine system *circulates* hormones.

Keeping the blood clean and flowing to your organs, tissues, and cells keeps you alive and functioning. Blood is carried through the body via arteries and veins. *Arteries* carry oxygen-rich blood away from your heart, while *veins* carry oxygen-deficient blood back to your heart. In graphics, this distinction is typically shown by color or shading. Red represents arteries (to indicate the transport of oxygen-rich blood), and blue represents veins (to indicate the transport of oxygen-depleted blood). In Figure 12-1, arteries are the shaded blood vessels; veins are the nonshaded blood vessels.

The one exception to the arteries carrying oxygen-rich blood and veins carrying oxygen-depleted blood is when blood is pumped to your lungs to get refreshed with oxygen. Here, the pulmonary artery transports oxygen-*deficient* blood into your lungs, and the pulmonary vein transports oxygen-*rich* blood back to your heart.

Whenever you hear about the cardiovascular system, think of the heart, lungs, and kidneys all working as one. Although it's easy to get confused, just know that even though these organs each have their own systems — heart (part of the circulatory system), lungs (respiratory system), kidneys (urinary system) — they all work toward the same goal: keeping your blood flowing and clean!

Keeping the beat: Your heart

At the center of the cardiovascular system is your heart. This muscle keeps blood pumping to the cells and tissues of the body. Your heart is absolutely critical to every single bodily function. Without flowing blood, you cannot live. Period.

The major components of your heart include the right and left atriums and the right and left ventricles (see Figure 12-2). Oxygen-deficient blood enters the right side of the heart and is pumped to the lungs. On the left side of the heart, oxygen-rich blood is received from the lungs and is pumped to the rest of the body.

The heart is quite an amazing organ. A very complex system of electrical pulses keeps it beating. These electrical pulses cause the heart muscles to contract and release in a coordinated fashion to create the pressure needed to pump blood through the network of arteries and veins. As the walls of the heart contract, blood is forced through the heart and sent to the lungs to get cleansed and replenished with oxygen, or it is pumped to the rest of the body where it supplies nutrients to your cells and tissues. Each contraction of the walls of the heart produces a sound that you recognize as your heartbeat.

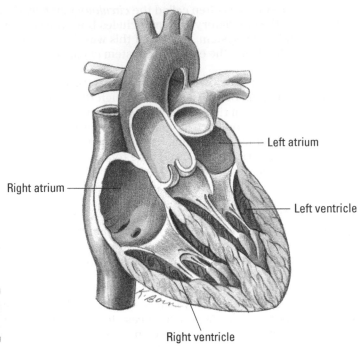

Left atrium

Right atrium

Left ventricle

Figure 12-2:
Your heart.

Right ventricle

Illustration by Kathryn Born, MA

Transporting oxygen and removing waste

Throughout your body is an intricate system of veins and arteries whose job is to move the blood where it needs to go. This system involves 20 major arteries that branch through your tissues, where they are further separated into smaller vessels called *arterioles* and *capillaries.*

Here's what happens (see Figure 12-3):

1. **Oxygen-rich blood flows from the arteries into *arterioles*, small branches of an artery that lead to capillaries.**

   Capillaries serve as the suppliers of oxygen to your cells.

2. **The capillaries supply the cells with nutrients, and then they pick up carbon dioxide and other wastes.**

3. ***Venules,*** **very small blood vessels that feed the veins, pick up the oxygen-deficient blood from the capillaries and send it back to the lungs and heart.**

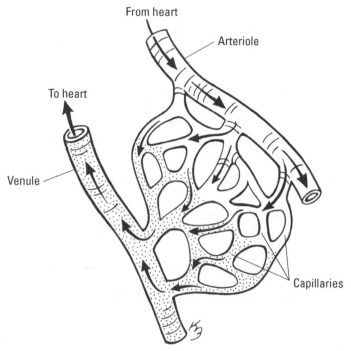

From heart

Arteriole

To heart

Venule

Capillaries

Figure 12-3:
Arterioles,
capillaries,
and venules.

Illustration by Kathryn Born, MA

If I told you that the length of your circulatory system's veins and arteries, if laid end to end, would stretch about 60,000 miles, or nearly 100,000 kilometers, would you believe me? You better, because it's true. The earth's equator is 25,000 miles around, meaning that your circulatory system could wrap around the earth more than twice. Mind-boggling!

Getting in on the bloody basics

Your blood supplies oxygen and nutrients to your cells and tissues. In addition, it removes waste and carbon dioxide from those parts of the body. But your blood does more than provide oxygen and nourishment; it also does the following:

- ✔ **Provides hormones and other essentials for proper growth, development, and maintenance:** These hormones stem from the endocrine system. Check out Chapter 13 for more on this topic.

- ✔ **Transports bodily wastes to the kidneys for removal from the body:** In Chapter 14, I outline the key functions of the urinary system. To find out what can go wrong, head to Chapter 9.

Read on to find out other important things to know about blood.

Components of blood

About five liters of blood are flowing through your body now. The primary components of blood are red blood cells, white bloods cells, platelets, and plasma:

- ✔ **Red blood cells:** These cells transport oxygen to your cells (via the protein *hemoglobin*) and remove carbon dioxide from the cells. Hemoglobin is what makes red blood cells red.

- ✔ **White blood cells:** White blood cells defend your body against infections. Essentially, these are the ground troops of the immune system.

- ✔ **Platelets:** These disk-shaped cell fragments help clot blood when you have a cut or a wound.

- ✔ **Plasma:** This yellow-tinted liquid suspends all the blood cells and platelets in the blood. It makes up over half of the total volume of blood.

Eating for blood type

Humans have four distinct blood types: A, B, AB, and O. Recently, some people have promoted a type of diet that has an individual "eating for his blood type." The idea is that people with different blood types have specific dietary needs due to the chemical composition of their blood. What does this diet suggest for the different blood types? Take a look:

- ✔ **Blood type A:** Type As work best on a vegetarian diet. Eating a diet full of whole grains, vegetables, fruits, and soy brings about the best results.

- ✔ **Blood type B:** Type Bs, according to this diet, should eat moderate levels of low-fat dairy, meat, fruits, and vegetables and should avoid eating corn, lentils, and wheat. In addition, people with type B blood should only engage in moderate activity.

- ✔ **Blood type AB:** For people with this blood type, a kind of pescetarian diet is recommended; that is, you should refrain from eating any meat other than fish. Type AB folks should eat soy-based foods, dairy, and most, but not all, fruits and vegetables. This group should also take part in meditation-like exercises to promote wellness.

- ✔ **Blood type O:** Type Os are encouraged to eat meats, poultry, and fish, and to cut back on grains and legumes. They also need to exercise vigorously.

If you are considering adopting this way of eating, be careful. First, according to nutritional scientists, no proper evidence exists supporting this diet's claims. Second, you may not be getting the necessary nutritional content. If this isn't enough to dissuade you from trying this diet, I strongly encourage you to speak to your doctor first.

Pressuring your blood

The pressure, or force, of blood against the walls of your veins and arteries constitutes your *blood pressure*. When you get your blood pressure reading from your healthcare provider, you get two values: One value represents the systolic pressure, and the other represents the diastolic pressure:

- **Systolic pressure:** The *systolic pressure* indicates the amount of force produced when the heart contracts. During this phase, blood pressure rises, and blood moves along in the vessels.

- **Diastolic pressure:** The *diastolic pressure* indicates the pressure created when the heart relaxes. In the diastolic phase, the heart relaxes, blood pressure drops, and blood fills the heart.

The systolic value is the first number noted (in printouts, it's the number on top) and the diastolic value is the second number noted (the bottom number on printouts). For example, if you're told that your blood pressure is "110 over 75" — represented as 110/75 mmHg (*mmHg* stands for *millimeters of mercury*) — the 110 value is the systolic pressure, and the 75 value is the diastolic pressure.

A healthy blood pressure usually falls within a range (see Figure 12-4). A normal systolic pressure can range from 90 to 120; a normal diastolic pressure ranges from 60 to 80. If your pressure falls above or below these ranges, you can be diagnosed as the following:

- **Pre-hypertensive:** Being pre-hypertensive means having a blood pressure measurement just below the hypertensive value and above the ideal blood pressure measurement.

- **Hypertensive:** If you are hypertensive, you have high blood pressure; your numbers are higher than average.

- **Hypotensive:** If you are hypotensive, you have low blood pressure; your numbers are lower than average.

Having high or low blood pressure presents unique health concerns, namely heart, brain, kidney and arterial damage. Even being pre-hypertensive may produce some similar negative physical effects on your body.

In previous chapters, I suggest that a diet high in salt/sodium (as well as some other high-fat, highly processed foods) is a very strong predictor of high blood pressure. I examine this connection again later in this chapter; head to the section "Staying away from sodium" for details.

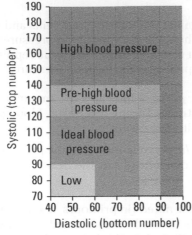

Illustration by Wiley, Composition Services Graphics

Figure 12-4:
Gauging
blood
pressure.

Hurting the heart: Cardiovascular disease

Cardiovascular diseases — heart attacks, strokes, atherosclerosis, and so on — account for the highest numbers of death and sickness worldwide, a trend that is, unfortunately, engrained in most Western countries, as well as some developing nations. Further, these diseases mostly stem from unhealthy behaviors that people can control rather than from genetic factors that they can't control.

Cardiovascular disease is often the result of poor health behaviors, such as the following:

- **Poor diet:** Eating too many refined sugars, too much saturated fat, and too much cholesterol

- **Not exercising enough:** Lack of or insufficient physical activity

- **Other lifestyle behaviors:** Smoking cigarettes, abusing alcohol, and suffering from too much stress

Any of these behaviors individually will probably lead to some form of cardiovascular disease. If you engage in two or more of these behaviors, your risk of cardiovascular disease is increased significantly. For a full discussion of the diseases that affect the cardiovascular system, refer to Chapter 7.

Eating Your Way to a Healthy Cardiovascular System

Ever heard of a *cardio-positive diet?* No? That's too bad. If more people thought of the connection between health — specifically heart health — and the foods that can promote a strong, healthy heart, there would perhaps be fewer instances of preventable heart disease.

A cardio-positive diet is one that assists in achieving positive health outcomes and includes the following key components:

- ✔ **Healthy food choices:** Low-fat foods, whole grains, lean meats, and lots of fruits and vegetables

- ✔ **Healthy behaviors:** Getting plenty of exercise and refraining from smoking and alcohol abuse

Sound familiar? This entire book is geared toward such a diet, mainly because this diet is the foundation of good health, not only for your heart but for every system in your body. However, to get the maximum benefit for you heart, this list needs to be tweaked a little. In addition to including whole grains and plenty of fruits and vegetables, a cardio-positive diets includes these things:

- ✔ **Omega-3 fatty acids:** Good sources of omega-3 fats are fish and flaxseed.

- ✔ **Soluble fiber:** Soluble fiber is a form of fiber that dissolves in water. It makes you feel full by slowing the emptying of your stomach, which helps regulate blood sugar levels by controlling the release of sugars into the blood. Good sources of soluble fiber include legumes, oats, barley, and flaxseed.

- ✔ **Black or green tea:** Tea has flavonoids, which are good for your heart because they help prevent blood clots and lower blood cholesterol.

- ✔ **Lean or non-animal protein sources:** Good choices include extra-lean beef and pork, skinless poultry, and soy protein.

- ✔ **Low-fat milk and yogurt:** Eating low-fat dairy helps eliminate a large amount of unhealthy saturated fats from your diet.

- ✔ **Monounsaturated fats:** As I explain in Chapter 7, fat is a necessary component of a healthy diet. The key is to eat healthy fats rather than unhealthy ones. Good choices include extra-virgin olive oil, canola oil, nuts, and seeds.

✔ **Supplements and functional foods:** These include multivitamins, fish oil, and so on. Supplements may not be necessary if you are eating a well-balanced, healthy diet. Nevertheless, omega-3 fatty acids are believed to be heart-healthy, and these supplements may help lower your risk of heart disease. Before taking any supplement, however, consult with your physician.

In addition, you must maintain a healthy weight and get 30 to 60 minutes of physical activity a day.

Your diet is one of *the* biggest predictors of cardiovascular health. Along with proper exercise, having a healthy diet can protect you from most cardiovascular diseases. Of course, no one can guarantee that you'll be 100 percent protected from heart disease; however, eating right and exercising regularly eliminates most of the risk — that I *can* guarantee.

Because diet, unlike family history, is a modifiable risk factor of cardiovascular disease (meaning it can be changed), you need to know which foods to eat and which to avoid. In the following sections, I provide details on a few key components of a cardio-positive diet, highlighting the things that you can do to help bring about positive health outcomes.

Keeping away from bad fats

A diet high in saturated fats, without question, increases your risks of developing cardiovascular disease. Here's why: Eating a diet high in saturated fats usually causes your cholesterol levels to spike. Cholesterol — specifically LDL cholesterol — is bad because it collects on the walls of your arteries, causing blockages. If eaten regularly, a high-fat diet begins to cause arterial plaque to form. This plaque is the root cause for a variety of cardiovascular diseases. (Refer to Chapter 7 for a list of these diseases and their biggest predictors.)

The fats to avoid are saturated fats and trans-fats:

✔ *Saturated fats* are found primarily in animal products: red meats and whole-fat dairy products like cheese, sour cream, ice cream, butter, and so on. They can also be found in some plant products, like coconut milk, coconut oil, palm oil, and cocoa butter.

✔ *Trans-fats* are, for the most part, man-made. (They result when liquid vegetable oil is processed to produce a solid shortening.) Trans-fats are used to enhance taste, texture, and shelf life of many processed foods, and they're a common ingredient in many of the foods you can find at convenience and grocery stores: shortening, potato chips, cookies and cakes, and margarine, to name just a few.

Trans-fats are just as dangerous, if not more dangerous, than saturated fats in terms of raising your cholesterol and thus your risk of cardiovascular disease. Figure 12-5 shows which foods are the most likely to have trans-fats (and probably saturated fats as well) in them.

One way to avoid trans-fats is to read the ingredients of any food you buy. In the U.S. and many other countries, trans-fats must be listed on the nutrition labels. Look for the term *partially hydrogenated vegetable oil*.

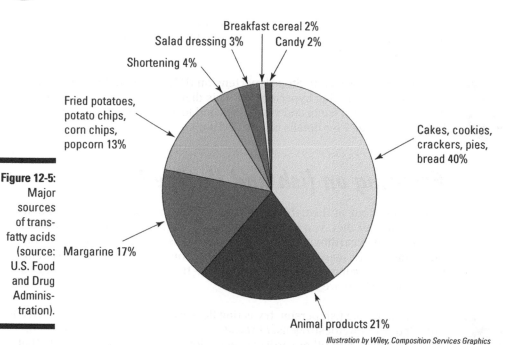

Figure 12-5: Major sources of trans-fatty acids (source: U.S. Food and Drug Administration).

Illustration by Wiley, Composition Services Graphics

For the best heart health, avoid saturated and trans-fats and control your total fat intake. Here are some research findings related to fat in your diet:

✔ If fat, even the healthy kind, makes up more than approximately 40 percent of your total daily calories, your risk of developing cardiovascular disease increases.

✔ A diet that's low in saturated fats, includes low-fat dairy and lean meats, and is filled with fruits and vegetables can lower the risk of a cardiovascular event, like a heart attack, by approximately 75 percent.

Staying away from sodium

High blood pressure (hypertension) is a major risk factor for cardiovascular disease. Eating a diet that includes lots of sodium contributes to hypertension. Why? Salt retains water. If you eat too much salt, this retained water is stored in your body and raises your blood pressure. Because hypertension contributes to more cardiovascular events, one way to lower your risk of cardiovascular disease is to eat a low-sodium diet.

If you reduce your sodium intake by one teaspoon of salt per day (about two to three grams of sodium), you can reduce the need to be treated for hypertension significantly.

 The Dietary Approach to Stop Hypertension (DASH) diet helps you reduce your risk of developing hypertension. This diet focuses on low sodium intake, coupled with fresh fruits and vegetables and low-fat dairy and lean meats. Head to Chapter 7 for details on the DASH diet.

Focusing on fish and flaxseed

If you take a look at the nations whose populations consume fish as a major portion of their diet, you find that the people in these nations have a low risk of dying of cardiovascular diseases. Japan is a perfect example of this phenomenon. Researchers attribute this outcome to diets that are rich in foods — tuna, salmon, and other seafood — that are packed with omega-3 fatty acids, which are cardio-protective.

 If you're not a big fish person, try eating flaxseeds for omega-3 fats. Flaxseeds are filled with phytoestrogens. *Phytoestrogens* assist in lowering the risk of stroke, clotting, and other cardiac events. Some research also suggests that phytoestrogens can also help regulate blood pressure. However, be sure you grind the flaxseeds up before eating them; otherwise, you'll just pass them in your stool instead of digesting them.

 In addition to being an amazing source of omega-3 fatty acids, flaxseed is also antioxidant rich, is the richest known source of lignans, is an anti-inflammatory, and is a great source of fiber. Flaxseed and flaxseed oil are good for your skin, hair, heart, immune system, mood, blood pressure, and cholesterol levels. They also help with weight loss and protect against radiation.

Going nuts for nuts

Nuts — almonds, walnuts, chestnuts, and others — are known for their protective effect against cardiovascular disease. Nuts may help lower cholesterol by replacing trans-fats and saturated fats with heart-healthy fats. Nuts are also packed with something called *arginine*. Arginine possibly assists with vein and artery health, keeping them functioning properly. Nuts are also a good source of magnesium, which helps to regulate blood pressure.

The challenge with nuts is eating enough to get the advantages of all their health benefits without going overboard in calories. You can easily eat more calories than you realize. To avoid eating too many calories and putting on weight, limit yourself to about two ounces of nuts a week.

My favorite nut, by the way, is the chestnut. Roast chestnuts for approximately around 15 minutes at 425 degrees Fahrenheit and enjoy! They are absolutely awesome.

Eating your fruits and vegetables

Simply put, fruits and vegetables protect your heart. In fact, a diet low in fruits and vegetables can increase the risk of dying of a cardiovascular event by nearly 25 percent. Here are just a few of the protective elements you can find in fruits and vegetables:

- **Phytochemicals:** *Phytochemicals* are elements in food that confer taste, color, and texture and are believed to have beneficial health qualities. (See Chapter 6 for more information on phytochemicals.) The thousands and thousands and thousands of phytochemicals in fruits and vegetables provide tons of protective effects. In fact, the phytochemicals are so numerous that they're almost impossible to name, at least in a book this size.

- **Carotenoids:** Carotenoids, like alpha-carotene, beta-carotene, and lycopene, are colorful plant pigments that convert into vitamin A. They are powerful antioxidants that can help prevent some forms of cancer.

  Foods that contain carotenoids are very colorful; they're usually deep orange and red; papayas, sweet potatoes, carrots, acorn squash, bell peppers, and tomatoes are just a few examples. To keep your cardio system working and working healthily, eat plenty of these colorful foods. The more colorful the fruit and vegetable, the better.

- **Vitamins B and E:** Fruits and vegetables are filled with vitamins B and E, which are super-antioxidants and are very cardio-protective. Specifically, vitamin B_{12} (folate) and vitamin B_6 reduce your risk of clotting (thrombosis) and atherosclerosis (the buildup of plaque in your arteries). Further, vitamin B_3 (niacin) elevates your HDL (good cholesterol) levels while decreasing LDL (bad cholesterol) levels. Vitamin E stops the production of *reactive oxygen species (ROS)*. ROS is formed when unshared electrons rapidly mix with oxygen. This is particularly troublesome when fat in your food undergoes the oxidation process.

Hopping on the whole grain bandwagon

Whole grains are cardio-protective for two reasons:

- ✔ **They are high in fiber.** Fiber helps your body get rid of excess cholesterol by binding with bile (made of body cholesterol) in the intestines and then excreting it out of your body as feces. Refer to Chapter 7 for further discussion on this topic.

- ✔ **They have high levels of B vitamins.** As I explain in the preceding section, B vitamins help ward off atherosclerosis and lower bad cholesterol while increasing good cholesterol.

Try eating oatmeal, brown rice, or whole-grain bread. These foods are great for getting tons of fiber and are filling, which may prevent you from overeating.

Enjoying wine and dark chocolate

Red wine and chocolate have flavonoids in them, particularly one called *resveratrol.* Flavonoids help lower blood pressure and improve HDL (good cholesterol) levels.

Moderate drinking can protect against cardiovascular disease. Having one to two drinks per day is shown to have a protective effect again fatal heart disease events. However, if you drink too much, the reverse occurs; strive to drink no more than five to seven drinks per week, unless you are pregnant or have a health condition that forbids drinking. In that case, avoid drinking altogether.

To get the most protective effect from chocolate that you can, choose dark chocolate (containing 70 percent to 75 percent cocoa), which has more flavonoids). Because chocolate is higher in fat and calories, be sure to eat it sparingly — limit yourself to no more than a one-inch cube of chocolate two to three times per week.

Chapter 13

Exploring the Endocrine System

*O*f all the body systems, the endocrine system is the one that people are often least familiar with. If they even know they have one, they often have no idea what it does. Yet the endocrine system is one of the most critical systems in the body. It's essentially your body's central command center. Functions that fall under the endocrine system include brain function, mood regulation, hormone production, and the body's growth and maintenance functions.

The word *endocrine* is of Greek origin. *Endo* means "within," and *crinis* means "secrete." Quite literally, the word *endocrine* means "to secrete within," and the primary purpose of the endocrine system is to secrete hormones that regulate bodily processes.

As with the other organ systems, you can forestall or even prevent chronic conditions by eating a proper, balanced diet rich with fruits, vegetables, whole grains, and lean protein. If you don't obtain the proper nutrition, however, endocrine system problems can cause fatigue, bouts of insomnia, body-weight changes, depression, and possibly even hair loss.

In this chapter, I cover how the endocrine system works, what it does, and how a healthily functioning endocrine system relies upon a healthy, nutritious diet.

Outlining the Basics of the Endocrine System

The endocrine system is essentially a group of glands that produce hormones. These glands and their hormones regulate body growth, sexual desire, metabolism, "adrenaline rushes" (the feeling produced when the hormone epinephrine is released in response to exciting, dangerous, or threatening situations), and a cadre of other, more complicated, functions of the body. In this section, I outline the key components of the endocrine system and the system's function.

Glancing at different types of glands

The major parts of the endocrine system include a bunch of different kinds of glands — adrenal gland, thyroid gland, thymus gland, pituitary gland, sex (ovaries and testicles) glands, pineal gland, and parathyroid glands — as well as the pancreas. Figure 13-1 indicates where these glands are in the body.

Each kind of gland has a particular job. In this section, I identify each of the glands and explain its role. Because the pancreas is also an important part of the endocrine system, I include it in this list, too.

Sex glands (gonads)

The sex glands include the ovaries and testes. These glands are what make you male or female — literally. The sex glands secrete sex hormones that influence the development of male-dominated or female-dominated physical characteristics.

Pancreas

One of the primary jobs of the pancreas is to produce the hormone insulin so that blood sugar (glucose) can be regulated. You can read more about the pancreas and insulin in Chapter 8, which covers diabetes.

Adrenal glands

The adrenal glands rest around your kidneys. The hormones secreted by the adrenal glands are most closely related to metabolism regulation and that "adrenaline rush" you may feel when facing an intense situation.

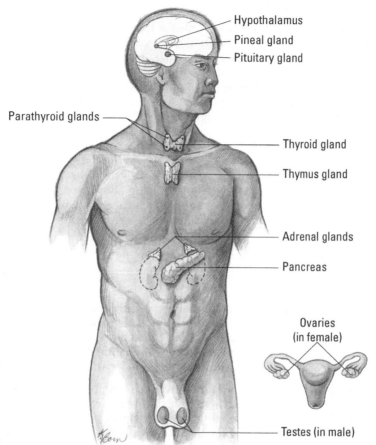

Hypothalamus
Pineal gland
Pituitary gland

Parathyroid glands

Thyroid gland

Thymus gland

Adrenal glands

Pancreas

Ovaries
(in female)

Figure 13-1:
The
endocrine
system.

Testes (in male)

Illustration by Kathryn Born, MA

Metabolism regulation

Among other hormones, your adrenal glands release the hormone epinephrine. The amount of epinephrine in your blood alters your metabolism. When epinephrine levels in your blood increase, your blood pressure and heart rate rise. Your respiratory system also adjusts by increasing blood flow and oxygen support to your muscles so that you can perform better and with increased muscular function.

When your body is in this state of readiness, your ability to burn energy more efficiently improves as a way to ensure that your system has what it needs to fuel any potential physical reaction you may need to make.

The adrenaline rush

Your adrenal glands are responsible for the adrenaline rush you feel when you experience stress, either good *(eustress)* or bad *(distress)*. In intense situations — like a grizzly bear crossing your path as you're out hiking, or a car veering into your path on the highway — adrenaline is secreted throughout the body. The adrenaline causes you to feel a sense of power and gives you strength that you can use to either engage the danger or flee from it (hence, the term "fight or flight").

This rush can be quite intense, and you may experience these symptoms:

- **Pain suppression:** You have a delayed, or no, sense of pain during the adrenaline rush. A delayed sense of pain allows you to handle an environmental situation without getting distracted by minor (and sometimes major) pain that may arise when you overexert yourself physically.

- **Surging energy:** This sensation results from a sudden dump of glucose into the bloodstream. This surge in energy allows your body to complete the required tasks rapidly. (Remember, glucose is the fuel your cells use to do their work.)

- **Increased strength:** An adrenaline rush allows you to complete tasks you normally cannot do without the epinephrine surge. You may have heard of the amazing stories of normal, everyday people completing some supernatural feats during an adrenaline rush, such as a mother lifting a car off her trapped infant.

- **Heightened nervous system function:** During an emergency, your survival instincts kick into high gear, and your actions and reactions are predicated on doing what you need to do — either fight or flee — to live. Your hearing, sense of smell, and eyesight get more focused and acute to any environmental changes that are occurring. Of course, you need your senses as sharp as possible, and your nervous system is the command and control center for all of this heightened awareness.

- **Elevated breathing and heart rate:** A response to a rapidly changing environment, faster breathing and heart rate elevate your blood pressure in order to fuel your muscles more efficiently, which lets you complete the necessary physical activity.

- **Increased clotting ability:** During this rush, your body's ability to clot blood is increased in preparation for a possible injury that could result from the situation. This chemical transformation in the blood allows your blood to clot more quickly, preventing excessive blood loss and preserving energy.

Thymus gland

The thymus gland is primarily associated with immune system function. It's responsible for producing *T lymphocytes,* the white blood cells that protect you from certain bacteria, parasites, and some viruses.

Thyroid gland

The thyroid produces the hormones that control how fast your body burns carbohydrates, fats, and proteins to produce energy. The hormones secreted by the thyroid gland primarily regulate the following:

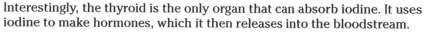

- **Metabolism and growth:** Thyroid hormones control the metabolism of every cell in the body. As such, they directly influence the efficiency of your metabolism, which in turn influences proper growth and development.

  Interestingly, the thyroid is the only organ that can absorb iodine. It uses iodine to make hormones, which it then releases into the bloodstream.

- **Body temperature:** Your thyroid controls your body's metabolism, which is responsible for the generation of body heat. Therefore, your thyroid is essentially in control of body temperature.

Parathyroid glands

Your nerve and muscle cells rely heavily on electrical charges to work properly, and calcium in your bloodstream goes into and out of cells, influencing the electrical charges of the cells. For this reason, blood calcium levels are very important for proper nerve and muscular function. Your parathyroid glands regulate your body's calcium levels.

Don't confuse the parathyroid with the thyroid gland. Their functions are very different, despite their very similar names. In fact, the word *parathyroid* is simply a combination of the Greek word *para,* meaning "beside" and the word *thyroid.* So *parathyroid* simply means "beside the thyroid." (Find out more about the thyroid gland in the preceding section.)

Pituitary gland

The pituitary gland is kind of like the shepherd of the endocrine system because it influences an array of different endocrine functions. Most notably, this gland initiates the production of hormones, most of which are protein-based, and the production of amino acid, without which you would not be able to survive.

Amino acids are the building blocks of proteins. Among their many functions, amino acids aid in digestion, growth, and repair and maintenance of the body.

Pineal gland

Sometimes referred to as your "third eye" because it has light-sensitive cells that function in the same way that retinal cells function, the pineal gland is primarily involved with functions such as the following:

- ✔ **Helping you fall asleep:** The pineal gland controls melatonin release. Melatonin is a hormone that assists with your sleep-wake cycle.

- ✔ **Helping regulate the endocrine hormones:** In this capacity, it impacts a variety of bodily functions, like sexual and physical development, among others.

The pineal gland resembles a pine cone, which is where it gets its name. *Pinea* is the Latin word for pine cone.

Hypothalamus

Just like the pineal gland, the hypothalamus assists with the sleep-wake cycle, but it does so much more as well:

- ✔ **It controls the overall function of the endocrine and central nervous systems.** The hypothalamus links the nervous system to the endocrine system via the pituitary gland.

- ✔ **It controls homeostasis within the body.** *Homeostasis* means maintaining a balance among interdependent systems. In the context of the endocrine system, it refers to keeping the body in a constant internal state of appropriate temperature, pH balance, blood pressure, water balance, and breathing.

- ✔ **It regulates food and water intake.** In tandem with the central nervous system, the hypothalamus regulates feelings of hunger, fullness, and thirst.

Truly, the hypothalamus is involved with so many crucial processes that it's impossible to imagine human functioning without it.

Some people consider the hypothalamus the "soul" of the body. The reason is that it's a central part of the body's limbic system. The *limbic system* is a complex network of connections within the brain responsible for basic emotions (fear, anger, and pleasure, for example), motivation, and memory. Many researchers and professionals consider the limbic system to be where personality and consciousness reside.

Shhh . . . It's a secret! Discovering how endocrine glands work

As the preceding section makes clear, the different glands that make up the endocrine system have their own jobs. Yet they all work in a similar fashion:

1. **The body receives some stimulus — either internally or externally — that triggers a reaction.**

2. **In reaction to this stimulus, the glands produce the components of amino acids, which are the basis for hormone production.**

3. **After creating the hormones, the gland secretes the hormone directly into the bloodstream.**

   Hormones are essentially chemical messengers that cause targeted organs or tissues to react in a certain way. They travel by way of the bloodstream to the organ or tissue whose function they control or regulate.

4. **The body structures react, based on the message the hormones deliver.**

5. **This process repeats constantly, as the organs and tissues adapt and the body receives new stimuli.**

As stated earlier, the endocrine system secretes different types of hormones that regulate metabolism, growth, reproduction and sexual function, regulation of mood, and sleep, just to name a few. Not only do these hormones regulate or control the function of key body systems, but they also enable you to react to, adapt to, and live in your environment. In so doing, these hormones create the connection between your mind and your body.

The health of the endocrine system affects all the other systems in the body, and for this reason, you can think of it as a type of command center for the body. In addition, the functions it helps regulate, like sexual functioning, are critical for human survival.

Taking Care of Your Endocrine Health

Disorders of the endocrine system can have a significant impact on your health and wellness. Given its ability to affect everything from your skeletal to your reproductive system, your endocrine system is vital to your overall well-being. When one of the glands begins to malfunction, it can affect a whole host of other organs and systems. For this reason, you need to know how your endocrine system is working and be able to recognize when it isn't working properly.

The major endocrine system issue is an imbalance of hormone levels. Such imbalances can result when a problem occurs in the production of the hormones or when your body doesn't appropriately respond to the hormones that are produced. An imbalance can result from these three very common situations:

- **An underlying disease or malfunction in a particular organ system:** Polycystic ovary syndrome (PCOS), for example, can cause hormonal imbalances that affect the endocrine system.

- **An infection:** Infections can disrupt the creation or delivery of hormones. Frequent vaginal infections can cause disturbances in the ovaries, for example.

- **Chronic stress:** Chronic stress can suppress the immune system, which can affect the function of the endocrine system.

Endocrine disorders include under- or overactive thyroids, diseases of the parathyroid gland, diseases of the adrenal glands, and PCOS (an ovarian health issue), just to name a few. Some examples of metabolic disorders include gout and rickets (called *osteomalacia* in adults). In this section, I briefly touch on a few common endocrine disorders and explain how to prevent them.

It's number 1 (unfortunately)! Diabetes

The most common endocrine disease worldwide is diabetes mellitus. As I explain in Chapter 8, diabetes is a condition in which the body improperly regulates glucose for one of two reasons:

- **There is an outright lack of insulin.** This lack results when the body — specifically, the pancreas — either doesn't produce insulin or doesn't produce enough of it. This type of diabetes is called *type 1 diabetes.*

- **The body does not respond to insulin (insulin resistance).** In this case, the body makes insulin, but the insulin doesn't do what it's supposed to do. Diabetes that results when the body doesn't respond to insulin is called *type 2 diabetes.*

Type 2 diabetes accounts for 90 percent to 95 percent of all cases of the disease, and it is quickly becoming one of the most prominent diseases in the world today. This type of diabetes is directly related to lifestyle. A sedentary lifestyle and a diet high in refined sugars and simple carbohydrates can, over time, produce insulin resistance.

If you have diabetes, you need to follow a diet that uses very strict guidelines in terms of what you can eat, how much you can eat, and when you can eat. Such a diet helps you control the amount of carbohydrates in your body, thus reducing the amount of glucose in the bloodstream. Head to Chapter 8 for a more detailed discussion of diet plans designed for people with diabetes.

Your best course of action is to talk with your physician about the diet plan that is best for you. Being in regular contact with your doctor and getting repeated checkups to keep the disease at bay is the most responsible thing you can do.

Getting gout

Gout is essentially chronic arthritis and inflammation in the joints. Over 50 percent of the cases occur in the big toes of sufferers. It is caused when an abundance of uric acid in the bloodstream causes crystals to collect in the joint. The buildup of crystallized uric acid flares the joint, a condition that can last for days or even months.

Uric acid builds up when purines are broken down by the body. *Purines* are chemical substances that naturally occur in your genes and in the genes of certain foods. Although all foods contains some purine, some foods have concentrated amounts of purine. For that reason, your diet can greatly affect the onset of gout attacks.

If you have issues with gout or are at high risk for the disease, avoid these foods, which are high in purines:

- Fish and other seafood
- Certain alcohols (beer, for instance, has the highest purine content of common alcohols consumed)
- Red meat
- Certain vegetables (cauliflower, peas, lentils, and asparagus, for example, contain higher amounts of uric acid than others)

A diet high in complex carbohydrates and rich with non-fat or low-fat dairy products and vitamin C–rich foods (citrus fruits, for example) is probably the best regimen to follow to control gout flare-ups.

Having a gout flare-up? Try eating 10 to 12 cherries (about a half cup) once or twice a day and drinking coffee. These foods have been shown to decrease the symptoms of gout and can be preventative as part of a well-balanced, healthy diet and lifestyle.

Polycystic ovary syndrome

Among women who are of childbearing ages, *polycystic ovary syndrome (PCOS)* is one of the most common endocrine disorders and also accounts for the most cases of infertility among women. Alarmingly, 10 percent to 30 percent of women may have this disease, and it can occur in girls as young as 10 years old.

Women with PCOS have higher-than-normal levels of *androgens* (often considered the "male hormone," even though women produce it as well), a situation that impacts the development and release of eggs during ovulation. Among other symptoms, PCOS often includes irregular menstrual cycles, increased hair growth, weight gain, and cysts on the ovaries (see Figure 13-2).

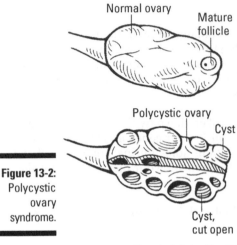

Figure 13-2:
Polycystic
ovary
syndrome.

Illustration by Kathryn Born, MA

Not only is PCOS itself an issue in terms of your health and wellness, but it can also increase your risk of developing other, potentially deadly diseases, such as diabetes and cardiovascular disease. Women with PCOS are at greater risk of developing diabetes because their bodies don't use insulin efficiently. As a result, they tend to have high levels of insulin in their blood, and high levels of insulin are linked to the over production of androgen.

To reduce your risk of getting PCOS or to increase your chances of fertility if you have it, follow these guidelines:

✔ **To prevent the disease:** Currently, there is no known way to reduce your risk of getting PCOS. However, considering that PCOS development has been linked with obesity, experts recommend keeping caloric intake under control and exercising regularly. A healthy lifestyle may reduce your risk. But the jury is still out on the direct link between diet and PCOS prevention.

✔ **To increase your chances of fertility if you have PCOS:** To increase your chances of conceiving, follow a well-balanced, healthy diet that is rich in whole, fresh foods. In addition, you must monitor insulin levels pretty closely, due to the link between insulin resistance and PCOS.

Researchers suggest that eating a large breakfast, a smaller lunch, and a snack-like dinner can raise your chances of conception when you are diagnosed with PCOS. Structuring your meals this way can also reduce your chances of diabetes and cardiovascular disease. When you eat a large amount of your energy in the morning, you have the entire day to burn the calories off, thus preventing excess energy buildup, which causes obesity, diabetes, and heart disease. In summary, don't skip breakfast — especially if you have PCOS and want to get pregnant.

Hormone imbalances can have a significant impact on the reproductive systems, particularly in women. If you have hormone imbalances and reproductive concerns, consider seeing an endocrinologist. These physicians treat patients with fertility issues and also assess and treat patients with health concerns surrounding menstruation and menopause.

Combating osteomalacia (rickets)

Rickets is a condition that affects children (the same condition is called *osteomalacia* in adults). With rickets, a vitamin D deficiency leads to calcification problems that can cause bones to soften and become malformed. The result is often bow legs.

To prevent rickets, you just need some good ol' vitamin D. To get enough vitamin D to make your bones strong and prevent them from softening, do the following:

- ✔ Eat a vitamin D–rich diet that includes appropriate amounts of dairy products, fruits, and vegetables.

- ✔ Make sure you get sufficient exposure to sunlight. Light-skinned people need at least 20 to 30 minutes per day in the sun; dark-skinned people need at least an hour. (The differences in pigment require more or less sunlight to achieve the same result.)

Hormonal imbalances can influence bone health. Rickets in children (or osteomalacia in adults) and osteoporosis, which involves loss of bone density (I discuss osteoporosis in the next section) are often discovered and treated by tests that determine whether the endocrine system is malfunctioning in some way.

Osteoporosis

With osteoporosis, your bones lose their density. Mainly older, post-menopausal women are most at risk for the disease. You may feel the effects earlier, but most people begin to experience symptoms when they are around 60 to 70 years old.

The disease affects different demographic groups differently as well. For example, older white women are more at risk than any other demographic group.

Although bone loss occurs naturally in most individuals, particularly women, strong bones are a key to mobility and good health as you age. For that reason, you want to do what you can to minimize bone loss and lessen its effects. The two keys to protecting your bones include eating a diet rich in calcium and vitamin D and remaining (or becoming) physically active. (You can read more about strategies to ensure good health as you get older in Chapters 17 and 18.)

By the time bone loss becomes a problem, it's too late to use diet to improve the situation. The time period when you should pay attention to your calcium and vitamin D intake is when you're in your preteens to late 20s. Ensuring you get enough calcium and vitamin D during these years can prevent early-onset osteoporosis from occurring later. Because bone mass reaches its peak at around the age of 30, girls (and guys) need to pack on as much bone mass as possible before then to prevent their bones from becoming brittle.

Noting health problems related to thyroid function

A number of health issues — ranging from hyperthyroidism to goiters to thyroid cancer — can stem from a malfunctioning thyroid. As you discover in this section, your thyroid is a very sensitive, but very influential, gland.

When your body is in a state of *hypothyroidism,* the thyroid does not produce enough thyroid hormone to meet the body's needs. When this occurs, many of the body's functions slow or shut down completely. Conversely, *hyperthyroidism* occurs when your thyroid overproduces the thyroid hormone. Symptoms of hyperthyroidism include emotional issues, like moodiness or impatience, body trembling, and a racing heartbeat. However, if you have a milder form of hyperthyroidism, you may not exhibit any symptoms at all.

Goiters, characterized by an enlargement of the thyroid gland (see Figure 13-3), form mainly as a result of iodine deficiency. They're associated with both hyper-thyroidism and hypothyroidism. Many people who lack access to fresh foods and vegetables develop goiters.

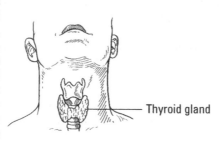

Figure 13-3:
The thyroid gland, shown here, becomes enlarged to form a goiter, usually due to iodine deficiency.

Thyroid gland

Illustration by Kathryn Born, MA

To promote a healthy thyroid, make sure you use iodized salt and eat whole grains and other high-fiber foods, fresh fruits and vegetables, and lean meats. Besides iodine, selenium and vitamin A are known to assist with healthy thyroid function. Selenium is found in oysters, sunflower and sesame seeds, and mushrooms. For great sources of vitamin A, look to cold-water ocean fish (like cod or haddock) and orange-colored fruits and vegetables (like carrots, mangoes, pumpkin, and so on).

Certain foods are *goitrogenic,* which means they can actually inhibit thyroid activity. Most goitrogenic foods are cruciferous vegetables, like cauliflower, cabbage, brussels sprouts, kale, and soy. Individuals who have hypothyroidism should avoid eating large quantities of these foods. Individuals who suffer from hyperthyroidism should eat more of these foods, being careful to not overconsume. Speak to your physician about dietary options to control any thyroid issue.

Interacting with the digestive system: The pancreas

Your pancreas works in tandem with your digestive system. These systems are so interlinked, in fact, that if something goes wrong with one system, the other is significantly affected. That's why keeping both systems working optimally is so important.

Here are a couple of examples that illustrate how the pancreas and the digestive system work as a team:

✔ **Neutralizing stomach acid:** The pancreas secretes enzymes into the stomach to help raise the pH of gastric acid — thereby reducing its acidity level — before the food empties from the stomach into your small intestine. Without being neutralized, the stomach acid can greatly damage the walls of your duodenum (the upper small intestine).

✔ **Aiding with digestion:** The pancreas secretes enzymes into the small intestine to help break down energy nutrients. For more information on the digestive system, refer to Chapter 11.

The pancreas is one of the most essential organs in the body. Not only does it assist with digestion, but it also helps with the regulation of insulin, which is essential for breaking down blood sugar.

As you can guess, eating a healthy diet can keep your pancreas healthy. In general, you should eat a low-fat diet rich in fruits and vegetables, lean meats, and low-fat dairy products. If you have *pancreatitis* (an inflamed, enlarged pancreas), it's particularly important that you don't eat a high-fat diet. Diets high in triglycerides and calories tend to irritate the pancreas and, if consumed over a long period of time, can result in a chronically inflamed pancreas.

Eating your way to a healthy endocrine system

In the preceding sections, I offer dietary recommendations based on each of the different disorders. You may have noticed that, in nearly all cases, my basic recommendations are the same:

✔ **Eat a healthy diet.** It should have these characteristics:

- Be low in simplified sugar and high in complex carbohydrates

- Be rich in fruits and vegetables

- Include lean meats

- Include low-fat dairy

✔ **Watch how many carbs you eat.** Many times, even if you have diabetes, you can eat simple sugars; you just can't eat too many.

✔ **Get plenty of exercise and sleep.**

✔ **If you have any concerns or questions, consult your physician immediately.**

For the most part, if you do the preceding four things, you'll keep your endocrine system healthy and happy.

Next time you are at your physician's office, make sure you ask about your endocrine system and how to verify that everything is working properly. Further, ask your physician to recommend some preventative things you can do to make sure you are operating at optimum health.

Chapter 14

The Ins and Outs of the Excretory System

In This Chapter

▶ Identifying the components of the excretory system

▶ Understanding the excretory system's purpose

▶ Establishing dietary guidelines for a healthy-functioning excretory system

*O*ne organ system that does not get nearly the attention it deserves is the excretory system. The amount of work this system performs for the body — and the sheer importance of its work — makes it one of the most critical body systems you have.

The kidneys, urinary bladder, ureters, and the urethra filter, process, and excrete a lion's share of whatever you put into your body (namely, your diet). Think about it: Along with the digestive system (which I cover in Chapter 11), the excretory system filters out most foreign substances (minerals, water, and so on) that you ingest either from your diet and or from other sources like medicines and pharmaceuticals. That's why maintaining a healthy, functioning excretory system should be of utmost importance to you; otherwise, you can end up facing very serious health consequences.

In this chapter, I describe the excretory system, explain how it works, and share how diet and nutrition play a vital role in keeping it healthy and strong.

Taking a Trip through the Excretory System

Your body has billions of cells. Each cell, from your scalp to your soles, produces waste. Naturally, that waste needs to be cleaned out of the body and disposed of. A number of major organs, such as your liver, your intestinal tract, and your lungs, assist in the dirty job of cleaning out your body.

The liver helps break down toxins that are then transported in the blood and filtered by the kidneys into the urine. Unused parts of your food (like fiber) remain in the intestine and are passed out of the body in feces. Your lungs breathe out the carbon dioxide (CO_2) waste. One system, however — the excretory system — rises above as your body's premier waste-removal system.

For the most part, your major organ systems work together to allow for healthy body functioning. The excretory system (specifically, the kidneys) is linked to both of these other systems:

✔ The circulatory system (primarily the lungs and the renal vein and renal artery), for oxygen and carbon dioxide exchange to cleanse the blood

✔ The digestive system (primarily the liver), for toxin exchange to be excreted via urination

This coordination is critical for your health and well-being.

Identifying the system's key components

The excretory system, whose job is to remove impurities and toxins from the blood, is primarily made up of the following parts (Figure 14-1 shows these parts):

✔ **The kidneys,** which filter blood and produce urine

Your two kidneys, which lie in the mid- to lower back, have two primary functions:

• To dispose of bodily wastes

• To regulate water and mineral (primarily sodium) content of the blood in response to bodily needs

Head to Chapter 9 to find out what happens when the kidneys fail to function as they should.

✔ **The renal vein and renal artery,** which supply the kidneys with oxygen-rich blood (renal artery) and carry away wastes (renal vein)

✔ **The ureters,** which transport urine from the kidneys to the bladder

✔ **The urinary bladder,** which holds the urine

✔ **The urethra,** which transports the urine from the bladder to outside the body

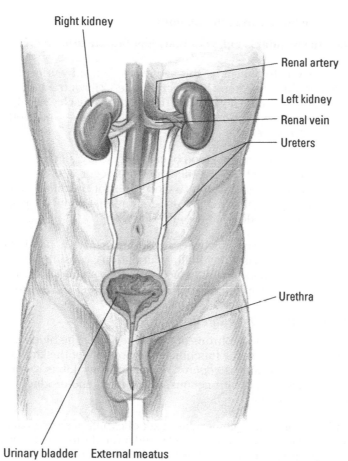

Right kidney

Renal artery

Left kidney

Renal vein

Ureters

Urethra

Figure 14-1:
The excre-
tory system.

Urinary bladder   External meatus

Illustration by Kathryn Born, MA

Watching the system in action

As the preceding section illustrates, removing wastes and toxins from your body is a vital function and involves a rather complex coordination between all sorts of different areas of the body. Here is a very simplified explanation of how the process works:

1. **The kidneys filter out bloodstream wastes.**

   Actually, it's the nephrons in the kidneys that are responsible for filtering waste. I explain what they are and how they work in the next section.

2. **This collection of wastes from the kidneys, along with amine group wastes from the liver, drain into the urinary bladder via the ureters.**

   Amine group wastes are residual compounds that result when nutrients are processed in the liver.

3. **The urine builds up in the bladder.**

4. **When the bladder is full, your body empties the urine out via the urethra.**

Here's an easy way to remember this sequence: A healthy urine flow occurs in this sequence: filtration (Step 1), collection (Step 2), contraction (of the bladder muscle; Step 3), and relaxation (of the urethral muscle; Step 4). Say it often enough — filtration, collection, contraction, relaxation — and pretty soon you'll be trying to *forget* it.

This process of cleansing the blood occurs every day, all day. Many urinary concerns happen when this sequence does not occur or is disrupted in some way. In the next sections, I give you a closer look at the different steps in the process and help you gain a deeper understanding of how the excretory system's various parts do what they do.

If you experience any issue, such as pain during urination, passing blood in your urine, or incontinence (involuntary urination), consult your physician immediately. If your kidneys don't function as they should and you don't resolve the problem, you can develop blood poisoning and eventually die.

Filtering the blood: The kidneys

As I mention earlier, the nephrons in the kidney filter the blood. *Nephrons,* shown in Figure 14-2, are the functional components of the kidney. (In fact, the Greek word for kidney is *nephros.*) The nephrons' job is to remove toxins, excess water, and *urea* (a nitrogenous, amine-filled end-product of protein metabolism sent by the liver).

Each nephron contains a glomerulus, a set of capillaries (microscopic blood vessels where veins and arteries meet), and a renal tube. As the waste passes from the capillaries, the renal tubes funnel it away from the blood.

If you consider how important the kidney's job is, you can count yourself doubly lucky that you have two of them, even though one, alone, can do the job. That's right. A human can function healthily and live a long life with just one kidney. It's one of the things that makes kidney transplantation (more on that in Chapter 9) relatively common and so successful. An individual can donate one kidney to a needy family member and live a completely normal life post-donation.

Filling up and flushing out: The ureters, bladder, and urethra

From the renal tubes in the nephron, the urine passes through the *ureters,* thin tubes leading to the urinary bladder. The muscles in the ureter walls constantly contract and release to force urine from the kidneys. About every 15 seconds or so, urine is transferred from the kidneys to the bladder.

The *bladder* is a muscular sac that stores urine. When the brain signals that it's time to empty the bladder, it simultaneously instructs the bladder walls and the urethra muscles to relax. This movement squeezes the urine out of the body, causing you to urinate.

Figure 14-3 shows this portion of the excretory system.

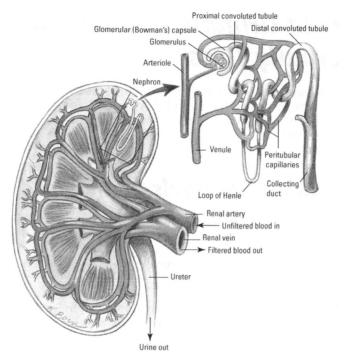

Proximal convoluted tubule

Glomerular (Bowman's) capsule

Distal convoluted tubule

Glomerulus

Arteriole

Nephron

Venule

Peritubular capillaries

Loop of Henle

Collecting duct

Renal artery

Unfiltered blood in

Renal vein

Filtered blood out

Ureter

Figure 14-2:
The nephron
in the kidney.

Urine out

Illustration by Kathryn Born, MA

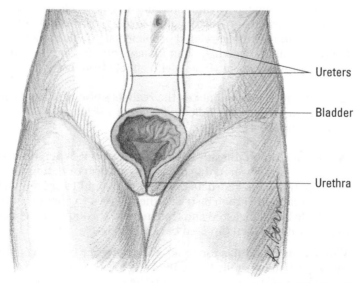

Ureters

Bladder

Urethra

Figure 14-3:
The ureters,
bladder, and
urethra.

Illustration by Kathryn Born, MA

Going beyond Urination: What This System Actually Does

If you asked people the question, "What exactly does the excretory system do?" many of the responses would probably focus on urination. That's fine, but it's incomplete. This system does so much more for you, and it's time we gave it its due. Read on.

Balancing water levels in the blood

The excretory system ensures the balance of water in the body. Essentially, it makes sure that your body doesn't lose too much water.

To perform this important role, the excretory system is in tune with body temperature and diet. If your body fluids drop — you're sweating excessively or eating foods that cause dehydration, for example — the excretory system compensates by helping the body retain water. How does it do that, you ask? Through less frequent urination, which preserves the existing water in the body.

People who live in warmer climates sweat more, on average, than people who live in cooler climates. No surprise there. If you live in a hotter climate, of course, you're going to sweat more. And as you would expect, your kidneys must be more efficient at regulating fluid levels to prevent overheating, dehydration, and other heat-related problems. If you live in a hot region, it's absolutely critical that you help your kidneys out: Be sure to maintain proper hydration to prevent any adverse health effects from body fluid loss.

The excretory system manipulates the reabsorption of water in your body, using a particular hormone, called *antidiuretic hormone (ADH)*. Here's how it works (see Figure 14-4):

✓ **When your blood doesn't have enough water:** When the water levels in your blood are lowered due to poor hydration or eating too much salt, the hypothalamus instructs the pituitary gland to secrete ADH into the bloodstream. ADH then instructs the kidneys to absorb more water from the foods being digested and transported throughout the body. This excess water is then directed back to the body.

✓ **When your blood has too much water:** If your blood has too much fluid, the hypothalamus tells the pituitary gland to reduce the amount of ADH in the blood. This action ramps up the excretion of urine, causing water levels in your body to drop.

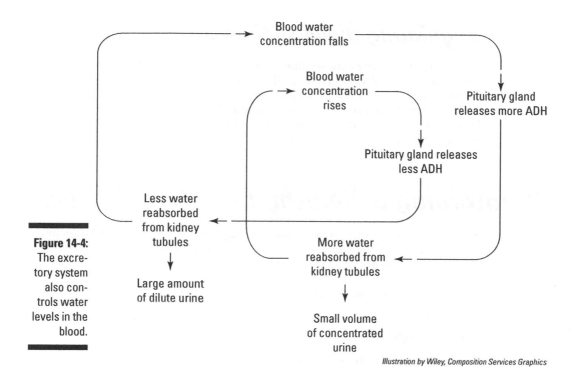

Figure 14-4:
The excretory system also controls water levels in the blood.

Illustration by Wiley, Composition Services Graphics

Drinking alcohol has a similar effect on AHD secretions as the hypothalamus does. When you're drinking alcohol, you may feel the urge to urinate more often. The reason is that the alcohol suppresses your body's production and secretion of AHD in the blood. (Remember, less AHD in the blood means more fluid left in your body.) The end result? You have to pee more.

Protecting your body from toxins

When food is digested, chemicals and other byproducts from the digestive process are released in the gut. Much of this byproduct gets excreted out with your feces, but whatever toxins remain could damage the walls of the colon and other sectors of the digestive system. These toxins include nitrogenous waste, including ammonia, which is the byproduct of amino acid digestion.

To prevent this kind of damage, the leftover toxins are redirected to the kidneys, which filter them from the digestive system and the rest of the body, to be excreted in the urine.

Regulating blood sodium levels

Your kidneys also regulate sodium (salt) levels in the blood. Akin to rising and falling levels of water (refer to the earlier section "Balancing water levels in the blood"), your kidneys adjust their filtering and excretion functions according to the fluctuations in the amount of sodium in the blood. When too little sodium is present in the blood, your kidneys extract more; when too much is present, they extract less.

Maintaining a Healthy Excretory System

To a large degree, you can maintain a healthy excretory system by following these general healthy-diet and healthy-living guidelines (you may notice that this list is *always* my go-to response):

✓ Refrain from smoking or using tobacco products

✓ Drink alcohol in moderation and responsibly

✓ Eat a high-fiber diet

✓ Eat a low-fat, low-calorie diet

✓ Get an appropriate amount of sleep

✓ Get an appropriate amount of exercise

In this section, I focus on diet, explaining the particular benefits certain dietary choices have on the excretory system, and provide a few other pointers that will help keep your excretory system hale and hardy.

Making good food choices

Your excretory system needs ample amounts of minerals, vitamins, and energy to maintain proper function of all major and support organs in the system. So naturally you're probably wondering what kind of foods you should be eating. Well, here's what you should eat to responsibly promote a properly functioning excretory system (again, you may notice that this list is pretty standard healthy-diet fare):

✓ **A variety of fruits and vegetables:** Your fruits and vegetables should make up approximately 50 percent of every plate of food you eat.

✓ **Whole-grain cereals and other complex carbohydrates:** Approximately 15 percent to 25 percent of your food plate should be whole grains. You can choose whole-grain breads and cereals for some options.

✔ **Moderate portions of dairy:** About 10 percent of your plate should be dairy foods. Cheese, milk, or yogurt can be a great choice for this food group. You must be careful of the amount you get, though, because these foods tend to be higher in fat and calories.

✔ **Lean proteins:** Opt for lean cuts of beef, skinless chicken, seafood, and fish. Or look to non-animal sources of protein instead. Your options include quinoa, lentils, chickpeas, tofu, avocados, and more. About 10 percent to 25 percent or so of your plate should be lean meats.

Think of the meat as a complement to your fruit and vegetables, rather than the star of the plate. Try to eat more vegetables and fruits than animal proteins at breakfast, lunch, and dinner.

✔ **Reduced amount of sweets, candies, and fast foods:** Notice I say that you should reduce the amount of sweets, candies, and fast foods. I didn't say you have to eliminate them entirely.

Can a person truly enjoy life without ice cream or pizza? I can most certainly say that I would not enjoy my life as much if I never ate those two foods. Of course, I am joking . . . a bit. My point? You can most certainly eat your favorite treats — pizza, chicken wings, chocolate, ice cream, and so on — and still have a healthy excretory system, but you need to eat those things in low or moderate amounts.

Eating meals like the one shown in Figure 14-5 will assist in keeping your excretory system working well. To find out more guidelines designed to help you eat a healthy diet, go to ChooseMyPlate.gov (www.choosemyplate.gov).

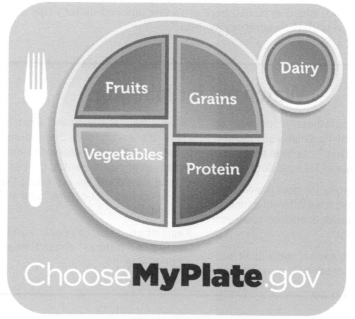

Figure 14-5:
A well-proportioned plate, Courtesy of Choose MyPlate.gov.

Illustration courtesy of USDA, www.choosemyplate.gov

Eliminating additives

As a rule, processed foods (fast foods and mass-produced food products) tend to have many different types of additives serving as significant ingredients. Additives confer taste, color, and texture to foods, and not all are harmful; some are perhaps even beneficial. Some additives, for example, contain phytochemicals or other substances to boost the nutrient value in a food. Still many additives are preservatives, and those can be an issue.

The problem with additives is that the excretory system has to work harder at processing additives and preservatives than it does to process other, more natural ingredients. Thus, the more additives you eat, the harder your system has to work. The harder your system works, the higher the chance you'll develop health issues later in life.

Your body can build up excess toxins even when you eat healthier, non-processed foods. Further, when you drink alcohol, use tobacco products, or take unregulated amounts of supplements, you build up even more toxins due to digestive byproducts. In addition, the lotions and creams you rub on your skin can introduce foreign substances into your bloodstream that, eventually, your excretory system has to filter out. Word to the wise: Be careful what you put in and on your body. Give your excretory system a break!

Following other dietary recommendations

Besides the obvious dietary recommendations to maintain proper functioning of major organ systems, here are a few tailored dietary tips and tricks that can assist with the excretory system.

Watch out for labeling

Processed foods aren't the only foods that contain additives, Many foods labeled "healthy," "natural," and "organic" may have additives as well. Why the confusion? For a couple of reasons.

First, different people (or governments and regulatory agencies) have different definitions of what *organic* means. Some may allow additives; others may not.

Second, words like *natural* really don't mean too much. What, for example, does the label "All-natural" really mean? Exactly. It's not clear. It's ambiguous. Sodium-nitrate (the mineral used as a preservative and a color-enhancer in cured meats), for example, is a natural ingredient. So a product that uses it can be labeled "All-natural" and still include this additive.

Remember, just because something is labeled "All-natural" doesn't mean that it's additive free.

Got thirst?

When you are thirsty, drink water. Drinking adequate amounts of water daily helps keep your urinary schedule regular and your excretory system flushed out. No real recommendation exists for how many glasses you should get in a given day, but many health professionals say eight 8- to 10-ounce glasses of water a day should do the trick.

Reducing your caffeine intake

Caffeine has been known to irritate your bladder, and if the caffeine isn't properly flushed out with adequate water intake, it can cause infections. Scientists suggest that increased amounts of caffeine may make you urinate more, but it can sometimes dehydrate you if you don't also drink enough water to balance out the increased urination.

Avoiding excess sugar

Having too much sugar in your blood forces the kidneys to work extra hard. They have to filter the extra sugar out, and it gets transferred into the urine. Some research suggests that an increased amount of sugar in your urine can spur bacterial growth in your urethra, thus increasing your risk of urinary tract infections (you can read more about this condition in the later section "Dealing with Urinary Tract Infections").

Exercising for the sweat

Exercise helps make your body strong and fit, better able to fend off infections, and less likely to succumb to a chronic disease of a major organ system. It also has an important role to play in maintaining the health of your excretory system.

When you exercise, you sweat. Sure, sweat helps you cool off, but it has another important function: It lets your body excrete toxins through your pores. The more toxins that are eliminated through sweat, the fewer toxins that need to be filtered by the kidneys and processed by the excretory system. This is a good thing. Less work for the system increases longevity.

Dealing with Urinary Tract Infections

Urinary tract infections (UTIs) occur when bacteria infect parts of the urinary system, and they can affect the lower (bladder) and the upper parts (kidneys). Many women and some men get UTIs. Symptoms include the following:

- Painful urination
- Frequent urge to urinate
- Fever

UTIs are no fun. First, they hurt. Worse, if left untreated, they can cause some very serious adverse health outcomes, including sterility. For that reason, if you have or suspect you have a UTI, talk to your healthcare provider.

Enjoying foods that prevent or reduce the effects of UTIs

Fortunately, you don't have to rely solely on medical professionals when it comes to UTIs. Several foods have been shown to help prevent and cure UTIs:

- ✔ **Cranberries:** Cranberries contain *hippuric acid,* a metabolic compound that prevents bacteria from taking root in the urethra and other parts of the urinary tract.

- ✔ **Yogurt:** Taking in enough of the *probiotic* (good) bacteria in yogurt crowds out and reduces the growth of bad bacteria, thus reducing the risk of infection.

- ✔ **Vitamin C:** Vitamin C makes your urine more acidic, thus lessening the ability of bacterial infections to take root.

- ✔ **Pineapples:** Pineapples contains an enzyme, *bromelain,* that may prevent bacterial growth. However, the most important feature of bromelain is its potential to decrease the irritation and swelling of a UTI.

- ✔ **Garlic and onions:** These help prevent bacterial growth in the urethra.

- ✔ **Blueberries:** These little superfoods have nearly the same effect on UTIs that cranberries do.

Taking other steps to avoid a UTI

Here are some other things you can do:

- ✔ **Drink plenty of water.** Doing so flushes your system out and prevents bad bacteria from infecting the bladder or other parts of the urinary tract.

- ✔ **Urinate before and after sex.** Doing so can help keep your urethra clear of bacteria that may have built up since you last urinated and lessen the chance of infections being spread between sexual partners. In addition, wiping before and after sex can also help keep bacterial transmission — and UTIs — between partners at a minimum.

- ✔ **Wipe thoroughly from front to back after going to the bathroom.** It's especially important for women to wipe thoroughly and from front to back when they poop. The anus carries a lot of bacteria. If you wipe from back to front, you run the risk of transmitting that bacteria into your urethra.

Part IV
Nutrition through the Lifespan

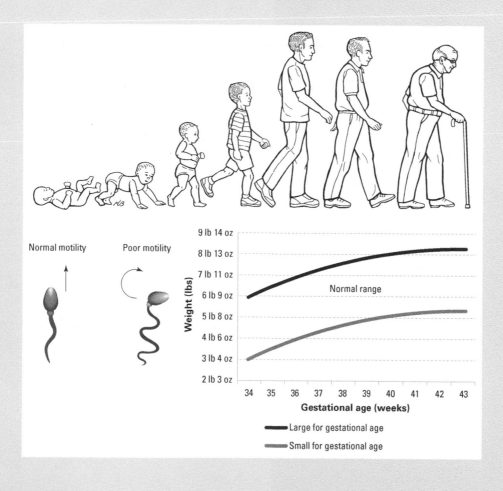

In this part. . .

✔ Understand the nutritional needs of expectant mothers and fetuses and how diet and exercise can promote a healthy pregnancy

✔ Learn the nutritional needs of children from infancy to the late teen years and get tips on how to ensure your children follow a diet that helps them grow up strong and healthy

✔ Discover the changes that occur during young adulthood and into middle age and how these changes impact your nutrition needs during the different periods of your life

✔ Become familiar with the nutrient needs of the elderly and how diet can help delay or prevent the onset of common afflictions

Chapter 15

Having a Baby? Pre- and Post-Natal Nutrition

*W*hether you are trying to get pregnant, you currently are pregnant, or you just had a baby, maintaining a healthy lifestyle for yourself can help ensure a healthy lifestyle for your child(-ren). It is essential that mothers (particularly expectant mothers) do what they can — eat a healthy diet, get enough sleep, and engage in exercise — to provide the healthiest environment possible for their babies.

Although mothers are often the focus, fathers aren't off the hook. They also have to ensure that they're leading the best lives possible before, during, and after the births of their children. Doing so is the best way to help shepherd in healthy lifestyles for their families. Just because dads don't physically carry or give birth to their babies doesn't mean their actions don't directly impact theirs babies' health.

It takes a healthy family to raise healthy children. If you have healthy behaviors and teach your children these same behaviors, your family has a great chance of achieving optimum health. Opting for healthy dietary and exercise habits early — even before you begin to have children — can help guarantee the best possible outcomes for you and your loved ones.

In this chapter, I present information on what you can do during conception and pregnancy to ensure a healthy pregnancy, a healthy baby, a healthy set of parents able to withstand the rigors of new parenthood, and the best possible health outcomes for your family.

Adopting Healthy Lifestyles during the Conception Period: The Basics

The *conception period* begins when you first get that twinkle in your eye and extends to the moment when you actually conceive your baby. During the conception period, both mother and father must understand that whatever they eat and drink, however they mitigate stress, whatever their exercise patterns are, and a whole host of other health behaviors can directly affect whether they get pregnant, how quickly they get pregnant, and possibly the overall health of the baby they eventually conceive.

In this section, I explain what both mothers and fathers can do to get their bodies ready to create and then nurture their little bundles of joy.

Not all people plan their pregnancies. If you're of childbearing age, are sexually active, and are not protecting yourself from a pregnancy, you're in this conception period whether you realize it or not. So follow the advice in this chapter to give any child that results the best head start in life you can.

Teaming up: Steps both moms- and dads-to-be can take

Unhealthy habits are unhealthy habits, whether you're pregnant (or trying to get pregnant) or not. Chances are the bad habits you need to overcome are the same bad habits everyone else struggles with. Here's a list of healthy things both women and men can do prior to conceiving to maximize their chances of a healthy pregnancy:

✔ **Eat a healthy diet.** In general, keep calorie consumption under control and eat a balanced, healthy diet in order to get the nutrients your body needs.

Specific nutrients help prevent birth defects, create a healthy pregnancy, and help support a healthy life post-birth. Getting appropriate amounts of iron, folic acid, and magnesium are crucial, especially during the conception period. Expectant mothers can usually get these in the form of prenatal vitamins.

You can find out more about the specific dietary needs for both men and women during this stage in the next two sections: "Identifying What Dad Can Do to Boost Fertility" and "What Mom can do: Preparing her body to sustain a healthy pregnancy."

✔ **Avoid hot tubs and hot baths.** Exposing reproductive organs (most alarmingly, testicles) to high temperatures for extended periods of time can affect fertility. If you love relaxing in a hot tub or taking hot baths, do so sparingly.

After they're pregnant, women should avoid hot tubs and baths altogether. The exposure to high temperatures can lead to miscarriage and/or birth defects.

✔ **Steer clear of drug and tobacco use, as well as alcohol abuse.** All three — drugs, tobacco, and alcohol — can affect fertility. Even more alarmingly, they can cause some very serious, debilitating birth defects. If you're taking medication and *before* you take any supplements, be sure to discuss the situation with your doctor.

✔ **Exercise!** Both men and women wanting to get pregnant should make exercising regularly a habit. As you know, regular exercise helps keep unwanted weight gain at bay and helps keep the body in optimum health. For couples trying to conceive, these factors are especially important, for these reasons:

  • Being overweight or obese raises the risk of not being able to conceive.

  • Exercise assists with healthy sperm production and menstrual cycles.

Consult your doctor to develop an exercise regimen that is best for you and your family.

Many of the benefits you'll experience by following the preceding suggestions are, to a degree, the same benefits everyone else experiences, too. But particularly for women, these changes are even more important because of the impact weight, blood pressure, and so on have both on the viability of the pregnancy and the health of the unborn child. Head to the later section "What Mom can do: Preparing her body to sustain a healthy pregnancy" for advice specific for moms-to-be.

Chatting with your doc: A checklist

If you plan on starting a family, consider having a chat with your physician, who can provide information and guidance and help you put together a plan for an optimally healthy pregnancy. Following are some key pieces of information or health checks you and your doctor will go over as you prepare for a future pregnancy:

✔ **Your reproductive life plan:** Be sure to discuss how many children you and your partner are planning to have.

✔ **Past reproductive history:** Share any information regarding past pregnancies, how long you've been trying to get pregnant (if you've already started), and so on.

✔ **Medical assessment:** Both you and your partner should get a total body physical to gauge your current health status. This assessment checks your overall physical health, as well as ensures you are of proper weight and eating healthily.

✔ **Infections and immunizations:** Be sure to keep your immunizations up to date and disclose to your doctor any past illnesses or infections.

✔ **Genetic risks:** You need to discuss with your doctor any possible genetic health risks you or your partner may have. He or she can advise you on whether genetic testing is advisable and how to proceed if it is.

✔ **Current diet and nutrition profile:** This assessment goes hand in hand with your medical assessment and addresses whether you're eating healthily and whether you should consider making any modifications to your diet to promote your general health, as well as your reproductive health.

✔ **Psychological and behavioral risks:** Understanding your mental health status and any adverse behavioral choices you are making can assist in planning for a healthy conception and pregnancy by creating plans on how to mitigate the unhealthy behavior.

✔ **Healthy environment:** Discuss with your doctor how to make the best possible environment for you and your future family inside and outside the home.

Identifying What Dad Can Do to Boost Fertility

The best chance to get pregnant is to have strong, healthy sperm. To produce healthy sperm, the father must be at the pinnacle of health and engage in healthy behaviors. What he chooses to eat, drink, smoke, and so on affects the motility and mobility of his sperm.

Sperm *motility* refers to the ability of sperm to propel themselves forward. *Mobility* refers to the rate of speed at which the sperm travel. Both are essential to increase the chances of conception. Sperm with poor motility don't move forward efficiently; they wiggle about without any clear sense of direction, as shown in Figure 15-1.

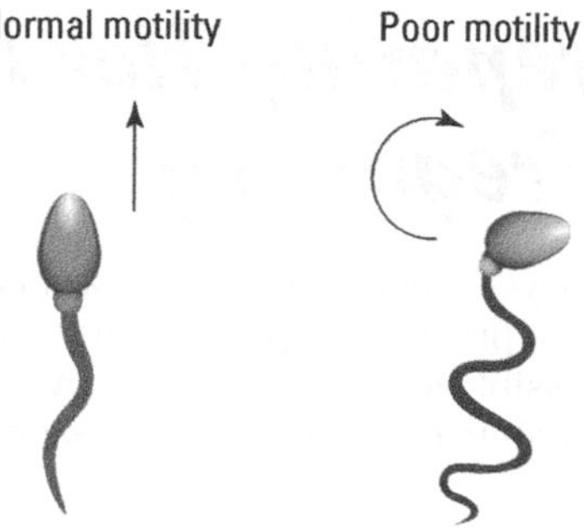

Normal motility   Poor motility

Figure 15-1:
Normal
sperm
versus
sperm with
poor motility.

Illustration by Wiley, Composition Services Graphics

Paying attention to diet

To give his sperm the best fighting chance possible, a prospective father should eat a healthy diet. Eating too few fruits and vegetables may reduce fertility.

Although no clear evidence identifies which foods can actually build healthy, strong sperm, some research suggests that the following foods can boost fertility:

- **Salmon:** Loaded with omega-3 fatty acids and protein, salmon may assist in building healthy sperm.

- **Tomatoes:** Tomatoes are rich in lycopene and may improve prostate health and function, which can assist in the effectiveness of sperm delivery.

- **Citrus fruits and berries:** These are high in vitamin C and may improve sperm quality.

- **Oatmeal and bran:** Both high in fiber, they can assist in lowering cholesterol (via digestion) and saturated fats (via taking the place of high-fat foods), which may affect sperm production.

Taking other steps to improve fertility

In addition to eating a healthy diet, a man can also do the following to improve his health and possibly fertility:

- **Exercise.** A sedentary lifestyle, when coupled with a diet that's higher in fat, salt, and sugar, can decrease vigor and may lead to conception difficulties.

- **Restrict (or eliminate) alcohol and eliminate tobacco use.** Both of these behaviors come with their own unique risks, but each promotes chromosomal damage in sperm and lowers sperm count.

What Mom Can Do: Preparing Her Body to Sustain a Healthy Pregnancy

Preparing for pregnancy is an exciting, yet crucial, period in a woman's life. During the conception period, she must practice responsible health behaviors, not only to make her body as fit as possible for carrying the baby to term, but also to develop responsible wellness habits that she will later teach her children.

Expectant mothers and women who are trying to conceive are about to enter a period of increased nutritional needs. After all, they are either currently nurturing or about to nurture a child in their wombs. That's why adopting healthy behaviors now is so essential. In this section, I outline some things women can do to prepare themselves.

During this period, whatever a woman does to and for herself, she is also doing to and for her child: eating, drinking, sleeping, exercising . . . you name it. Healthy behaviors help the developing child; unhealthy or dangerous behaviors can lead to some very serious, often debilitating, effects for the child. Consider, for example, the case of fetal alcohol syndrome. This terrible condition causes severe mental and physical defects in the baby and is directly linked to the mother's alcohol abuse.

Expectant mothers should always consult their monitoring physicians before adopting any diet, exercise habit, or other behavior that could potentially affect their babies.

Regulating your weight

Every woman, no matter her age, must strive to achieve a healthy body weight. However, during the conception period, a woman's body weight is particularly important because it can impact whether (or how easily) she can get pregnant, and unhealthy weight (too high or two low) has serious implications for the growing baby.

Understanding the perils of being underweight

Underweight women (whose BMI is below 18.5; refer to Chapter 5 for more on BMI), for example, are at particular risk. If they don't gain the appropriate amount of weight during their pregnancies, they are more likely than normal-weight mothers to give birth to a baby with low birth weight (LBW).

An infant's birth weight is a significant predictor of future health outcomes for that child. In fact, a child born with a LBW is at more than 35 times greater risk of dying in the first year of life than a baby of normal weight. In addition, LBW babies are at a higher risk than normal weight babies of developing other health issues, such as obesity, high blood pressure, type 2 diabetes, and heart disease throughout their lives.

The chart in Figure 15-2 shows the range of birth weights for varying gestational ages.

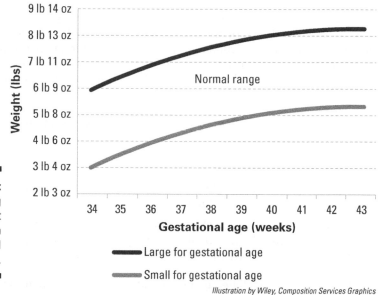

Figure 15-2:
Evaluating birth weight based on gestational age.

Illustration by Wiley, Composition Services Graphics

Identifying the perils of being overweight

Women who are obese during the conception period should try to reduce their body weight as they prepare for pregnancy. Being at a healthy weight *before* pregnancy can assist in your efforts to become pregnant. Obese women can have a more difficult time trying to conceive than women of normal body weight.

Perhaps more importantly, being at a healthy weight before pregnancy can reduce the risk of complications during the pregnancy, as well as reduce the risk of serious health problems with the developing fetus. Compared to normal-weight mothers-to-be, obese women are also at higher risk of experiencing difficulties during their pregnancies. Read on for the details.

Due to the acute risks their weight status may pose to their pregnancies, obese women who are planning to become pregnant or who are already expecting should consult with their monitoring physician to determine what a healthy weight during gestation is and to receive advice on how to achieve that body weight. They should pay particular attention to eating a balanced diet to ensure that they 1) get adequate amounts of key vitamins and minerals that will promote the growth of a healthy baby and 2) achieve optimal states of wellness for themselves throughout their pregnancies.

Having larger babies

Children borne to obese mothers are often larger in size than children born of normal-weight mothers. Although this may not be an issue for full-term babies, it can be problematic for babies born prematurely because they appear to be of normal weight and fully developed, which may not be the case. Premature babies have special health concerns that must be cared for; a premature baby that looks fully developed may not get the medical attention he or she needs.

Premature babies are at high risk for these health problems, to name just a few:

- ✔ **Apnea:** In these babies, breathing stops for 20 seconds or more.

- ✔ **Respiratory distress syndrome (RDS):** These babies lack a protein that keeps the air sacs in their lungs from collapsing.

- ✔ **Necrotizing enterocolitis (NEC):** NEC is an intestinal problem that can lead to diarrhea, which in babies is a very significant health concern because of how quickly they can become dehydrated.

To protect the overall well-being of the child now and into the future, these conditions must be addressed.

Developing gestational diabetes

Pregnancies in obese women are considered high-risk due to the increased likelihood that they will develop gestational diabetes or hypertension. *Gestational diabetes* is a form of diabetes that occurs during pregnancy, when the mother's body produces insufficient amounts of insulin. Symptoms include the presence of sugar in the urine (revealed by a test done in the physician's office), excessive thirst, frequent urination, fatigue, nausea, consistent infections, and difficulties with vision.

Typically, gestational diabetes goes away after the baby is born; however, women who develop this condition are more likely to develop type 2 diabetes later in life.

Upwards of 5 percent of expecting mothers develop gestational diabetes, and certain subgroups — namely obese women — are at particular risk. In these at-risk groups, the incidence of gestational diabetes can be around 10 percent.

Being at greater risk of having babies with serious health issues

Babies born to obese women are at higher risk of developing neural tube defect (NTD) and heart abnormalities than those born to normal-weight mothers. The reason is that obese mothers often develop gestational diabetes or hypertension during pregnancy.

The *neural tube* (brain, spinal cord, and other key structures of the nervous system) is formed during the first three months of pregnancy. NTDs are birth defects of the spine, brain, or spinal cord. The two most common neural tube defects are *spina bifida* (in which the fetal spinal column doesn't close) and *anencephaly* (in which most of the brain and skull do not develop). Babies born with spina bifida often experience nerve damage leading to at least some paralysis; babies with anencephaly are usually stillborn or die shortly after birth.

The diabetic status in the mother can contribute to poor glucose regulation in the fetus, which is hypothesized to raise the risk of NTD. Researchers hypothesize that high blood glucose levels in the mother exposes the fetus to excess glucose, causing the baby to put on weight (see Figure 15-3). Coupled with possible folic acid deficiencies in the mother's diet due to an imbalanced nutritional regimen, these babies are at an even higher risk of developing NTD.

Figure 15-3:
How gestational diabetes in the mother causes problems for the growing baby.

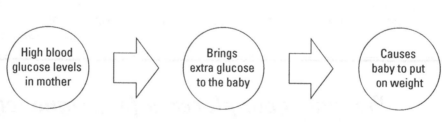

Illustration by Wiley, Composition Services Graphics

Therefore, if you are trying to get pregnant, think you want to get pregnant some time in the future, or are sexually active and of childbearing age, take a women's multivitamin or ensure that you are getting enough folic acid in your diet, usually by consuming dark leafy greens, legumes, and enriched grain products.

A positive trend for a terrible defect

Neural tube defects are terrible, and although researchers don't really know why they occur, they do know that certain people — mainly women who are obese and those who do not get sufficient folic acid in their diets — are at greater risk of having children who suffer from these potentially debilitating and deadly defects.

There is some good news on the neural tube front, though! NTD has been on the decrease ever since grain products started being enriched with the B vitamin, folate. The incidence of spina bifida, for example, fell dramatically between 1991 and 2005 (see the following chart).

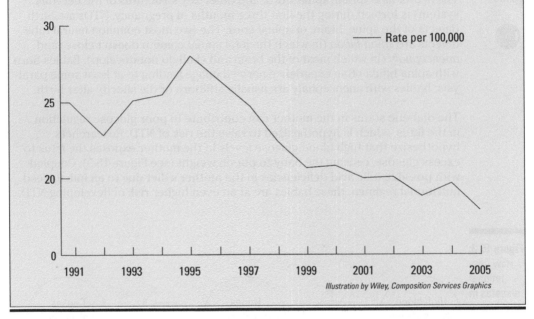

Illustration by Wiley, Composition Services Graphics

Prepping your placenta for pregnancy

When they think of caring for their babies, many pregnant women envision rocking the baby to sleep, walking the floors at night to soothe a colicky infant, and so on. Well, until you can actually hold that baby in your arms, you need to make sure your biological "nanny" — your placenta — is as healthy as possible. After all, your placenta is the structure that nourishes and "cradles" your baby through nine months of gestation. The health of your placenta is directly dictated by the health of your uterus during the first month of pregnancy.

The placenta provides nutrients and removes wastes for the baby. It is the only way you have to nourish your baby during pregnancy. If the placenta isn't working sufficiently or if it was underdeveloped during the first month of pregnancy, the fetus suffers from at least minimum levels of malnutrition — a situation that can lead to potentially serious, adverse health outcomes for the baby.

Getting your placenta up to snuff

Properly nourished women develop the healthiest placentas. To get your placenta up to snuff, eat a well-balanced, nutrient-packed diet. In addition, getting sufficient amounts of rest and developing effective relaxation strategies can relax the muscles, particularly abdominal muscles, which can assist in maximizing placental blood supply.

Here are some dietary suggestions that can improve placental health; be sure to discuss these with your monitoring physician:

- ✔ **Get enough iron.** Iron is necessary for expanding blood volume. The blood volume in pregnant women increases by an average of about 50 percent; this extra blood ensures that sufficient levels of hemoglobin get to the baby. Also, without proper blood flow, expectant mothers may experience *lethargy* (extreme tiredness). You can get extra iron from your diet by eating lean meats and dark green, leafy vegetables, like kale or salad greens.

- ✔ **Get enough zinc.** Zinc is stored in the placenta and assists in producing the healthiest weight possible for the child.

- ✔ **Get enough vitamin E.** Vitamin E is thought to improve blood supply and also helps with the proper growth of the placenta.

Problems with an underperforming placenta

Even though you may be eating nutrient-packed foods to get the proper amount of key nutrients to your baby, your baby may still become undernourished if your placenta did not develop properly. A healthy placenta ensures that nutrients can move easily across the placenta; in an unhealthy placenta, the nutrient transportation becomes insufficient.

If your baby is malnourished in utero due to an unhealthy or underperforming placenta, nothing after birth can make up for this deficiency. Throughout your child's life and into adulthood, he or she may be at higher risk of developing a wide range of health problems, such as developmental problems, including learning disabilities, physical limitations, and so on.

You're Pregnant — Now What?

During pregnancy, a woman's body experiences numerous changes, all of which are essential to produce the best possible environment to nourish her baby throughout the pregnancy. In this section, I explain how to ensure you're getting proper nutrition to sustain the nourishing environment your baby needs through each trimester of your pregnancy.

Understanding the process of trimester development

Human pregnancy lasts about 40 weeks, and these weeks are divided into three distinct periods of gestation, called *trimesters*. Each trimester lasts three months and involves distinct physical developmental changes in the baby. A mother's nutritional choices can directly influence the physical growth of the fetus during these phases.

Understanding the importance of the first trimester

A lion's share of fetal development occurs during the first two to three months of pregnancy. Although minimal growth occurs during the first two weeks after fertilization, crucial development occurs. After the second and third weeks, dramatic changes occur in the fetus. By the time you get to week ten, the baby has fingers, toes, a heart, digestive organs, and a brain and nervous system. He or she has also undergone external physical development and now looks like a baby.

The beginning weeks of pregnancy are essential to proper development. Without adequate folic acid in your diet, your baby can suffer enormous adverse health outcomes, including neural tube defects (refer to the earlier section "Being at greater risk of having babies with serious health issues" for information on NTDs). This is why it's so crucial to get enough folic acid in your diet *before you get pregnant*. By the time you realize you're pregnant, these systems are mostly formed. If you don't build up your stores of these nutrients early, by the time your developing fetus needs them, it'll be too late for you to help.

This period of time also helps determine uterine — and, therefore, placental — health. How healthy the placenta is is a big determiner of how healthy the child will be (see the earlier section "Prepping your placenta for pregnancy" for details).

Second and third trimesters

The second and third trimesters are defined by substantial growth in length and weight. The organs are also growing and perfecting themselves, becoming more and more complex. The eyes, bones, organs, brain, and lungs are developing, and with that rapid growth, their nutritional needs increase. Specifically during the third trimester of your pregnancy, the baby grows rapidly. Therefore, your diet must be as nutrient-packed as possible.

Eating while pregnant: A trimester guide

Here are some common questions many first-time moms ask:

> "What — and how much — should I eat during my first (second and third) trimester?"

> "How much weight should I put on throughout the pregnancy?"

> "Can I drink alcohol?"

A well-balanced diet is the ultimate key to developing a healthy pregnancy, and eating healthily should start during the conception stage and continue throughout gestation and beyond. In this seciton, I outline some things to think about as you consider your diet during your pregnancy. Consider this information a starting point for your discussions with your monitoring physician, who can give you guidance tailor-made to your health and pregnancy.

During the first trimester

Early in pregnancy, many women experience nausea (morning sickness) that makes adhering to a healthy diet difficult. Some women even lose weight during pregnancy due to morning sickness.

You must do what you can to keep eating and eating healthily during the first trimester. Here are some dietary tips that can help with morning sickness:

- ✔ **Eat ginger.** Doing so calms the stomach.

- ✔ **Avoid spicy foods.** Spicy foods can aggravate the stomach.

- ✔ **Eat smaller portion sizes.** Smaller portions are less likely to overwhelm your digestive system.

- ✔ **Sniff herbs.** Yes, this is an an odd tip, but basil, oregano, and rosemary can assist in alleviating some of the symptoms of morning sickness.

During the second trimester

In the second trimester, food choice is even more essential. During this stage, your growing baby has low energy needs (approximately 100 more calories than you would normally eat in a day), but the mineral and vitamin needs are high. Your challenge is consuming enough nutrients without consuming too many calories. Foods like fruits and vegetables, whole grains, and lean proteins give you more nutrient-dense, less energy-dense meals.

During the third trimester

This is the trimester when the baby packs on the pounds. That doesn't mean you should pack on the pounds, too. You cannot "eat for two." In fact, you need only a few hundred more calories for the child to ensure its health. You absolutely should *not* double your caloric intake during this trimester. Instead, focus on eating whole-grain bread and cereal products, a variety of fruits and vegetables, lean sources of protein, and low-fat dairy products.

A word about prenatal vitamins

Should you take prenatal vitamins to supplement your diet? Consult with your monitoring physician to see whether you need one. Prenatal vitamins are often necessary during the first and second trimesters, but you may not need one in the third trimester. As long as you eat a healthy, balanced diet, there would be little reason why you would need a supplement, unless iron deficiency is still a problem. But, as always, check with your doctor.

Managing calories and weight gain during pregnancy

As I say earlier, even though you're pregnant, you should not buy into the idea that, as a pregnant woman, you're eating for two. Too many women believe they have to eat for two fully grown human beings to get through pregnancy. Nothing can be further from the truth. You have a tiny little infant in your womb, not a sumo wrestler.

In the first trimester, you should gain only a small amount of weight. In total throughout the pregnancy, you should put on only between 25 and 35 pounds (your doctor can give you a more precise target weight based on your biology and health status).

To avoid excessive weight gain, choose nutrient-dense, not energy-dense, foods. And remember that you barely need any more calories than what you needed pre-pregnancy (if you were at a healthy conception weight), until you reach your second trimester when growth begins to accelerate.

Use this chart as a guideline of how many extra calories you should consume each trimester to sustain a healthy pregnancy:

Trimester	*Additional Calories per Day*
First	100 extra calories
Second	250–350 extra calories
Third	450–500 extra calories

Getting the right nutrients

During pregnancy, you need a good balance of energy nutrients to ensure that your body has the energy it needs and that your baby develops normally. Follow these guidelines:

- ✔ Foods like low-mercury fish, lean proteins, whole grains, nuts, avocados, seeds, and olive oil are all great sources of energy.

- ✔ Plenty of low-fat milk, yogurt, and cheese ensure adequate calcium intake, which is necessary for your baby's growing bones.

  Be careful when eating certain cheeses and meats to avoid those that are prone to microbial contamination. Avoid undercooked meats, softer or raw milk cheeses, non-pasteurized dairy, or eggs that are not well done (say good-bye to soft-boiled eggs or eggs sunny side up until after your baby's birth!).

- ✔ Eat iron-rich foods, like lean meats (red meat particularly) and some whole grains (or take a prenatal vitamin to ensure you get the iron you need). During pregnancy, particularly during the first trimester, additional blood is needed to support the growing baby during this crucial development phase. Iron assists with oxygen delivery to your baby. You also need ample amounts of calcium and iron to help support proper bone growth and blood flow in the baby. Yogurt and fortified cereals do wonders for supplying such demand.

  Consuming vitamin C with iron from eggs and plant sources helps your body more efficiently absorb the iron.

- ✔ Eat DHA-rich foods. *DHA* is a form of fat that is great for brain and eye development of the baby. You can get DHA through a prenatal vitamin, or you can get it by eating eggs marketed as high in omega-3 fatty acids and salmon.

  Try eating healthy sources of fish with high omega-3 fatty acids (healthy meaning low-mercury fish) to help fetal brain development, especially during the final trimester.

Usually, the smaller the fish, the lower the levels of mercury. Stay away from king mackerel, shark, swordfish, and tilefish, which have high levels of mercury. But check with the EPA's fish consumption advisories (`http://water.epa.gov/scitech/swguidance/fishshellfish/fishadvisories/`) and your monitoring physician for more specific guidelines and advice.

Some women experience an aversion to certain foods during pregnancy. If you find a particular nutrient-dense food distasteful, find an alternative food that can provide the same nutrients. If you just avoid the foods you don't like without replacing them with suitable alternatives, maintaining proper nutrition will be more difficult and could be harmful to both you and your baby.

Salt, alcohol, and smoking: Do you or don't you?

Excess salt in the diet may lead to ankle swelling and water retention. So next time you find yourself tempted to overdo it on the salt, don't. Put it away. Cutting down on salt can reduce the swollen feeling during pregnancy.

Should you drink alcohol? Some say yes. Some say no. I say no because we have no way of knowing what the tolerable intake levels of alcohol are versus what intake levels cause damage to the growing fetus.

Yes, alcohol may alleviate stress for the mother (a benefit). It may even be that red wine confers some benefit on the fetus itself. Who knows? The problem is we don't because it's impossible to do any type of experimentation on a growing fetus. In other words, no one has any idea how much alcohol would be damaging to a fetus or what amount, if any, would be harmless.

With tobacco, definitely stay away. Nothing good comes from tobacco use, particularly while pregnant. There are several reasons why tobacco use is absolutely terrible for a healthy pregnancy; here are two primary ones:

- Thousands of chemical additives are in cigarettes; when inhaled by the mother, these chemical additives can affect the fetus.

- Cigarette smoking — specifically the combined work of nicotine and carbon monoxide — interrupts oxygen transport to the fetus.

Chapter 16

Caring for Kids, from Infancy through the Teen Years

I sometimes think how cool it would be to be a child — or even a teenager — again. Most of the time, however, I am completely glad I never have to relive those ages. What strikes me most when I look back at those years, however, is how choices I made then still influence me today. And all of this pondering of my diet and exercise habits during my youth gets me wondering how those choices will affect me as I move into middle age. When I take this line of thought a few steps further, I imagine my future children and wonder how my choices — then and now — will influence what they'll eat, how much they'll exercise, and how happy and healthy they'll be.

In this chapter, I outline things parents can do to guide their children to pick up healthy diet and exercise habits. Although the task may seem daunting, several of the suggestions are straightforward, easy, and effective. I also explore and explain myriad strategies you can use to promote the best possible health outcomes for your children. By the end of this chapter, you'll know how to positively influence your children's choices related to diet and exercise as they age.

Bottom line: Whether you're planning a family, are in the throes of raising your family, or are simply trying to better understand how the things you learned and did in your own childhood still affect your diet and nutrition choices today, you'll find helpful information and insight in this chapter.

The Building Blocks of a Healthy Diet for Children

At no other point in an average person's lifetime is it more important to have healthy diet and exercise habits than in childhood. In fact, you would be hard-pressed to identify another time when practicing wellness to ensure proper growth and development is more crucial. (Of course, during pregnancy, nutrition and healthy behaviors are key. For details on how to ensure you and the developing fetus receive the nutrients needed, refer to Chapter 15.)

Unfortunately, in the United States, approximately 80 percent of children eat diets that are ranked as either poor or needing improvement. That figure is repeated (give or take a few degrees) worldwide. In short, the vast majority of children around the world are either malnourished or undernourished. Although exceptions exist, the fact that so many children are at risk for adverse health outcomes due to poor diet and nutrition is at best alarming; at worst, it's a travesty.

All is not lost, however. We can get our children to the level of optimum healthiness. Doing so just takes understanding what needs to be done and then implementing proper eating habits.

Being aware of the changing dietary needs as children grow

At no time in life does the human diet change faster than it does between a child's second and third birthdays. True, children switch from breast milk or formula to solid foods at the end of their first year; however, milk remains a key source of fat, protein, vitamins, and minerals during this time period.

Between the second and third birthdays, however, milk is slowly replaced by other foods as the main sources of these nutrients in a child's diet. This time period is your window of opportunity for creating health dietary habits for your children, and it matters what foods you introduce because you're beginning to establish their dietary preferences.

Introduce your children to fresh foods first, before introducing them to artificial, canned foods. Doing so helps you reinforce a preference for natural tastes and makes these foods seem more appealing as your children get older.

Facing common challenges when making the transition to solid foods

During this stage of rapid growth and development, as infants and young children transition between a milk-dominated diet and a solid food–dominated diet, it's vital that they get the nutrients they need. Yet the task becomes more difficult as children move away from breast milk/formula, for these reasons:

✓ **After their first birthday, children's appetites tend to fluctuate.** Although this fluctuation is normal, it can be a little disconcerting to parents who may interpret the finicky behavior to mean that something is wrong or that their child is being malnourished. Yet a little bit of disinterest in food, or even increased attention to certain foods, is normal. Just like us, young children go through phases.

Still, if you notice intense disinterest or an unusual interest in certain foods, make an appointment with your pediatrician just to make sure an underlying health problem isn't causing this fluctuation.

✓ **Around 2 to 3 years old, children's external environments begin to influence what they want to eat.** Even toddlers are influenced by television, social media, other toddlers in their play group or nursery school, and adults other than their parents. To counteract forces that may undermine your focus on healthy, natural foods, do the following to reinforce to your child that a healthy diet is a good diet:

- Present healthy foods to your child enthusiastically.

- Eat — and enjoy — the healthy foods yourself.

- Have members of your family consistently support the diet you are introducing to your child.

Many times, children want to eat foods that are too high in sugar, salt, and fat because they see others eating these foods, not necessarily because they physically desire them. Friends, television and media, and family can most certainly drive this desire for unhealthy foods. Be careful. If you provide a positive environment in your home, your child is more apt to stay the course with a proper diet.

Identifying good sources of nutrients for infant and toddler diets

Early childhood is filled with opportunities for children to try new foods. It's also a time when children begin to be influenced by people other than their parents about what they should be eating. Many times, you'll discover that the "good diets" that others endorse don't necessarily match up with your views on what constitutes an appropriate diet. Navigating these issues can be a challenge, but it's nothing a diligent, consistent parent can't handle.

Infants and toddlers need the same nutrients older children and adults do. Read on to discover the kinds of food that provide those nutrients. Use this information as an guideline of what to feed your child to help him or her transition from infant into toddler years:

- ✔ **Infants (0 to 6 months):** Infants at this age get all of their nutritional needs met through breast milk or iron-fortified formula.

- ✔ **Infants (7 to 12 months):** Infants at this age get much of their nutritional needs met through breast milk or iron-fortified formula, in addition to these foods:

  - Broccoli

  - Grain products (whole grain and enriched)

  - Infant cereal (iron-fortified)

  - Avocado (mashed)

  - Fruits (mashed)

  - Fruit juices (vitamin C-rich)

  - Beef

  - Orange and yellow fruits and vegetables

  - Vegetable-, soybean- and canola-based oils and spreads

  - Spinach

  - Yogurt

- ✔ **Toddlers (1 to 3 years):** At this age, the main source of nutrients comes from foods other than breast milk or formula:

  - Avocado

  - Broccoli

  - Dairy

  - Dark green, leafy vegetables

  - Eggs

  - Enriched and whole-grain products

  - Fortified cereals

  - Juice (calcium-fortified, vitamin C-rich)

  - Legumes

  - Margarines

- Meats (beef, chicken, and so on)
- Oils (vegetable, corn, safflower, and soybean-based)
- Orange and yellow fruits and vegetables
- Whole milk
- Yogurt

These lists are particularly helpful when you're looking for food and snack alternatives that ensure your child is getting proper nourishment without too much fat or sugar. (Head to the later section "Fitting In Healthy Snacks" for guidelines to ensure healthy snacking.)

Getting the proper amounts and right kinds of energy

The energy sources in your child's diet include proteins, carbohydrates, and fats — items that need to be carefully monitored to ensure that they're coming from whole, fresh sources. Too often, children get their energy from overly processed, high-calorie, and high-fat foods. As a result, they end up eating entirely too much sugar and fat in the form of simple carbohydrates and bad fats, like trans-fats.

Children that develop habits of overconsuming food during their formative years run the risk of holding onto those habits throughout their lifetime and may end up facing a lifelong battle of body weight issues, including obesity and obesity-related diseases.

In this section, I explain how to monitor the carbohydrates, proteins, and fats in your child's diet to ensure he or she is getting the energy needed from the healthiest sources possible.

Carbs for the kiddies

Carbohydrates are the primary energy source for the brain. Because infants have larger heads in proportion to the rest of their bodies compared to children over 1 year old, their needs for carbs are higher. The recommended levels of carbohydrates for infants are as follows:

- ✔ **Infant (0 to 6 months):** 60 grams per day
- ✔ **Infants (7 to 12 months):** 95 grams of carbs per day
- ✔ **Toddlers (1 to 3 years):** A child's daily intake of fiber should be equivalent in grams to his or her present age plus 5. For example, your 2-year-old should have 7 grams of fiber per day.

Breastfeeding is a great source of carbohydrates for infants. It's quite sweet comparatively to other milks and foods available, and it should be the primary source of carbohydrates in infants between 0 and 6 months. Other good sources of carbohydrates for babies who are transitioning to more solid foods (infants 7 months and older) include softened vegetables and fruits (carrots and bananas are always a favorite), bread, and yogurt.

Make sure that your child is eating the right type of carbohydrates — whole grains. Eating whole grains ensures that his or her diet has an adequate amount of fiber. This is especially important for children who may not be getting enough in their diet due to poor dietary choices outside of the home environment.

Getting the right amount of fat

Fat is an essential part of a child's diet. It is absolutely necessary for proper brain and nerve development and function, and it helps your body process certain nutrients, like the fat-soluble vitamins A, D, E, and K. In times of food scarcity, fat is a source of energy that your body relies on to function.

Depending on age, upwards of one-third of a child's daily energy needs should stem from fat sources. The dietary reference intake (DRI) recommendations suggest the following (to find out about DRIs, refer to Chapter 3):

- ✔ **For children ages 1 to 3:** Approximately 35 percent of daily energy needs should come from fats.

- ✔ **For children 4 years old and into their teens:** Approximately 25 percent to 30 percent of daily energy intake should come from fat.

Fat intake needs to be carefully controlled, and the sources of the fat need to come from proper places. Whole milk (and its great fat), for example, does do a body — especially a child's body — good. Cupcakes and sugary, fatty foods do not, especially with toddlers. Be sure to check out Chapter 12 for more discussion on different types of fat.

Choosing the right proteins

Proteins are the building blocks of the body — literally. They are the foundation for body tissue and organs. They also serve as a source of energy and conduct most cellular functions. Getting enough protein in your child's diet is absolutely critical. Children between 1 and 3 years old need about 16 grams of protein per day per kilogram of body weight. Children 4 to 6 years old need approximately 24 grams of protein per 1.1 kilogram of body weight.

The key is to choose the right kinds of proteins. Here are some guidelines:

- **Choose protein sources that are lean but not too tough.** Good choices include soy products, particularly tofu, beans, and slow-cooked, roasted meats (so that their muscle fibers can break down).

- **Avoid greasy, fatty meats, like fried chicken, hamburgers, or chicken wings.** These are usually high in salt and calories. As a general rule, you want to steer clear of these foods because they promote overeating and unneeded weight gain.

- **Make sure you thoroughly cook any meat to avoid food poisoning as well as choking.** The more thoroughly cooked, the less chance of microbial contamination and the more the protein *denatures,* or breaks down, making it easier to chew and much less of a choking hazard.

Getting your vitamins and minerals

Children grow fast, and their need for vitamins and minerals is ever increasing. To ensure proper height and weight growth, their diets needs to be loaded with nutrient-dense foods. Refer to the earlier section "Identifying good sources of nutrients for infant and toddler diets" for good sources of nutrients for infants and toddlers. For older children, a healthy diet — one that includes plenty of vegetables and fruits, whole grains, healthy fats, low-fat dairy, and lean protein sources — ensures they're getting the vitamins and minerals they need.

If you want more detailed information on the upper intake levels by age for the different nutrients, check out the Health Canada site: http://www. hc-sc.gc.ca/index-eng.php.

Taking care with iron and lead

Parents need to be mindful of two minerals in particular in their children's diet: iron and lead. Usually, children are at risk of getting too little iron and too much lead. In this section, I explain how to address both of these issues.

Addressing iron deficiency

Approximately 10 percent of toddlers in the U. S. have an iron deficiency. This deficiency usually stems from unstable food sources (hunger) and/or switching to unfortified milk and milk products.

To ensure your children get enough iron, try incorporating some of the following foods into their diet. These foods are great sources of iron (as always, be wary if your child is allergic to any of these foods):

✔ Iron-fortified breakfast cereals

✔ Seafood (clams, oysters, and mussels, for example)

✔ Beans and legume (navy beans and lentils)

✔ Tofu

✔ Seeds and nuts (pumpkin seeds, walnuts, and so on)

✔ Molasses (believe it or not, molasses is a good source of iron)

Getting the lead out

More than one-quarter of a million children in the U.S. have issues with lead toxicity — a number mirrored worldwide. Although there have been dramatic decreases in lead poisoning in the past few decades, it remains a pressing issue because of the health issues associated with lead poisoning.

About 310,000 U.S. children between 1 and 5 years old have elevated blood lead levels, which can accumulate over months and years and cause serious health and cognition problems, such as the following:

✔ Learning disabilities

✔ Behavior problems

✔ Malformed bones

✔ Slow growth

✔ Seizures, coma, and death at very high exposure levels

Although lead exposure is dangerous to both children and adults, kids face the greatest risk because they are more likely to be exposed. In fact, children make up about 70 percent of lead exposure cases, whereas adults and teens make up the rest.

Sources of lead exposure include the following:

✔ Lead-based paint and contaminated dust in homes built before 1978

✔ Drinking water from lead pipes

✔ Contaminated food

✔ Soil (lead doesn't biodegrade)

✔ Toys (old toys, as well as new toys from China)

Lead exposure often goes undetected and causes no obvious symptoms. To avoid lead exposure, do the following:

- Have your child screened if you're concerned about lead exposure.
- Frequently wash your child's hands, toys, and pacifiers.
- Use only cold tap water for drinking and cooking.
- If your home was built before 1978, have the paint and dust from your home tested.

A word about supplements

If fed a proper diet — one that includes a diverse variety of fruits and vegetables — your child should not need any type of supplement, unless a physician directs you to do otherwise. This applies to adults as well. Such supplements can be expensive, and if they're not taken properly, they can be dangerous.

Keep these points in mind:

- **Well-nourished children do not need supplementation.** Consult with your physician before giving your child any dietary supplement or changing his or her diet drastically.

- **Be careful of supplements that are marketed to children.** These tend to look and taste like candy. Having these materials on hand and readily available can invite higher risks of toxicity due to overconsumption. Your child may confuse the supplement with candy and eat a handful of the pills. This mistake can pose substantial risks to the child's welfare if it occurs regularly. Iron is the biggest danger; ingesting as few as four chewable tablets exceeds the threshold for safe levels. Although not all children's chewable vitamins contain iron, the ones that do are required to have a warning label that states the following:

  > Accidental overdose of iron-containing products is a leading cause of fatal poisoning in children under 6 years old. Keep this product out of reach of children.

- **If you do keep children's vitamins on hand, treat them as you would any medication: Keep them out of reach and dispense them yourself.** Look at the label on the bottle of children's vitamins. You can see how eating multiples of these supplements can put your child in a very dangerous position in terms of vitamin and mineral toxicity.

Fitting in healthy snacks

What would childhood be without being able to enjoy a snack at school, home, or with friends? Snacking is an inherent part of being a kid, no? Therefore, if you're wondering whether you should let your child eat snacks, the answer is "Of course!" Snacking should be a healthy and happy experience for children.

Notice the word "healthy" in the preceding sentence? Therein lies the crux. Snacking is great for kids if it's healthy. Snacking is bad for kids if it's not. The challenge of parents, dieticians, nutritionists, and school lunch ladies everywhere is how to get kids to eat healthy snacks when snacks are supposed to be fun, and fun foods tend to be bad for you.

Here are some rules for snacking you can follow to ensure your children are getting the nutrients they need without the bad stuff (excess sugar, salt, and fat) that can cause problems:

- ✓ **If you are thinking of giving vegetables, serve baby carrots or snap peas.** Baby vegetables in general tend to be sweeter than full-grown, ripe vegetables, and these varieties in particular tend to be a bit sweeter than all other vegetables. The added sweetness may make the snack more appetizing.

- ✓ **If you're thinking of giving fruits, give ripened fruits, not young, unripe fruit.** Fruit is at its sweetest when it's at the peak of ripeness.

- ✓ **Control the amount of fried, processed, and highly salted and sugared foods.** Too much sugar, non-nutrient-dense foods, and calories can lead to nutritional deficiencies and possibly obesity.

- ✓ **Have snacks readily available.** Kids get hungry often. After all, they're growing and need the energy for proper growth and maintenance. So when your child is hungry, have healthy snacks — fruit slices, baby vegetables, applesauce, whole-wheat crackers, and so on — on hand.

   But be careful! A fine line separates giving snacks when they are warranted (that is, it's been awhile in between meals, for example) and encouraging unhealthy snacking. If you don't carefully monitor the snacks your child eats, you could unwittingly encourage obesity.

- ✓ **Be consistent with the type of snacks you give.** Make healthy snacks (fruits, vegetables, milk, and so on) the snacks you give regularly, and give the unhealthy ones (cakes, cookies, baked goods, and so on) sparingly.

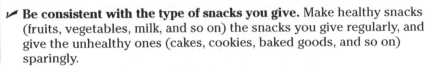

Fun with definitions

Toddlers and young children eat too few fruits and vegetables. Part of the problem is that the terms *fruit* and *vegetable* have been redefined a number of times by a number of different people. Governmental organizations, for example, allow pizza sauce and french fries to be labeled vegetables — usually to attain some policy objective (like balancing school budgets while addressing, on paper at least, dietary concerns of health professionals and parents). You can argue semantics, but not many people would equate a french fry with fresh broccoli or steamed peas on the nutrition scale.

Guess what the most popular fruit and vegetable snacks are among children in the developed world. Answer: bananas and french fries. Although bananas, being real fruit, are fine, they are little more than sugared fiber and potassium. You can't just eat bananas and be healthy. A child whose only fruit serving is bananas isn't getting the nutrients she needs.

And french fries? Sure, they come from potatoes, but calling them a vegetable isn't much different than calling vodka vegetable juice. French fries should be eaten sparingly because of the salt and fat content. In addition, the potato starch is little more than glucose, meaning that it's high on the glycemic index, a measure of how rapidly blood sugar level rises after eating. For a discussion on hypo- and hyperglycemia, head to Chapter 8.

Patrolling What Your Children Eat

You have a tremendous influence on your child's diet, and this is never more true than when they're young. Although not every mealtime needs to be turned into a battle — sometimes it's not worth the fight over the uneaten cauliflower on your child's plate — you can't just let them eat whatever they want either. Children need consistency in terms of the type of diet you expose them to.

The childhood years are the last time you will have supreme power over what your child eats, so make the most of this opportunity! In this section, I explain how you can make a healthy diet appealing to even the pickiest eaters.

Providing an inviting environment

Let's face it, children can be extremely picky when it comes to what, where, when, and how much they eat. Don't worry; there are some things you can do to help influence them to eat properly in healthy amounts. In this section,

I start with some basic things you can do to nudge your children in the right direction when it comes to choosing — and actually eating — healthy foods. Who knows? Maybe they will actually begin to enjoy it!

You are the gatekeeper for what your child eats. If you're having trouble getting your children to choose healthy options, the following suggestions may help you spur interest:

- ✔ **Let your child play an active role in selecting what the family eats.** You can use meal planning time to teach kids about healthy options and what they do for the body.

  Preselect four or five healthy options and then have your child select from those. In this way, you still choose what's for dinner while giving your child some ownership of the decision.

- ✔ **Have your child help prepare the meal.** Kids can do any age-appropriate task: They can mix, dice (with plastic knives, of course!), add ingredients, taste, or perform any number of other tasks. Letting them help in the actual meal preparation helps them feel involved. Plus they're more likely to want to eat what they've helped prepare.

- ✔ **Keep food portions on the smaller size.** Remember, kids don't need to eat the same amount adults do. In addition, children are adverse to eating portions of food that are many times larger than their heads. If you think small (portions), you tend to get big results!

- ✔ **Don't force your children to eat if they don't feel like it or if they don't want the food you're providing.** Force-feeding may encourage overeating, which may lead to obesity and related diseases later in life.

  If one of the rules in your house is that kids have to clean their plates before they're done, make the portions extra small (a teaspoonfull, for example), especially for foods you know they don't care for or for foods that you're just introducing. Doing so is a way to enforce the rule without forcing a child to eat a large portion of food she doesn't want, and it's a way to get reluctant eaters to try new things.

- ✔ **Don't bribe your child to eat.** Don't think you offer bribes? Have you ever told your child that she can have dessert if she eats her vegetables? The problem with bribes is that kids tend to learn the wrong lesson: that they need to eat healthy foods only when offered some type of compensation. Try to avoid this implication at all costs because, as a general rule, a child's price for compliance tends to grow more and more unreasonable over time.

After the meal, if you notice your child didn't eat too much or steered away from eating her vegetables (which should be the biggest portion on the plate!), ask her if she would like to finish her meal before you put the food away. Then remind her that nothing else will be served until the next meal (or snack time).

If your child isn't turning her nose up at food due to stubbornness, she will quickly catch on that hunger isn't a good feeling and will choose to eat what's served rather than go without. If she doesn't eat a food because she genuinely doesn't like it, no worries. Next time, don't cook that food or offer some options to choose from. If you have a large family where eliminating food choices can be problematic, perhaps alternate when you serve certain foods so that everyone gets his or her favorite meal or side dish on certain days of the month. Or you can also offer a bigger snack to compensate for the smaller meal.

If your child never seems to want what you've prepared and you find yourself preparing two meals, you may be reinforcing her picky behavior by providing an alternative. Rethink your approach of just giving in and have a talk with your child about her behavior and what's expected at mealtime.

Avoiding choking hazards

One of parents' biggest fears is having a child choke on her food. This fear is especially pronounced as small children move from breast milk and formula to solid foods. To minimize the risk of choking, following these four primary rules:

- ✔ **Be careful when introducing solid food to toddlers.** You don't want to introduce the foods too early. Toddlers may not possess the tools necessary (teeth, proper motor function of chewing and swallowing, and so on) to effectively chew their food.

- ✔ **Make sure children are seated properly when eating.** Children should sit up while eating; they shouldn't be in a reclining position or lying on their backs.

- ✔ **Make sure your child is supervised by an adult.** This is one of the reasons why you should not let your kids eat in moving cars. If you're watching the road, you can't be watching them.

- ✔ **Avoid certain foods.** Before a certain age, round foods (cherries, candies, grapes, cut up hot dogs, and so on) and hard-to-swallow foods (many animal meats) pose a particular threat to children. Avoid or eliminate these foods from your menu.

    If you do decide to serve foods that pose a choking danger, make sure they're cut up into appropriately sized pieces and that a responsible adult is around to supervise the child as she eats.

Table 16-1 lists a number of foods, dividing them into two groups: those that are kid-friendly and those that pose choking hazards.

Table 16-1	Kid-Friendly Foods or Choking Hazards?
Kid-Friendly Foods	*Choking Hazards*
O-shaped cereals	Hot dogs, sausages
Toast with crust removed	Hard, gooey, or sticky candy
Eggs	Peanuts, nuts, seeds
French toast cut into pieces	Whole grapes
Canned or well-cooked fruit	Chunks of meat or cheese
Cooked pasta pieces	Marshmallows
Avocado dip or chunks	Globs of peanut butter
Canned or well-cooked vegetables	Popcorn
	Chunks of raw fruit or vegetables

You are not being a bad parent for not giving in to your child's demands. Kids will test you and your patience. I cannot stress enough how important it is for you to stand your ground and offer healthy options and portion sizes. Don't be swayed by pouting, crying, or stomping feet. You must know the difference between stubbornness and true hunger/discomfort from food choices, that's for sure. But don't worry if your kids get mad at you just because you say no. They'll get over it soon enough.

Beyond pickiness: Identifying food intolerances, aversions, and allergies

Some kids just won't eat certain foods, and usually, there's a reason why. Perhaps he has a friend who won't eat certain foods, and he is influenced by this friend's choices. Perhaps he just doesn't like the food's taste, texture, or smell.

Sometimes, however, your child may have a physiological response to a food. Milk makes his stomach upset, for example, or shellfish makes his throat feel funny. In these cases, you're probably looking at a food allergy or intolerance (shellfish allergies and lactose intolerance are both very common, for example). These responses may make a child reject certain food items, even though he may not be able to articulate the reason with anything more specific than "I don't like it."

Your task is to determine what exactly the issue is so that you can take the necessary steps to address the issue or help your child overcome it.

In general, the biophysical reasons why children steer clear of certain foods fall into three categories: food aversions, food intolerances, and food allergies.

Food aversion

With food aversion, an individual dislikes certain foods because of that food's taste, color, or texture. Food aversions can also be brought on by social influences — your child's friends teasing him for bringing certain foods in his school lunch, for example.

If your child shows extreme dislike for a food — telling you forcefully and seriously that he doesn't like the food, making awkward faces after eating the food (a grimace, for example, or a shudder), or avoiding touching the food or having it touch other foods on the plate — talk to your child to try to get to the bottom of the issue. You may discover a larger problem than just not liking the taste of a particular food. Perhaps you can help your child find solutions to the problem, whatever that may be.

Food intolerance

With a food intolerance, an individual has an adverse physical reaction to food. Examples of food intolerance include shellfish and nut allergies, lactose intolerance, celiac disease (wheat gluten allergy), and so on. You may be dealing with a food intolerance if your child consistently feels uncomfortable or sick after eating the food product.

To uncover a food intolerance, keep track of what your child eats and how he feels after eating. If a problem persists or if you notice a pattern developing, visit an allergist, immunologist, or a gastroenterologist for an official diagnosis.

Food allergies

As I indicate in the preceding section, a *food intolerance* is a situation in which your body has difficulty digesting certain foods. A food intolerance is different from a food allergy, in which your immune system mistakes your food for something dangerous and begins to react as if it is fighting an infection. Food allergies can be life threatening, unlike food intolerances.

Pay close attention to any complaints or adverse health reactions to certain foods from your children. Also watch to determine whether eating certain foods produces particular effects, such as the following:

- Rashes
- Coughing
- Inflammation
- Intestinal discomfort

If you see such a pattern develop, contact a physician immediately. Your child may have an allergic reaction to certain types of food. Because some reactions, particularly upon subsequent exposures, can be especially dangerous — even deadly — you need to be very careful.

Following are some of the most common foods that cause allergic reactions:

- Eggs
- Fish and shellfish
- Milk
- Peanuts
- Soy
- Tree nuts
- Wheat

The next time your child eats these foods, keep tabs on her bathroom habits, her physical appearance, or any complaints from the child herself. A food allergy may be at work.

Some food allergies are quite deadly, particularly those associated with clams, shrimp, lobsters, mussels, oysters, and other shellfish. Discuss this health issue with your doctor to learn how to protect your child if she is affected by allergies.

Deciding on school lunches

Parents are the gatekeepers for their children's diets, but at school, the kids are at the mercy of whatever is being served that day in the cafeteria, unless they pack their lunches. As you can imagine, this situation creates a number of concerns for parents who carefully monitor their children's diets. The two big concerns? The quality and nutritional value of the food served and whether children will make the right decisions when choosing their lunches.

The quality of the food being served

The food provided in school cafeterias can sometimes be of questionable nutritional value. This concern is exacerbated by recent food recalls from the beef and agricultural industries related to foodborne illness. (For more on foodborne illnesses, refer to Chapter 10.)

The fact is that schools are supposed to provide at least one-third of the recommended nutrients needed by children in a given day. Schools attempt to meet these requirements and do so with varying degrees of success.

You can contact your child's school district to inquire about the nutritional guidelines used in serving school lunches. In the United States, both state and federal governments determine the rules and regulations given to school districts on what and how to serve foods. You may have to do some investigating, but if you ask enough questions, you'll begin to get answers. Try starting your search by viewing Nutrition.gov's website on school lunch and breakfast programs at `http://www.nutrition.gov/food-assistance-programs/school-lunch-and-breakfast-programs`.

Whether kids will make healthy choices when left on their own

School cafeterias tend to serve food in one of two ways:

- **A la carte meals, in which children can choose their entrees and sides from the options provided.** These options generally include healthy choices (salads, fresh fruits and vegetables, and so on) and not-so-healthy choices (cheeseburgers, fries, and so on) side by side.

- **Pre-set meals, in which children's choices, if they have any at all, are limited.** These options are set by the school district or governing agent in charge of developing school nutritional policy.

Which do you think produces a more nutritious meal? Not surprisingly, children who have a choice regarding what to eat generally eat fewer fruits and vegetables than those who are given a set plate of food. Although that scenario isn't ideal, it can be — and in some school districts is becoming — much worse. Fast food is beginning to be offered in many school lunchrooms. In addition, soda and snack machines compete for access to your child's stomach.

One dark and stormy afternoon . . .

Here's an urban legend that has probably surfaced (or resurfaced) everywhere: Supposedly, a person — usually a parent — just happens to be around when boxes of school lunches are taken off the delivery truck. On the side of one box is a label that reads "Grade F, but edible."

Given the way school cafeteria food tends to taste, this story just keeps getting traction. Does the fact that people tend to believe it stem from the perception that school cafeterias use low-quality food? Is it a sign of the paranoia of parents (or their kids) about what the lunch ladies are actually serving? Or do the storytellers just like to add to the hysteria? Maybe it's a combination of all these factors.

True or not, this story reflects the concern parents and children have about what, exactly, is served in school cafeterias.

Taking action

If you are in doubt about or dismayed by the quality of food and the choices your children have at school, you can take the following actions:

✔ **Start packing your children's lunches.** Doing so may be beneficial in a few different ways. Two important benefits: One, you'll know what your child is eating that day (or at least what they're *taking* to eat). Two, you get to spend time with your child planning the meal and choosing healthy options together.

✔ **Get involved.** Parent groups are springing up all over that deal specifically with nutrition issues at schools and address the content of the lunches themselves, the choices offered by vending machines in the schools, and so on. Great strides are being made to ensure that kids aren't bombarded with unhealthy, non-nutritious foods throughout the school day. Getting involved in these efforts lets you influence what your children are served.

Understanding the Effects of Diet on Your Child's Health

As you know and as I've made clear throughout this book, diet is directly and intimately related to health outcomes. In terms of your child's health, here are some other topics that link diet and children's health.

Eating breakfast: The most important meal of the day for children

Breakfast is, without doubt, the most important meal of the day for your child; therefore, it should also be the largest. Unfortunately, most people treat dinner as the most important meal of the day — which is completely the wrong tack to take, for these reasons:

✔ **Breakfast, as the first meal of the day, comes just as your body leaves a brief period of fasting.** This is the time when you need energy to get up and going and to sustain you into the afternoon. By eating your largest meal in the morning, you're providing your body — and your children's bodies — a sustained source of energy through midday.

✔ **The majority of your protein should be served in the morning.** Try having your child eat a serving or two of almonds or walnuts on their granola with a glass of low-fat milk and/or a side of reduced-fat bacon.

The day's other meals (lunch and dinner) should be divided proportionally to meet the remainder of your caloric needs for the rest of the day. In addition, both later meals should primarily be created from fruit and vegetable platters. Carbohydrates, fats, and proteins should lessen as the day progresses. Here is an example of a balanced menu for the rest of the day's meals that is ideal for your child:

- ✔ **For lunch:** A medium-sized sandwich (whole-grain bread with natural peanut butter and jam) with a side of vegetables and fruit juice

- ✔ **For dinner:** Vegetable stir-fry with brown rice, a modest side of meat, and fruit for dessert

Think of it this way: You should eat like a king for breakfast (largest portion), a prince for lunch (medium portion), and a pauper for dinner (smallest portion of the day).

Gimme some sugar: Addressing the causes of hyperactivity

Ask most parents whether eating too much sugar makes their children hyperactive, and overwhelmingly, they'll answer a resounding *"Yes!"* Then, at least in my experience, they offer tips on how you shouldn't feed a child any sugar a few hours before bedtime because the sugar "makes them all crazy" and unable to fall asleep. This story and the experience behind it are so common and shared by so many different sets of parents that the idea that sugar causes hyperactivity and that the only way to control hyperactivity is to control sugar has become a common trope in parent circles.

Interestingly, no scientific evidence links the amount of sugar a child eats and that child's level of activity, either *hyperactivity* (being abnormally active) or *hypoactivity* (being abnormally sedentary).

So are the parents wrong? Quite the contrary. They know their children better than anyone. Perhaps your child *does* get hyperactive when he eats candy and sweets, and perhaps a bit of that hyperactivity stems from a little burst of energy (however fleeting) produced by carbohydrate sugar in the sweets. I would bet, though, that the primary source of that hyperactivity stems from something social, not physical. Perhaps your child gets hyperactive after eating sweets, but the cause isn't the sugar; rather, it's the excitement of receiving a treat. Maybe the excessive energy you see is due to your child being very happy at being rewarded. In fact, all children get more active after eating a meal with carbohydrates; this is normal and appropriate — children should be active.

Children should be able to enjoy cakes and candies. What's a childhood without ice cream on a hot day or going to the local candy store to buy some licorice or taffy? Sweets are an integral part of being a child. Still, you need to ensure your child doesn't get too much — not because of the hyperactivity, but because of diabetes and obesity problems that can arise later in life.

According to American Heart Association (AHA) guidelines, the amount of added sugar that a child should consume on a daily basis depends on the child's age and caloric intake. Table 16-2 lists these amounts. To put these values into perspective, one store-bought cupcake has five teaspoons of added sugar, about 20 grams.

Table 16-2	Recommendations for Added Sugar	
Age	*Daily Caloric Intake*	*Limit Added Sugar to This Amount*
Preschoolers	1,200–1,400	16 grams (about 4 teaspoons)
Children 4–8 years	1,600	12 grams (about 3 teaspoons)
Pre-teens and teens	1,800–2,000	20–32 grams (5–8 teaspoons)

Source: American Heart Association

Popping those pimples

Can food cause pimples? Chances are your mother told you that eating greasy foods and chocolate, among other things, causes massive outbreaks of pimples. I, myself, was terrified to eat these foods, and many of my classmates were obsessed with avoiding them as well for fear of getting acne or some other type of skin disorder.

You may be surprised to know, however, that no particular type of food actually causes sporadic breakouts or even full-blown acne. The majority of pimple breakouts and acne stem from the following:

- **A genetic or hormonal issue:** Girls (and women as well) tend to get acne and pimples during menstruation, pregnancy, and/or menopause. The hormonal changes tend to cause flare-ups on your skin.

- **Clogged pores:** If you touch or rub your skin with hands that are full of grease from the foods you eat, you can clog your pores and trigger a breakout. In other words, greasy foods *can* contribute to pimples — but not in the way you (or your mother) probably assumed.

Some research suggests that certain dietary factors that trigger higher amounts of sugar in the blood may trigger acne. Foods that may have this effect include highly sugared foods, carbohydrate-filled foods like bread and bagels, and some milk products. Research is ongoing on this link.

The best way to help teens avoid breakouts and acne is to make sure they eat very balanced meals, ones that are not too high in fat and carbohydrates. Also they should keep stress low, drink plenty of water, exercise, and regularly wash their faces. This regimen ensures that their bodies are at their optimal point of healthiness — a state of wellness helps them fend off unwanted pimples.

Caring for those cavities

Dental problems are a serious issue. Gum disease, for example, has been linked with heart disease! Amazing, right? The best time to ensure that children develop strong, healthy teeth is when they're young, and a dietary and lifestyle regimen that fosters healthy tooth and gum development should extend throughout the formative years, from infancy into the teen years. This regimen should include the following:

- ✔ **Drinking appropriate amounts of milk and/or calcium-fortified orange juice.** The calcium and added vitamin D help keep teeth strong.

- ✔ **Eating a diet of healthy foods that are packed with nutrients.** Nutrients that promote healthy teeth and gums include calcium, phosphorus, and other important vitamins and minerals. All are needed to build strong teeth that will last a lifetime.

- ✔ **Developing good teeth-cleaning habits.** Regular brushings, flossing, and dental checkups and cleanings promote healthy teeth.

Developing bad habits when you are younger — like eating tons of sugar; drinking little if any milk; avoiding foods packed with calcium, phosphorus, and other key vitamins and minerals that your teeth need; and not brushing regularly — can lead to a the following dental problems:

- ✔ **Cavities:** The combination of poor diet and not brushing regularly creates an acid that attacks your teeth. Over time, the tooth enamel wears down, and your teeth begin to decay. If the decay continues chronically, you begin to develop dental *caries,* or cavities.

- ✔ **Serious tooth degeneration as you age:** The lack of calcium in your child's diet when she is younger can lead to some serious tooth decay later in life because softer teeth are prone to infections and decay. And the earlier these problems set in, the worse it is for tooth health.

Chapter 17

Making Sense of Middle Age

You're only as young as you feel, right? Well, for people in the their 20s, youth is as much a physical property as it is a mindset. Face it, you're still young. You still have loads of energy, your abs are still tight, your skin is still firm, your hair hasn't begun to gray . . . you get the picture.

And then a funny thing happens. Starting in your middle to late 20s and continuing into your early 30s, you begin to see and feel the effects of aging, and there is *nothing* you can do about it. You're going to get older, and as you do, your body is going to change.

But that's life. It happens to everyone. And that's what I cover in this chapter. Read on to gain knowledge about, make sense of, and hopefully come to terms with how your body will change as you move from young adulthood into middle age.

Coming to Grips with Your Changing Body

In your 20s, you're in the proverbial prime of your life. You rule your world. You spend 10 to 15 hours a week at the gym. You stay up late and perhaps wake up even later. Maybe your alcohol intake is a bit less monitored than it should be. For the most part, you can eat and drink whatever you want and stay the same weight. In short, you work hard and play hard and burn the candle at both ends, and your body, being the remarkable machine that it is, sustains all these demands with nary a complaint.

Think this will last forever? I'm here to end that dream right here, right now. Youth — and the energy and metabolism that come with it — doesn't last. No matter how much you bench press, how fast or far you run, how many pints you can tip back without getting sick, or how invincible you feel, the first gray hair you find can bring you crashing back to earth quickly.

At a certain point, you become acutely aware of your own physical limits. You understand that you're not Superman or Superwoman. You *can't* eat an entire pizza at 2 a.m. and then expect not to feel bloated and lethargic or suffer a supreme case of indigestion the next day at work. You can't run on three hours of sleep a night all week and then expect to be the life of the party on the weekend.

Some people may find this realization a good thing; for others, it may be a terrible one. Whether you view it as good or bad, however, there is absolutely nothing you can do to stop the aging process. But you can make it enjoyable. Maybe you'll even find these changes something to look forward to rather than dread.

In this section, I outline some examples of how your body may change as you go from young adulthood into middle age. Most of these changes are unavoidable. However, they don't happen all at once. They occur gradually and can even be slowed down a bit with a healthy lifestyle that includes regular exercise (both physical and mental) and a well-balanced diet.

Paying attention to changes in body shape

At about age 30, you'll begin to lose lean tissue, and your bone mass will begin the process of degeneration. The process continues as you grow older.

You will actually begin to shorten as your get older, as well, for three primary reasons: First, as your muscle mass decreases, particularly in your abdominal area, your posture becomes less than perfect. Second, your spine begins to compress due to fluid loss between each vertebrae. Third, the arches of your feet begin to fall, which makes you more flat-footed.

On average, expect to lose about a half-inch (just over 1 cm) every decade after you hit 40. Figure 17-1 illustrates the physical changes that occur over the course of a lifetime. Notice how, in adulthood, the upright posture gradually grows more stooped and, as a result, shorter.

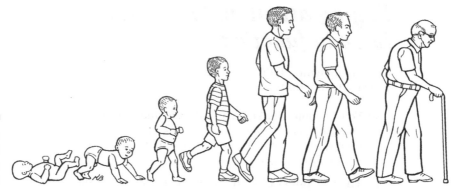

Figure 17-1:
Aging's toll
on the body.

Illustration by Kathryn Born, MA

Your body fat percentage begins to increase as fat replaces lean muscle tissue. This switch results in weight loss, even though the percentage of body fat is increasing. Men often gain weight until about 55 years old and then, due to lowering levels of testosterone, begin to lose weight. Women, on the other hand, usually gain weight until they're 65 years old. Weight loss in later life occurs in part because lean muscle tissue is replaced with fat.

Noting how body movement changes

The free movement you enjoy today may be gone tomorrow. Because of a loss in lean muscle (see the preceding section), getting around may become a bit burdensome as you age. Plus your joints stiffen as you age, making even simple movements potentially quite painful.

How limited your movement becomes depends on the extent of muscle or bone degeneration. When physical activity decreases as you get older, you lose muscle mass and your bones become weaker. As a result, you experience more pain due to the bone loss or due to tissue breakdown (joint, tendon, and/or ligament damage) and are inclined to exercise even less, further weakening your muscles. When coupled with weight gain, movement becomes even more difficult.

Not only can excess weight put more pressure on your joints, thus impeding movement and causing discomfort, but it can also make you move differently and in a way that actually causes pain. For example, people who are obese tend to use a different gait when they walk. This gait alters the way in which the body moves. Specifically, it causes the back to sway more with each step, and this movement places stress on the spine. Excess weight places extra stress on the lower spine and on the knee joints. In fact, many of the knee replacement surgeries are done on people who carry extra weight.

Paying attention to changes in body function

As you move into middle age, you can expect the following changes in how your body functions:

- ✔ **You become weaker.** This effect is due to the reduction of lean muscle and the loss of bone density. Tasks such as lifting objects, pushing or pulling heavy objects, and even sometimes simply walking can be a chore. Bone loss can also result in fractures.

- ✔ **The sharpness of your vision decreases.** Multiple things can go wrong with your eyesight as you age. For example, your lenses can lose their elasticity, which can cause you to become more farsighted, and the pressure inside your eye can increase, causing glaucoma.

- ✔ **Mental function and cognitive development generally tends to decrease with age.** As you age, you become more forgetful and lose the ability to think quickly and remain acutely aware of your physical surroundings. This change is caused by multiple factors, including reduced brain volume (size), neuron degeneration, and weakened signaling between brain cells, causing lapses in decision-making ability.

- ✔ **Sexual desire rises and then falls as you age.** Usually the decrease of testosterone in men and estrogen in women can greatly affect sexual desire. Further, erectile dysfunction and menopause can alter the course of sexual relations between couples. Finally, underlying mental health concerns, like depression or anxiety, can be the root cause of these sexual health issues.

Taking action to offset the effects of aging

The preceding examples of how your body may change as it ages are only a few of the many changes that may occur. For some, the list of changes may be longer; for others, it may be shorter. Which of these effects you'll experience — and the degree to which you experience them — depends on the following:

- ✔ **Genetic predispositions:** Some examples of age-related genetic predisposition include male-pattern baldness, certain cancers, and diabetes. Genetic predispositions are considered *non-modifiable* because you can't do anything about your genes.

- ✔ **Lifestyle choices:** These factors include things like high-fat, low-fiber diets, low water intake, lack of exercise, tobacco use, alcohol abuse, and other risks that can cause adverse health outcomes later in life. These factors are modifiable because you have the power to increase or decrease your risk by changing your behaviors.

To help prevent negative aspects of aging, you can take these steps:

✔ Eat a healthy diet that includes appropriate amounts of fruits and vegetables, whole grains, and lower saturated fats.

✔ Stay active and get a sufficient amount of daily exercise.

✔ Curb alcohol abuse and quit smoking.

✔ Engage in mental exercises to keep your brain active.

Bottom line: Aging happens to everybody. You can't avoid it. What you can do, though, is make aging a healthy, positive experience. The key to turning aging into a positive experience is to eat properly, exercise regularly, and limit stress and bad habits, like smoking and alcohol abuse.

Paying Extra Attention to Your Diet

As I mention earlier in this chapter, life for young people is often looser. They stay up late, eat pretty much whatever and whenever they want, and there's no Piper to pay. Now fast forward a few years (or decades!). You're a professional and working hard (hopefully!). Perhaps you're married or have children. You go to bed early. You wake up earlier. You're on a tight schedule for breakfast (which you eat only if you have time), lunch (which you eat at your desk or at the job site), and dinner (which, if you're lucky, you can sit down to enjoy, provided the kids don't need to go to orchestra or football practice).

Your life is like clockwork, and the added responsibilities you have push away time for anything else, including activities like exercising and relaxing that are good for both your body and your soul. Being so pressed for time can definitely affect how and what you eat. Yet this is one area of your life that you can't run on autopilot. You need to pay attention.

With all of the responsibilities adulthood brings, you need to be wary of forming unhealthy habits, like eating or drinking too much, not exercising enough, and so on. Sometimes a lack of time and task management skills can also bring on stress and anxiety, which can contribute to your choosing unhealthy behaviors (such as overeating, smoking, and alcohol abuse). These behaviors are dangerous not only to *your* physical and emotional well-being but to your family's as well. By managing stress and anxiety appropriately, you can dramatically decrease your risk of death and disease.

Nutritional needs change over a lifespan, and they vary, depending on age, sex, activity level, and health status. In this section, I take a look at some dietary changes that may come as you shift from young adulthood to middle age. Before you change your diet or lifestyle pattern in any significant way, discuss such a change with your physician. Sometimes the changes you want to make can actually be more harmful than helpful.

Minding your vitamins and minerals

As you age, you need to become more aware of your particular dietary needs to avoid deficiency or toxicity issues. Consult with your physician on what nutrients you specifically need to pay attention to in your diet. Your doctor can provide dietary suggestions to ensure you eat a well-balanced diet and recommend supplements, if needed. Here are some things to think about:

- ✔ Although you need the same amount of nutrients as you age compared to when you were younger, your body loses its ability to efficiently process the nutrients from your diet. For example, many older people have trouble absorbing vitamins B_{12} and D. As a result, you may need more of certain vitamins and minerals.

- ✔ The kinds of vitamins and minerals and the amounts needed often differ by gender and depend on body composition and the rate of absorption and processing, information you can get from your doctor. For example, as women age, their bones lose a large part of their mass, thus making them brittle and increasing the risk of fractures. To offset this change, women typically need vitamin D and calcium supplements to help prevent osteoporosis, or at least slow it down. Men, on the other hand, need to get more selenium in their diets because it helps prevent the onset of prostate cancer.

Getting enough of the energy nutrients

Although age isn't a key factor in how much of each of the energy nutrients you should get, activity level is (the percentage of carbohydrates, fats, and proteins are pretty similar for adults and children; revisit Chapter 2 for a refresher on recommendations on these nutrients). Your energy needs increase or decrease as you become more or less sedentary. It's probably no surprise, for example, that active teenagers and young adults need more energy nutrients than older adults, not only for energy needs, but for body repair and maintenance purposes.

As you move into middle age and your activity level dwindles, you typically need to eat less energy (that is, consume fewer calories) while being careful to ensure that you get the appropriate amount of nutrients.

Revisiting taste

Your tastes change over time. You may end up loving certain foods now that you swore you would never eat when you were a child or young adult. On the flip side, you may find that foods you loved as a child are now extremely unappealing. The reason for these changes could be that your palate has just grown more sophisticated over time, or it could be that you're losing taste buds.

Yes, that's right. As people age, their taste buds begin to wear out and become less sensitive, changing their perception of foods. In addition,

your sense of smell may change, also affecting your ability to taste. Smoking and eating scalding hot foods can also affect how well you taste.

My own little anecdote: When I was a child, I ate slices of bread with spoonfuls of mayonnaise. That's it. Just bread and mayo. I called it *mayonnaise bread*. How original, right? I loved it. There wasn't a better snack for me. Now I get borderline nauseous at the thought of eating that again.

Racing to Save Your Exercise Habits

The older you get, the harder it is to exercise, both physically and socially. Physically, your body begins to wear down; warming up, recovering, and even performing exercise itself takes longer. Socially, things can get even more complicated because of all the obligations you have. In this section, I explain the challenges you face in staying active and offer strategies that can help you incorporate exercise into even the busiest schedule.

Recognizing the challenges to maintaining an exercise routine

A number of physical changes can restrict your exercise patterns. Here are just a few:

- Joint pain and muscle aches and pulls
- Nerve damage
- Decreased lung capacity
- The slowing down of motor skills
- Diminished vision

The physical limitations can be a difficult thing to come to terms with, but at least they are predictable. The social limitations, on the other hand, can be even more complicated because they are ever-changing and sometimes erratic.

Marriage, children, long hours at work . . . just the everyday, ordinary obligations of life take time away from your ability to exercise. To continue your exercise regimen, you need to be able to adapt it. Whereas you may have worked out from 3 p.m. to 6 p.m. with your friends when you were young, now you work until 5 p.m. and then have to go home and take care of your family.

Incorporating exercise into a busy schedule

Sure, you can work out in the evenings — provided you aren't too tired — but you probably have to say goodbye to being able to devote two to three hours a day to working out. For many, the solution is to work out in the morning instead. Many have to get up at 4:30 a.m. in order to have the time to drink a cup of coffee, get to the gym to workout, shower, dress, and get themselves to work on time. Rinse and repeat.

This kind of schedule is a challenge in itself because of how tempting it is to stay in bed rather than get up. Nevertheless, as difficult as it may be to find the time, you have to. It's for your own good. Exercise helps you retain muscle mass, slows bone loss, improves cardiovascular fitness, helps you maintain a healthy weight, and so on and so forth. Other than eating a healthy diet, exercise is the single best thing you can do for your body and your health.

If you're open to getting up earlier or working out at odd times (like 10 p.m.), you may find that the added responsibilities of adulthood don't have to undermine your commitment to staying active. And if finding time to dedicate to exercise eludes you, find little ways to incorporate exercise into your daily regimen.

Try to incorporate exercise in your everyday routine. Due to an intense work schedule that makes keeping a regular physical fitness schedule difficult, I incorporate little bursts of exercise into my daily routine. One of my favorites: Doing dips at my kitchen counter as I wait for the morning coffee to brew. I do about 50 each morning. It's great for strengthening my shoulders, upper back, lower neck, and triceps. I also do squats and lunges as I brush my teeth, I do push-ups in between 30-minute intervals of writing this book, and I do abdominal crunches in bed at night before I go to sleep. You've got to find what works for you and what doesn't. Get creative! Head to the next section for more suggestions.

Some Final Tips for Mastering Middle Age

So are you looking for the magic bullet? Fat chance on finding one here, but what I can do is to provide you with some easy-to-follow tips and tricks that can help your body adjust to middle age and help you live in a way that lets you enter your senior years in optimum health:

- **If you're smoking anything (cigarettes, hookah, marijuana, and so on), *stop now.*** Setting aside the current debate on medical purposes of marijuana, rarely does anything good come out of inhaling environmental smoke into your lungs. The overwhelming amount of evidence suggesting links between smoking and cancer, heart disease, stroke, and a plethora of other chronic diseases is staggering. So pass on even thinking about lighting up.

  If you're currently smoking and you're addicted, seek assistance with smoking cessation. Evidence suggests longer life, tastier food, and a better quality of life when you're smoke free. Not to mention, your children won't pick up the habit and won't be exposed to your second-hand smoke.

- **Cut down on the alcohol.** Alcohol abuse results in numerous negative side effects that have immediate and future consequences: vehicular crashes, violent behaviors, addiction, *cirrhosis* (irreversible scarring of the liver), and even cancers, including liver, oral, larynx, and esophageal cancer, among others.

- **Ensure you are keeping your calorie intake in check.** Now is a crucial time in your life to control your calories. As you get older and more sedentary, your body's ability to efficiently burn up extra energy lessens. If you overeat, you may pay a heavy price in terms of weight gain (pardon the pun, please). For more information on how to keep calories in check, head to Chapter 2.

- **Balance it all out.** You don't have to eat cabbage on Monday, carb load on Tuesday and Thursday, eat tuna and celery on Wednesday, sleep all day Friday, and so on. Nothing good ever came out of overindulgence or extreme behaviors. My lovely mother and dutiful father *always* told me that "too much of anything is no good."

  You don't need a strict diet or a crazy exercise regimen at any point in your life. Just eat and exercise normally — even during the bustle of being middle aged. Yes, life is busy, but don't let that affect your health. You can find that happy medium of enjoying your job, your kids, your changing body, and living a long and fruitful life.

Finally, as my father says to me almost each and every time I speak to him: "Michael, two words in this world can make you live the healthiest life possible . . . *common sense.*" I can't tell you how many times in my life this has been true. I have two words for him: *Thanks, Dad.*

Chapter 18

Retiring into the Golden Years

· ·

In This Chapter

▶ Keeping a positive attitude as you age

▶ Recognizing the risks associated with growing older

▶ Discovering what nutritional regimens are best for aging

· ·

Your later years in life are supposed to be the "golden years." The term itself puts a positive spin on growing older, as do the things people associate with these years: retirement and no more deadlines, contracts, or rush hour traffic; leisure pursuits like golfing, fishing, and watching sunrises — in short, freedom to do what you want with your time. No wonder it's called "golden."

However, growing older has a definite downside: worsening health, diminished range of movement due to the effects of bone and muscle decay, and perhaps even physical, social, or emotional limitations that dampen your zeal for tasks and hobbies you once enjoyed. It can seem like a cruel joke that, just when you finally have the time to do everything in life you wanted, your ability to actually do those things is diminished. Hopefully not, but possibly so.

This chapter is about growing older and what you can do nutritionally to hold the negative effects of aging at bay. True, doing some of the things you did in the past may be a bit more difficult, but with a healthy lifestyle and positive attitude, anything is possible.

Accepting the Changes That Age Brings

Getting older is inevitable. The key to keeping an optimal level of health is to understand and accept the fact that your body composition is changing. You'll lose bone density and muscle mass and experience digestive issues — two major changes seniors experience as they age. If you're a woman, you have menopause to look forward to, and many older people face mental health issues. In this section, I discuss these changes and tell you what you can expect.

As your body changes, your diet needs to change as well because the manner in which your body digests, absorbs, and transports nutrients changes as you age. If you don't adapt your diet to compensate for these changes, you may experience deficiency issues that can lead to other adverse health issues, such as an actual deficiency disease (getting osteomalacia [called *rickets* in children] from a lack of vitamin D, for example), lethargy, weakness, and so on. Now more than ever you must be vigilant about your diet to ensure you're getting the nutrients you need.

Losing muscle mass and bone density

You'll experience two very noticeable changes as you enter into your older years: the loss of lean muscle mass and the loss of bone density. A decline in muscle mass associated with aging begins at age 35 and advances steadily. Table 18-1 outlines the progression of this loss.

Table 18-1	Age-Related Effects on Body Composition		
Population	*Muscle*	*Adipose (Fat) Tissue*	*Bone*
Healthy young people	30% of body weight	20% of body weight	10% of body weight
Seniors, by age 75	15% of body weight	40% of body weight	8% of body weight

A real problem with these changes is that they're not easily observable. And if people can't see it, they assume it's not happening. This can be very dangerous in the context of body alterations due to aging. Mobility, balance, and physical stability are all key health issues for older people and, if impaired, can have huge consequences on quality and length of life. To help curb the effects of aging upon your freedom of movement, remember that you may not observe every change your body is experiencing.

Try to become more sensitive to changes in your body, such as weight gain or loss, bloating, irregular or intense feelings of fullness and/or hunger, frequent constipation, acid reflux, changes in your senses (hearing, sight, taste, smell, and touch), and so on. Doing so can help you detect changes that come with aging. When you're aware of these changes, you can consult with your physician about ways to adjust your lifestyle to stay healthy and fit.

Losing muscle mass

When you are around 40 years old, you begin to lose muscle mass. After about age 50, this loss really picks up speed. In fact, you typically lose more muscle mass than gain it after the age of 50, which puts you on a slow but sure decline the rest of your life. Not only do you lose the number of muscle fibers, but you also see a decline in how well the muscles actually work. (***Note:*** Although this kind of muscle loss is a natural process that everyone goes through, it can also be the result of underlying health issues, such as problems with the endocrine system.)

When you lose muscle mass (in a process called *sarcopenia*), you tend to put on or develop more body fat. Basically, fat fills in where the muscle used to be. Subsequently, you may not notice this switch from muscle to fat because your body size or shape may not change. However, you can possibly perceive this switch by noticing the following changes:

- You feel that you are losing strength.
- You have more difficulty performing physical tasks without becoming winded or exhausted.
- You feel a constant heaviness or dragging feeling in your abdomen or hip/buttock areas.
- You notice a looseness (jiggling) in those areas.

Figure 18-1 illustrates how losing muscle mass makes you more prone to physical injury and accidents that can lead to restricted movement, fractures, and a whole host of physical limitations.

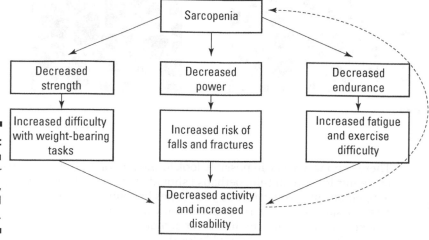

Figure 18-1: Sarcopenia affects your endurance, stability, and strength.

Illustration by Wiley, Composition Services Graphics

Losing bone density

Loss in bone density occurs naturally when you age. Up until your late teens and early 20s, you have active bone growth, including growth spurts. You retain the bulk of this bone mass throughout the rest of your 20s and into your early 30s. After your 30s, you begin to lose bone density due to the aging process.

As you age and more and more bone loss occurs, you gradually develop *osteopenia,* a health issue in which bone mineral density falls below average levels. If the loss continues, osteopenia develops into *osteoporosis,* adult bone loss. Figure 18-2 shows the difference between healthy bone and osteoporotic, or brittle, bone.

Millions of people (mostly women) have osteopenia, or are at risk of it. Osteopenia can be reversed with a good diet rich in calcium and phosphorus, as well as certain prescription drugs. The same is not the case with osteoporosis. Although the effects of osteoporosis can be lessened dramatically by getting enough vitamin D and calcium in your diet when you are young, your bone health is mostly determined by genetics, and there is little you can do to cure yourself of this disease.

Normal healthy bone   **Bone with osteoporosis**

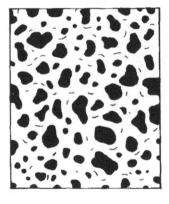
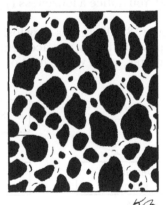

Figure 18-2:
Healthy
bone versus
brittle bone.

Illustration by Kathryn Born, MA

There is no way you can possibly look in the mirror and say to yourself, "Wow, my femur looks a bit thin; perhaps I should eat more calcium." Not going to happen because you can't see your bones becoming less dense without an X-ray or similar procedure. Even scarier, you can't feel this loss of bone density, either. But the fact of the matter is that as you age you begin to lose bone density. In fact, it is quite possible for the bone to lose so much density that it breaks because it can no longer support even the weight of your body.

Which comes first — the fall or the break?

Many times elderly people with osteopenia or osteoporosis experience fractures. A common fracture in the elderly is a hip fracture. Here's what most people suspect happens: A person with brittle bones falls, and the brittle bone easily breaks under the force of the fall. Yet many health professionals argue that what *really* happens is that the brittle bone breaks first and causes the fall.

That being said, you still need to be careful and be on the lookout for any symptom, however minute. Pay attention to the following:

- ✔ Increasingly poor posture
- ✔ Back pain (vertebrae), as well as pain in bones
- ✔ Lessening of height over time

Gender makes a difference in the degree of bone density loss a person experiences over his or her lifespan. Women are more at risk than men and are also at higher risk for bone fracture as they grow older. As Figure 18-3 shows, women have less dense bone to begin with, and they enter the dangerous fracture threshold nearly two decades earlier than men.

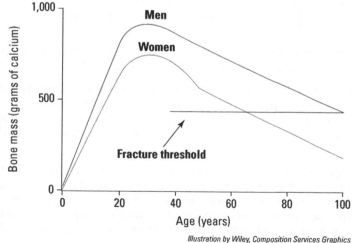

Figure 18-3: Gender differences in bone mass.

Illustration by Wiley, Composition Services Graphics

The severity of adult bone loss is often dictated by the amount of calcium and vitamin D a person gets during his or her formative years of growth and development. To make sure you have the strongest bones possible, be sure to get sufficient calcium and vitamin D during your formative teenage years and into your 20s. Head to "Vitamins, minerals, and water" later to find out how much vitamin D and calcium you should take.

Simply put, you need to build up strong bones *before* you reach peak bone mass. After you hit that point (in your late 20s and early 30s), you can no longer add bone. The stronger your bones are then, the healthier your bones will be as you age. Conversely, if you have brittle bones at peak bone mass, the process of degeneration is hastened.

Disappearing digestive ability

As you grow into retirement age, your digestive tract will undergo a few changes:

- ✔ **Your appetite may change.** Often this is the result of your body's changing sensory ability. The way you taste, smell, see, or physically perceive food can alter your appetite. For example, your ability to taste and smell, which are intricately linked, may change and certain foods may taste different or unappealing. Chapter 17 has more on this phenomenon.

- ✔ **You may produce less salvia.** If your body experiences a decrease in saliva, you may experience difficulty chewing, which can interfere with both food choices and the amount of pleasure you receive from eating food.

  Having difficulty chewing (from weakening teeth, loss of strength, or the lack of saliva) can raise your risk of choking.

- ✔ *Peristalsis* **(the actual movement of food through your digestive tract) may slow down, and fluid intake may decrease.** These events can lead to constipation and a decrease in stomach acid production, which, in turn, can lead to indigestion and/or malabsorption of key essential nutrients.

  A diminished ability to digest food can lead to malnutrition. Physical factors, such as decreased efficiency of digestion or inability to eat (chew) certain foods, puts seniors most at risk for this adverse health outcome. Seniors can easily avoid malnutrition by following a few simple rules, which I explain in the later section "Addressing the nutritional needs of the elderly."

Managing menopause

Menopause, the cessation of a woman's reproductive ability, usually begins in her late 40s and early 50s and can last for a few years. This natural change causes substantial changes in a person's body. In a sense, you're in hormonal flux. As uncomfortable as menopause can be for some women, it's totally normal. Here's what you can expect, all of which are attributed to hormone changes:

- ✔ Hot flashes (A hot flash is a sudden feeling of warmth over the body, but mostly involving the head, neck, and shoulders. For some women, hot flashes are accompanied by a flushed appearance and/or sweating.)
- ✔ Diminished sex drive
- ✔ Mood swings, irritability, and possibly depression

During menopause, you are at greater risk for bone density loss, as Figure 18-4 shows. The body's ability to replace old bone with new bone diminishes greatly with age. Women going through menopause have to take particular care of themselves because they also experience a drop in estrogen levels. Estrogen helps with calcium absorption, and a drop in estrogen contributes to the bones getting weaker.

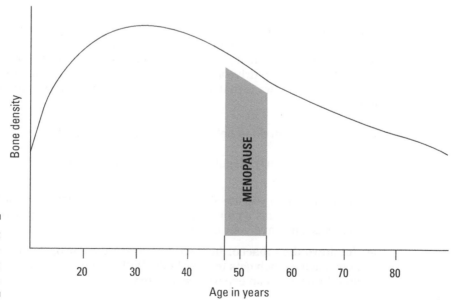

Figure 18-4: Bone density during menopause.

Illustration by Wiley, Composition Services Graphics

Discuss menopausal change with your physician. She can monitor exactly what your body is going through and can perhaps tailor specific remedies to assist with the transition.

Everyone knows that menopause affects women, but some researchers now claim that men also go through a "change of life" similar to menopause. This event happens for men around the same age at which women experience menopause — their late 40s and into their 50s. The changes men experience include fatigue, weakness, depression, low testosterone, and erectile dysfunction.

Paying attention to your mental health

Verbal skills, like speaking and vocabulary, may be strained as you age, but not nearly as much as memory. Memory decreases each decade of your life after you reach 40 due to physiological changes in the brain, including decreased brain volume and other neurological changes. You can take steps to remedy this memory loss, like reading and keeping both mentally and physically active, but for the most part, this happens to everybody in some fashion as they age. Currently, there are millions of people globally that are affected by memory loss. How severe the memory loss is depends on a number of things, including the ability to preserve mental functioning.

What does memory loss look like? You may forget where you put your glasses or what you went to grab in the kitchen (everyone has probably done this a few times!), but for some it gets progressively more profound. For example, you may forget how to drive a car, what your spouse's name is, or something similar. The good news is that such debilitating memory loss is not inevitable for everyone.

Some things you can do to help preserve your mental ability:

- **Exercise regularly.** Regular exercise encourages the development of new brain cells.

- **Chill out!** When you are stressed, you secrete cortisol. Cortisol leads to memory problems if constantly present in your body. So put your feet up, relax, and save your brain.

- **Put down the tobacco.** Smoking increases vascular problems, affecting how much oxygen gets to your brain. Without enough oxygen going to your brain, you can experience memory issues.

✔ **Eat right.** Keep your body (and brain!) well nourished. Did you ever hear that fish was "brain food"? It is! The omega-3 fatty acids in fish are great for boosting memory retention.

✔ **Stay social.** Social interaction becomes limited for many seniors as loved ones pass away or move away, or they become isolated. Social isolation can introduce mental health concerns, like anxiety and depression, which can affect physical health.

✔ **Seek help when needed.** The entire process of physical change can bring about a term of adjustment for the individual. Losing your ability to see or hear clearly, taste properly, walk and run as fast and as long as you once did, and so on can introduce negative feelings. If left untreated, these feelings can lead to depression.

If you notice that your memory issues are becoming progressively more frequent or that you are having difficulty remembering things that you can't blame on simply being distracted (you can't remember what month it is, for example, or you get lost even traveling a well-known route), set up an appointment to talk with your doctor. Head to the later section "Protecting yourself from Alzheimer's disease and dementia" for details.

Addressing the Nutritional Needs of the Elderly

After you pass a certain age, perhaps the mid- to late 60s, your nutritional requirements don't change too terribly much. What does change is the amount of energy needed to sustain a healthy life. This change in energy requirements alters the type and amount of food you should eat as you age. In this section, I take a look at some of the main areas to pay attention to as you plan your diet.

Curbing your energy intake

As you age, the combination of bodily changes (decreasing metabolic rate) and diminished physical activity creates a situation in which your body demands less and less energy to get through the day. In other words, you don't need to eat as much. At the same time, your nutrient needs don't change. In short, you need less energy (translation: fewer calories) but the same amount of nutrients — a situation that presents quite a challenge to maintaining a healthy weight.

To balance the diminished need for energy with the continuing nutrient demand, seniors must do the following:

- **Consume nutrient-dense foods.** These foods — fruits, vegetables, and lean protein sources — provide the proper nourishment without the excess calories that can cause you to gain weight.

- **Limit energy-dense foods.** Eating calorie-dense foods regularly, when coupled with a diminished (or nonexistent) exercise regimen can cause you to gain weight easily.

Table 18-2 lists how many calories senior men and women should consume per day.

Table 18-2	Daily Calorie Consumption for the Elderly	
Activity Level	*Senior Men*	*Senior Women*
Physically active	2,400–2,600 calories/day	2,000–2,200 calories/day
Moderately active	2,000–2,200 calories/day	1,600–1,800 calories/day
Sedentary	1,800–2,000 calories/day	1,400–1,600 calories/day

Planning for protein

Generally, protein intake should remain the same for seniors as they move from middle to old age. They should consume 0.03 ounces of protein for every 2.2 pounds of body weight, which is nearly the same amounts recommended for middle-aged and young adults.

Table 18-3 lists some healthy sources of protein to consider when planning your next meal.

Table 18-3	Healthy Protein Foods for Seniors	
Protein Source	*Serving Size (Grams of Protein)*	*Examples*
Beans and peas	1/2 cup (~6 grams)	Kidney beans, red beans, black beans, pinto beans, white beans, chickpeas, green peas, soybeans, tofu
Nuts and seeds	2 tablespoons (~2–6 grams)	Peanuts, almonds, walnuts, sunflower seeds, pecans, pumpkin seeds, cashews
Fish	1 ounce cooked (6–7 grams)	Tuna, salmon

Protein Source	Serving Size (Grams of Protein)	Examples
Lean poultry	1 ounce cooked (6–7 grams)	Skinless chicken and turkey
Lean meat	1 ounce cooked (6–7 grams)	Lean cuts of beef, pork, and lamb
Eggs	1 ounce cooked (6–7 grams)	Whole eggs, egg whites, and egg substitute
Dairy	1 cup (8 grams)	Low-fat or nonfat milk or yogurt

Many people believe that you should increase the amount of protein in your diet as you age to help prevent muscle mass loss. Although increasing protein in your diet provides the resources for muscle mass, it alone doesn't do the trick. You need training and exercise to build muscle mass. What often ends up happening is that seniors increase their protein but not their exercise. This strategy not only does not build muscle, but it may put certain individuals at higher risks of diseases stemming from eating too much protein or gaining too much weight.

The only time seniors should increase the protein in their diets is if they are healing or recovering from surgery or if they need a bit more strength. Consult with a physician before making any substantial changes to your diet, especially regarding energy nutrients.

Fitting fats into your diet

Seniors need to keep calories under control as their need for energy decreases with age (refer to the earlier section "Curbing your energy intake"). Fat intake, on the other hand, should be monitored but not substantially decreased.

There is one type of fat, however, that seniors should eat more of: omega-3 fatty acids. Omega-3 fats have been proven to reduce inflammation, which is a causal factor of heart disease, cancer, and other major chronic diseases that plague the elderly.

You can find omega-3 fatty acids in these foods, among others: salmon, mackerel, anchovies, sardines, and other types of fatty fish; flaxseed oil; and walnuts and chia seeds. Usual recommendations range from between two and three servings per week.

Should you take fish oil supplements? Some very early research is floating around professional nutrition circles that indicates that fish oil supplements may be ineffective at protecting against adverse health events, such as heart disease. Although taking fish oil pills to augment your diet isn't too much of a concern currently, consult with your physician first before taking them. You may be able to get the appropriate amounts of omega-3s in your diet alone.

Concerning carbohydrates

When you get older, it's all about fiber. Fiber. Fiber. Fiber. Fiber is found in plant matter (grains, vegetables, and fruits). You need fiber to assist with preventing constipation. Further, fiber helps regulate blood cholesterol levels, which helps protect against heart disease and other cardiovascular events. Be sure to check out Chapter 14 for more about this topic.

As you age, your intestines do not function as efficiently as they did when you were younger. Couple this with prescription drugs that affect bowel habits, and bowel movements often become irregular for many older people. For that reason, seniors must be particularly mindful of getting sufficient amounts of fiber. High-fiber foods help move digested food and feces through the gastrointestinal (GI) tract. High-fiber foods also supply much needed vitamins and minerals (particularly B vitamins). Older adults should eat around 25 to 35 grams of fiber per day.

Eating prunes is a great way to stay regular. Try cutting some into your morning whole-grain cereal. Not only will you get a great dose of fiber, but you'll also be getting a good amount of needed vitamins and minerals as well. When you add some milk to that breakfast . . . wow! . . . what a fantastic way to start your day.

As you increase the fiber in your diet, keep these points in mind:

- ✔ **Getting fiber from food sources is better for your body than getting it from a supplement.** Who wouldn't prefer fresh produce to those gritty, orange-flavored powders you mix into drinks?

- ✔ **Incorporate increased fiber in your diet slowly.** You won't have as much gas. Trust me.

- ✔ **As you increase your fiber intake, you must drink enough water.** Yes, fiber assists with constipation and keeps your bowels regular, but if you don't increase the amount of water in your diet as you increase fiber, you'll actually just make yourself more constipated.

Vitamins, minerals, and water

For the most part, nutritional intake should remain stable as you age. No substantial increases or decreases in the types of foods or supplements you ingest are necessary unless your physician directs you otherwise. However, the elderly do need a bit more of some vitamins and minerals than other people do, including the following:

- ✔ Certain B vitamins (namely B_{12})
- ✔ Vitamin D
- ✔ Iron
- ✔ Calcium

In the next sections I go into more detail on a few of these nutrients.

Vitamin D and calcium

The increased need for vitamin D and calcium is primarily geared around preserving bone health:

- ✔ **Calcium:** Seniors should be getting approximately 1,200 to 1,400 milligrams per day of calcium, which is equivalent to four cups of milk or dairy per day.

  One added benefit of calcium is that it helps to lower blood pressure. Therefore, ensuring you get enough calcium in your diet when you are a senior can help preserve bone health and promote heart health at the same time!

- ✔ **Vitamin D:** Vitamin D works with calcium to help preserve bone integrity. Elderly people usually have a lack of this nutrient due to a deficient diet or because they don't spend enough time outside in the sunlight without sunscreen. People 51 to 70 years old should be getting approximately 15 micrograms of vitamin D, and those over 70 should get about 20 micrograms.

Vitamin B_{12}

Seniors need to get enough B_{12}. Vitamin B_{12} is needed for DNA/RNA production, red blood cell creation, and nerve cell health. A diet chock-full of low-fat dairy or plant milks, vegetables, fruits, and lean meats can supply an ample amount of B_{12}. Consult your doctor if you need a supplement.

B_{12} deficiency is common among the elderly due to poor intake from the diet and reduced absorption from an aging digestive system. Plant milks such as almond or soy are fortified with B_{12} and therefore help adults older than 50 meet their RDA.

Sodium

Because many elderly people have high blood pressure, a low-sodium diet is recommended. Although salting your food can contribute to increased sodium in your diet, you need to pay particular attention to prepared foods. Foods like canned goods, frozen dinners, fast food, and so on have significant amounts of sodium, which is the primary influence in the level of sodium in the blood.

Opt for foods low in sodium, like fresh fruits and vegetables, lean meats, and whole grains. Try to find new and innovative ways to incorporate these foods into your diet to ensure you don't get more than 2,300 milligrams a day. For example, replacing seasonings containing salt (like garlic or seasoning salt) with other spices and herbs provides lots of opportunities to experiment with new flavors!

Water

If I told you that seniors don't generally feel as thirsty as younger people, would you believe me? Maybe not. But as people age, they don't feel thirsty as often as people half their age do. This situation can be very dangerous. Not feeling thirsty doesn't decrease the body's need for hydration. In other words, their bodies still need that water, but seniors sometimes don't drink enough to fulfill that need.

Considering the lack of thirst and the potential lack of hydration, seniors should check their urine. If the urine is dark yellow and has a pungent smell, they are not hydrated enough. Urine needs to be clear or light yellow with little or negligible odors — a sign that your body is well hydrated.

Fighting Common Diseases of the Elderly with Diet

Prostate and breast cancer are primary concerns for seniors. Millions have been affected by these diseases. How can you use nutrition to help prevent these diseases? Keep reading. I offer food tips for each of these diseases. Following these recommendations may help you lower your risk for developing these conditions.

Protecting yourself from prostate cancer

Prostate cancer affects millions of men worldwide and is the number-one cancer killer among this population. Although prostate cancer is highly preventable, men are still dying unnecessarily every year. There are certain factors that can help prevent the disease, many of them dietary:

- ✔ **Eat a low-fat diet.** Be particularly careful to avoid trans-fats, which are man-made fats from unsaturated sources of fats artificially hydrogenated. Refer to Chapter 7 for more on types of fats.

- ✔ **Eat more omega-3 fatty acids.** Get your omega-3s from fresh fish, but avoid flaxseeds, which may encourage prostate growth. For more information on omega-3 fatty acids, refer to "Fitting fats into your diet" earlier.

- ✔ **Eat more fresh fruits and vegetables.** Especially good for you are tomatoes, walnuts, blueberries, olive oil, cabbage, and kale. These foods are the super cancer fighters. Use them to plan many of your meals.

- ✔ **Don't eat too many pickled foods.** The high salt content can contribute to adverse health outcomes, particularly stomach and esophageal cancers, and possibly even prostate cancer, but more research is needed.

- ✔ **Eat red grapes or drink red wine and green tea.** Grape skins have antioxidant effects. Green tea can also provide a great antioxidant boost. (*Antioxidants* prevent the oxidation of cells by hyperactive electrons, called *free radicals*. Refer to Chapter 6 for more information on cancer manifestation.)

- ✔ **Try to get more selenium in your diet.** Selenium is essential for immune system health. Foods like mushrooms, whole grains, and certain nuts can give you that extra boost.

Protecting yourself from breast cancer

You would be hard-pressed to find a disease, save HIV/AIDS, that has gotten more attention in recent years — and for good reason — than breast cancer. Breast cancer affects millions of women every year, and it has links to dietary habits. Recent research links high-fat diets to this disease, but what is most alarming is that the research suggests that high-fat diets eaten during puberty may lead to breast cancer later in life (read more about it here: http://www.medicalnewstoday.com/articles/269441.php).

Following are some things you can do now to help prevent breast cancer:

✔ **Increase fruits and vegetables in your diet, particularly cabbage, broccoli, whole grains, tomatoes, garlic, onions, melons, and soybeans.** The fiber and phytochemicals (refer to Chapter 6) in these foods help eliminate free radicals and waste in your body that may potentially cause cancer.

✔ **Limit trans- and saturated fats in your diet.** A diet high in fat and calories leads to an increased risk for breast cancer because it affects cell growth, particularly in the immune system.

✔ **Increase lean meats in your diet to get good sources of protein.** Fatty meats contain saturated fats, which are bad (as I explain in the preceding item on this).

✔ **Drink alcohol in moderation or not at all.** Although moderate red wine intake can be protective against certain diseases and possibly even cancer, alcohol abuse is linked with an increased cancer risk.

✔ **Eat plenty of omega-3 fatty acids, particularly from fresh fish sources.** Although omega-3 fatty acids are primarily known for heart health, some research suggests that eating these fats in place of other, more "dangerous" fats can decrease your chances of developing cancer.

Protecting yourself from Alzheimer's disease and dementia

Few diseases are as scary as Alzheimer's disease or other forms of *dementia* (the decline in mental acuity, alertness, memory, and/or decision-making to a degree that affects daily life). Alzheimer's disease is the most common form of dementia, making up to 80 percent of all cases of diagnosed dementia. Affecting up to 30 million suffers globally, this disease is a very real and very serious health concern for seniors. There is no cure. Currently, prevention of the disease is your best defense.

Research suggests that certain dietary regimens can help protect against this disease. Researchers point to the Mediterranean Diet (a diet inspired by Greek, southern Italian, Spanish, and Portuguese cuisines that revolve around olive oil, moderate fish and seafood intake, fruits, vegetables, whole grains, moderate dairy intake, moderate wine intake, and low amounts of red meat) as being protective against the disease. Generally, though, eating a "brain health" diet is best. What is a brain health diet? Avoiding large quantities of saturated and trans-fats, eating omega-3 fatty acids, controlling calorie intake, and eating nutrient-dense foods. Such a diet can lessen your risk of developing Alzheimer's disease.

Keeping It Simple and Structured

Getting older is difficult. Not only are you experiencing physical changes, but you are also undergoing mental, social, and emotional changes as well. Use the following suggestions to help ease the burdens of aging through eating healthily:

✔ **Don't be afraid of change or to try new things!** You want diversity in your diet. One way to broaden your foods is to incorporate new items slowly into your diet.

Many seniors have diabetes and need to consume a consistent amount of carbohydrates to help them regulate their blood sugar. To incorporate new sources of good carbs slowly into your diet, add oatmeal or whole-wheat toast to your breakfast a few times a week, for example. As you develop a taste for these new foods, increase them accordingly and appropriately.

✔ **When in doubt, make a smoothie out of your meal.** Seniors may have difficulty remembering to eat, or they may have difficulty chewing their food — situations that put them at risk for malnutrition. One way to overcome this is to make smoothies whenever possible. Smoothies are easy to swallow, and you can fit many types of foods into them.

Turning breakfast into a smoothie usually works a bit better than turning other meals into smoothies. But don't be afraid to experiment with different combinations. You may be surprised how many delicious fruit and vegetable combinations you can concoct!

✔ **Exercise responsibly.** Moving freely becomes harder as you get older, but that shouldn't stop you from staying active. Taking short walks daily is a great way to introduce healthy exercise into a responsible wellness program.

Getting older should be a rewarding experience. If you keep a positive mindset and eat healthily, there is no reason you can't continue to do many of the things you used to do in your 20s. Here's to the good times in the years to come!

Part V
Theoretical Foundations of Health Behavior

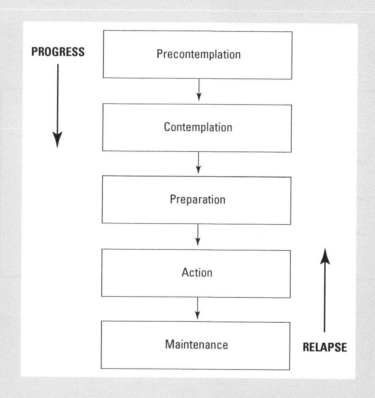

In this part. . .

- ✔ Recognize how personality, culture, and social norms influence health behaviors
- ✔ Discover different models of health behavior that enable you to uncover the key factors influencing patient choices
- ✔ Find out how to influence an individual's health behavior through persuasive, targeted messaging

Chapter 19

Modifying Health Behaviors

*I*n the first three parts of this book, I provide a pretty extensive introduction to the tenets of clinical nutrition in terms of *content,* the information itself: nutritional guidelines, the link between diet and health outcomes, how nutritional needs change over the course of a lifetime, and so on. In this chapter, I introduce how to convey that information to others.

This and the next chapter may be the most important chapters in the whole book for people who are interested in clinical nutrition. Why? For the most part, anybody can find nutritional information in a number of places, such as this text, and be able to grasp how to eat healthy, exercise, avoid tobacco, drink in moderation, and so on in order to live a long, healthy life.

But knowing how to effectively and efficiently communicate that information to someone else in a way that lets that person understand and comprehend the information and then successfully adhere to those recommendations is an entirely different set of skills. Knowing and mastering these skills is crucial to effective clinicians.

As a health professional, you have an obligation to help others alter their behavioral choices to improve wellness. Ranging from physicians persuading a patient to quit smoking to clinical nutritionists promoting the consumption of fresh fruits and vegetables, altering behaviors is a core function of these professions. In this chapter, I present the foundational elements of health behavior theory and help you understand how to apply that knowledge when trying to change human behavior.

Grasping the Theoretical Foundations of Health Behaviors

The term *health behavior* represents an interesting concept — that how you behave can (and most certainly will) affect your health outcomes. In other words, sooner or later, the decisions you make now determine your health and wellness status well into your future. The term encompasses a collection of many variables unique to each individual: his or her perceptions, values, personality, beliefs, habits, cultural influences, family history, and other psychosocial variables that can affect disease prevention, health maintenance, and treatment choices.

In this section, I explain how, to be effective as a clinical nutrition, you must recognize and then be able to reach through to help your client.

Reaching through people's differing opinions, ideas, and notions

All people have their own perceptions of life, love, liberty, health, death, happiness, illness, wellness, favorite baseball team, best ice-cream flavor, and so on. You must account for these differing opinions when you're attempting to alter their behaviors. You must attempt to understand how they define the world you're trying to influence.

How would you measure whether a patient of yours is happy? Would you count how many times he smiles during the day? Would that day be during the week or on a weekend? My guess is that people are more apt to smile on the weekend. Or would you measure your patient's laughter? How would you even do that? By loudness? Duration? Tonal quality?

And then the challenge becomes even more complicated when you realize that people laugh and/or smile for a whole variety of reasons, many of which have nothing to do with happiness. For example, have you ever smiled, giggled, or laughed when you were nervous? Sure you have. You probably didn't even notice it. Some people resort to laughter when they are scared or frightened. Perhaps it's a defense mechanism.

So counting smiles is unreliable, as is measuring laughter. Again, how would you determine if a patient is happy? How about asking him straight up? Sure, you could, but how would you define happiness? What if your patient has a different notion of what being happy means? What if your definition of "very happy" is someone else's version of "somewhat happy"?

Consider this example, which is more relevant within a clinical nutrition context. Imagine that you're researching the effects of manic depression on overeating. First, how would you *operationalize,* or define/measure, depression? After you determine how to measure manic depression and its gradations, you have to determine how to figure out whether your different groups of people are over-eating. Seems like a simple enough task. Just ask study participants whether they overeat, which you define as eating more than 2,200 calories per day, right? But what if they don't answer accurately because they don't know how many calories they eat in a given day? What if they don't answer accurately because they're too embarrassed? Tricky, right?

If you overcome these challenges and identify a manically depressed person who overeats, how would you get that person to change his behavior? Tell him to stop? Good luck with that. The most difficult part of any health professional's job is getting the client/patient/participant to listen and then follow guidelines.

This same narrative can play out in a number of other situations, ranging from trying to get children to drink more milk at school, having overweight elderly women reduce their caloric intake by 30 percent, or having children opt for more vegetables at the dinner table than desserts. Changing someone's behavior is a difficult task. However, it's a necessary skill for health professionals, especially nutritionists and medical clinicians.

Getting familiar with the terminology

As you dive deeper into the concept of health behavior change, you need to be familiar with the terminology. Keep in mind that the following are just a fraction of what health behavior theorists and health professionals have defined over the course of time. However, they serve as a good foundation:

- ✔ **Attitude:** A general feeling, or evaluation, of something. In this case, your attitude on broccoli may be that it tastes delicious, and you love the bright green color when you cook it.

- ✔ **Normative beliefs:** The generally held beliefs in a society. If you're concerned what others will think if you perform or don't perform a specific behavior, you're being influenced by normative beliefs. For example, what would your mother think if you threw your broccoli in the trash instead of eating it?

- ✔ **Behavioral beliefs:** An assessment of a specific behavior's consequences. Think of it as an internal evaluation process in which you assess how — or whether — your behavior choices will affect your health. Would chronically skipping out on eating broccoli or other vegetables be detrimental to your health?

✔ **Self-efficacy:** The sense of control an individual has over his behaviors and surroundings. In other words, you assess whether you have the ability to go buy broccoli, have access to a stove or microwave in which to prepare it, or can eat it. Self-efficacy relates to *perceived behavioral control,* defined in the next item in this list.

✔ **Perceived behavioral control:** A person's perceptions of his ability to perform a given behavior. Your assessment of whether you have the skill to actually cook the broccoli is an example of perceived behavioral control. Do you know what preparing and then properly cooking broccoli takes?

✔ **Perceived severity:** The negative outcomes associated with a disease or a particular behavior. Perceived severity has a more powerful influence on behavior than actual severity. If you perceive that smoking cigarettes isn't dangerous, for example, you'll smoke, despite how dangerous they really are.

Another example is type 2 diabetes. Because it occurs so gradually and doesn't affect them until later in life, many people discount it as being severe. They think, "Oh, I can change tomorrow and be okay. It won't affect me for a bit, so as long as I make healthy changes in the next few years, I don't have anything to worry about." As a result, they tend to put off making changes because their perceived severity of the disease is low.

The perceived severity can impact the changes people are willing to make. For example, in your opinion, which is a more serious disease: the common cold or terminal cancer? Most people would think that terminal cancer is a bit more serious than a cold. Therefore, if you don't care for broccoli but find out that it is protective against a cold, would you eat it? Probably not. But if I told you that broccoli is protective against terminal cancer, would you be more apt to eat the broccoli? Probably.

✔ **Perceived vulnerability:** Your belief about how likely you are to contract, or acquire, a certain disease. What is the likelihood that you will develop cancer because of a poor diet? Pretty high, actually. However, some people don't believe that to be true; therefore, their perceived vulnerability is low.

✔ **Cues to action:** A system of reminders that spur you to act on a certain behavior. For example, if you need to be reminded to eat broccoli, which helps prevent terminal cancer, you can add "Eat broccoli on Thursday!" to your weekly menu plan, or you can tape a picture of broccoli to your refrigerator. These kinds of cues may sound silly, but they work.

✔ **Barriers:** The perceived physical, mental, spiritual, or economic challenges that prevent an individual from achieving certain objectives. For example, fresh salmon that costs $13.99 a pound would be an economic barrier to a parent whose grocery budget is very tight.

✔ **Intention:** The presence or absence of desire to perform or not perform a particular behavior. Do you intend to eat broccoli if I told you all the great benefits of eating it? Intention is key in making health behavior changes. Without intention, changes don't occur. One of the most impactful things you can do as a clinical nutritionist is to get a patient to state an intention to make a change. For details, head to the later section "Intending to Perform Behaviors: The Key to Action."

✔ **Perceived social support:** A subjective judgment that your social group (friends, family, colleagues, partners, and so on) will provide aid to you in times of stress. Will your parents support you as you begin a new diet? Will they provide encouragement to you to help you get through the cravings? Sadly, many people wanting to make a change are often undermined by key people in their social support group.

Keep these terms and their definitions in mind. They all exert some influence on people's behaviors. In addition, I've peppered these terms throughout this and the next chapter as a way to reinforce your familiarity with them.

Examining the Influence of Personality

Typically, people's personalities are consistent throughout their lives. In addition, personality is highly associated with behavioral choices, particularly regarding health and wellness. For example, a person with a *narcissistic personality* (someone who is vain and has a grandiose view of his own talents) would be less apt to take advice from others than a person with a more passive, less bullish personality.

It is possible to predict health behavior choices based on personality profiles. And because personalities are consistent throughout a person's life, you can use what you know about a particular personality type to tailor your message in a way that can be heard and acted upon. If you know how to deliver a message designed to persuade a narcissist to adopt a better diet when he's 35 years old, for example, you know how to communicate with him when he's 40, 50, 60, and older.

Personality traits are so constant because they stem from a person's genetic makeup. Unless you know of some easy way to manipulate gene expression to alter personality traits, you're pretty much stuck with whatever personality you were born with.

Any clinician or behavioral scientist can tell you that patients' abilities to adhere to dietary, medical, and behavioral regimen changes rely heavily on personality type. As you would expect, some people are harder to convince than others to follow behavioral, and in this book's case, dietary, guidelines. Two well-known personality assessments are the Myers-Briggs test and the Locus of Control model. I explain each in this section. In Chapter 20, I offer some strategies to help you communicate with different personality types.

A person's personality is predictive of the types of dietary habits he exhibits. When you prescribe changes to an individual's diet or you counsel someone about making alterations to what he is eating, your message has a better chance of getting through if you tailor it to the personality type.

Myers-Briggs personality assessment

The Myers-Briggs test was developed in the 1920s. This test is given in the form of a survey, and it measures psychological preferences related to how individuals view the world around themselves and how they navigate society.

According to Myers-Briggs, people can be fall into 16 different types, based on where they fall along four axes. These axes are

- **Introversion/Extroversion:** In this axis, the survey questions determine whether you are an *introvert* (inward-turning person, meaning that you tend to be passive and more reclusive than an extrovert, and seek interaction with thoughts and ideas) or an *extrovert* (outward-turning, meaning that you are more sociable and seek interaction with people and objects).

  If you tell an introvert to eat broccoli, he would self-reflect and make a decision based upon his own ideas and perceptions of broccoli. An extrovert would be more apt to seek peer information or approval before making a decision to eat broccoli.

- **Sensing/Intuition:** This axis is the information-gathering axis, and it indicates where an individual tends to gather new information and how he perceives it. If you tend to fall more into the sensing category, you are much more likely to listen and adhere to information that is tangible, concrete, and could be gathered with your five senses. If you are more intuitive, you tend to have more trust in abstract information. You are more future-focused that the sensing people, who are more present-focused.

  If you tell a sensing person to eat more broccoli, he would use his senses (sight, taste, smell, and touch) to examine the broccoli and focus on the benefits that broccoli will give him in the short term (increased fiber to help with constipation, for example). An intuitive person will perceive that broccoli is part of a larger scheme of healthy living and can help prevent cancer 30 years from now.

- **Thinking/Feeling:** This axis represents the judging area of a personality. "Thinkers" tend to be more detached from the topic at hand and view it from an objective, non-personal perspective. "Feelers" look at a topic from a more subjective perspective and are more likely to rely on personal feelings about a topic.

For example, if you tell a "thinker" to eat broccoli, he might perceive the information as simple factual data: if he eats this plant, he'll gain needed nutrients to help keep himself healthy. A "feeler" is more apt to have personal sentiments attached to the decision or idea of eating broccoli. His mother used to make him eat broccoli, and so thinking about eating broccoli has a certain nostalgia attached to it, spurring him to eat the broccoli partially because of his subjective feeling toward the food.

✔ **Judging/Perception:** This axis refers to how you want to live your outer life. If you are more judging personality, your life tends to be more structured and your life choices more predictable. If you are more perception-oriented, you're more flexible with your decisions and are more likely to want to alter your lifestyle.

If you tell a judging personality to eat broccoli, he would be more likely to consider how to fit broccoli into his more regimented diet. A perception person, on the other hand, would view eating more broccoli as an exciting challenge to incorporate new things into his diet.

Health professionals use these four axes to create a series of sixteen differing personalities. Each has its own disposition toward how information is perceived and then how decisions are made, based upon the presented information.

Looking at the Locus of Control model

The Locus of Control model was developed in the mid–20th century to help explain different types of people and how much power, or influence, they have in controlling events, people, and other situations around themselves. Participants are given a survey and then placed into one of two groups, according to the score their responses received. The groups are internal and external (see Figure 19-1):

✔ **Internally dominant:** Individuals who are internally dominated believe that they have more power and control in the events that surround them and in how those events unfold. Internally dominated people would have to be persuaded that, when they eat broccoli, they are taking charge and making themselves healthier. Doing so makes them more likely to adopt a behavior.

✔ **Externally dominated:** Individuals who are externally dominated believe that other forces — God, fate, karma, luck, chance, or something else — have more control over them and their actions than they themselves do. This type of person is more apt to adopt a behavior promoted by a trained dietary professional (such as a clinical nutritionist) than to adopt some self-initiated idea.

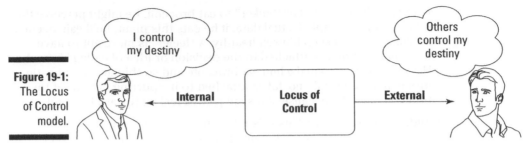

Figure 19-1: The Locus of Control model.

Researchers are now breaking down personality types into more than the two types defined by the Locus of Control model. (You can see this with the Myers-Briggs test, which I discuss in the preceding section.) Matter of fact, my earlier work with these personality concepts broke Locus of Control into four subgroups: unrealistic externals, realistic externals, realistic internals, and unrealistic internals. By more precisely defining the type of person who is receiving the message, we can target the message in a way that increases the chances that he or she will alter behavior. In other words, the more that a message is tailored, or specifically designed for, an individual, the more apt that individual is to follow directions or guidelines.

Examining Environmental Influences

People don't live in vacuums. The environments in which they live have a significant impact on their health behavior choices, particularly their diets: what they eat, when they eat, what foods they perceive as good and bad, and so on (refer to "Reaching through people's differing opinions, ideas, and notions" earlier for a discussion of how important personal perceptions are in understanding dietary choices). In this section, I introduce these environments and tell you how you can apply this knowledge in your work as a clinical nutritionist.

Understanding the three different environments

You may have noticed that I use the word *environments,* plural, in this discussion. That's because the physical environment in which a person lives is not the only environment that influences health behaviors or dietary choices. Two other environments are important factors as well: a person's social environment and his intrapersonal environment. Here's what you need to know about each of these environments. Keep in mind that some overlap exists between these different environments.

Physical environment

The physical environment is the external geographic space or situation in which the individual or group resides or interacts. In other words, it refers to the physical setting and how a person's interaction with his physical setting affects his health behaviors, particularly dietary choices. Examples of the physical environment include things like how far a person has to travel to go to a supermarket, his ability to purchase food, his ability to cook food, and the availability of fresh fruits and vegetables.

Several variables impact how an individual's physical environment influences his dietary choices: self-efficacy, perceived behavioral control, accessibility (how available services or goods are to an individual), cues to action, fear (whether he's afraid that an event or thing will cause an adverse health event), and threat (if an event or thing causes an adverse health event, what he can do to lessen his risk; this relates to perceived severity). Refer to the earlier section "Getting familiar with the terminology" for more on these terms.

Social environment

The *social environment* refers to the external societal space or situation in which the individual or group resides or interacts and how this interaction affects health behaviors, particularly dietary choices. In other words, it's the social setting in which an individual finds himself. Examples of the social environment include cultural norms, societal expectations from its citizens, and local customs and beliefs. For example, if you grew up in a household that never ate tofu (if you even knew what it was) and scoffed at the idea of anyone actually eating it as a substitute for red meat, you would think twice about talking to your parents about serving it at Christmas dinner. Peer influence is highly predictive of what behaviors are adopted, particularly with dietary changes.

Several variables impact how an individual's social environment influences his dietary choices: normative beliefs, accessibility, cues to action, fear, and threat. However, the social environment is primarily influenced by an individual's peer group (normative beliefs). Refer to the earlier section "Getting familiar with the terminology" for more on these terms.

Intrapersonal environment

Whereas both the physical and social environments are external — that is, they represent outside influences — the intrapersonal environment is within an individual. This environment refers to the internal thoughts, feelings, and emotions that affect a person's health behaviors, particularly dietary choices. Fear of trying new foods, the eagerness to adopt different behaviors, and the confidence in oneself to alter diet are all part of the intrapersonal environment.

Although these feelings and perceptions may be influenced by the physical and social environments, the final determiner of what action a person takes resides within that person. If my family has always avoided new foods, for example, I may turn down invitations to go to lunch with co-workers when the destination is an ethnic restaurant. This demonstrates the link between peer influence and whether — and how — you choose to engage in certain behaviors.

Several variables impact how an individual's intrapersonal environment influences his dietary choices: attitude, perceived vulnerability/perceived severity, benefits/barriers, perceived behavioral control, fear, threat, and intention. Refer to the earlier section "Getting familiar with the terminology" for more on these terms.

Putting these environments together: Reciprocal Determinism

As I mention earlier, these three environments overlap in various ways, and the interplay between them can be represented by the *Reciprocal Determinism model* (see Figure 19-2). Albert Bandura, the famous behavioral psychologist, developed this model, which suggests that the social and interpersonal environments interact with each other, which then influence someone's behavior. In Bandura's construct, the social environment includes the physical environment.

Say that you grow up in a close-knit neighborhood where residents don't have a lot of money but have pooled resources to create an urban garden (physical environment). The families work the plot together, the produce is harvested and shared, and the entire enterprise, in addition to being work, is also a lot of fun (social environment). Chances are you'll grow up valuing fresh foods, not only because of their nutritional benefits but because of the good feelings you associate with the experience (intrapersonal environment). When you get out on your own and start your own family, chances are you'll ensure that fresh produce is a key ingredient in the meals you prepare (dietary choices).

Another example is highlighted in something called the Roseto Effect. This phenomenon suggests that traditional cultures (in this example, Italian) value highly social relationships and incorporate the community into making each other healthy. Through support systems and a large emphasis on family values (eating dinner together as a family, respecting parents and elders, reciprocal respect, and so on), this community was able to protect its members from the effects of major chronic diseases, like diabetes and heart disease. When this social support system breaks down, the protective effects disappear. It's a great example of how social environments can influence your physical health. You can read more about the effect at http://ajph.aphapublications. org/doi/pdf/10.2105/AJPH.82.8.1089

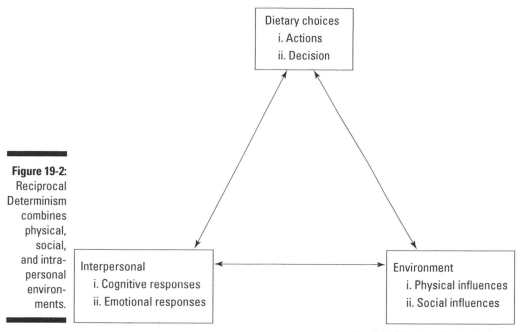

Figure 19-2: Reciprocal Determinism combines physical, social, and intrapersonal environments.

Too often medical and health professionals promote health as if it were taking place in a vacuum. Their messages are generic and don't take into account the environmental influences that impact their patients' choices. If you use this impersonal approach, your patients may not listen to you. When delivering health information, keep these general guidelines in mind:

- ✔ **You must take into account all three environmental realms to effectively alter others' dietary behaviors.** Although you can just tell patients that sweet potatoes are good for them because of the abundant beta carotene, that may not be the most effective way to compel them to eat more sweet potatoes. Because personality and environment influence how a person feels about certain health behaviors, particular dietary guidelines, and impact how receptive a person is to medical and health advice, you can use this knowledge to determine which approach will most effectively compel your patient to alter his behavior.

- ✔ **You must make your message resonate with your patient.** Achieving this objective depends on how you present the information. If you share information in a monotone, non-interactive manner, using complicated language and an indifferent attitude, chances are your patient will barely want to listen to you for five seconds, let alone adopt the behavior you recommend.

As a health promoter you must be as effective and efficient as possible when you counsel patients. In the next chapter, I offers lots of tips, tricks, and strategies that can help you communicate important information with patients in a way that spurs them to take the needed action.

Intending to Perform Behaviors: The Key to Action

Have you ever intended to do something? Of course you have. You intended to read this book today, and now — look, you're reading it. You intended to get up in the morning, brush your teeth (hopefully!), and perform your daily activities. You intend to do things all this time.

In the context of clinical nutrition, *intention* is defined as a person's readiness to perform a specific behavior. Whereas intentions in general usage don't always result in action, in clinical nutrition, a person who intends to perform a behavior will perform it. *Behavior* itself has been defined as the interplay between intention and perceptions of behavioral control. Perceived behavioral control refers to the effect your perceived ability to mentally or physically perform a behavior has upon your intention to adopt a certain behavior (such as eating broccoli). A positive intention (the intention to cook and eat broccoli) is produced from a positive perceived ability to perform the behavior (your ability to cook and eat broccoli). (Refer to "Getting familiar with the terminology" earlier in this chapter for a quick review of these and other key terms.)

When you design a dietary plan that you want someone else to adopt, attempt to get your patient to intend to perform the behavior. Following are some ways to spur intent:

- **Setting up a reminder system:** Have clients write down on a piece of paper and post on their refrigerator that they will eat five servings of fruits and vegetables each and every day. This trick sounds very simple, but little reminders can go a long way to spur intention.

- **Getting family and friends involved:** When people have strong support systems around them, they are more apt to intend to do something than when they feel they're alone in performing a behavior. So get clients' spouses involved in planning and cooking meals. This support system and interaction makes a person more likely to try new foods.

- **Empower the patient:** Giving people the strength and desire to change their lives for themselves (for their health or their family's well-being) can spur in them the desire to change. Giving clients information on how easy broccoli is to prepare and then telling them just how beneficial broccoli is for them and their loved ones empowers them, and they'll be more likely to intend to eat broccoli.

You don't necessarily have to wait until patients actually perform the behavior. Behavior change may take longer than you expect. As long as they truly intend to make the change, they most likely will.

Many models and theories use intention as a key variable because it is so predictive of making an actual behavioral change. In the next and final portion of this chapter, I discuss some major health behavioral theories and models in more depth to illustrate just how important different variables are in altering behaviors.

Modeling Behaviors with Behavior Models

Changing behaviors, as I explain earlier, is difficult. In my experience, altering dietary habits is even more difficult than making other types of changes due to the many variables that can alter the decisions you make in regards to your health and the overwhelming amount of stimuli that can amend the choices you make about the food you eat.

One way to get a handle on all these variables is to put them into models. These models can help you map out which variables are the most important ones influencing the choices your patient makes.

Many models and theories attempt to explain human behavior. I cover three of the most popular in the next sections: the Health Belief model, the Theory of Planned Behavior, and Transtheoretical model. These models have been used to predict and alter health behaviors in areas ranging from HIV prevention (getting patients to participate in needle exchange programs) to programs to reduce osteoporosis risk (persuading 25-year-old women to get proper amounts of calcium and vitamin D).

Every individual has a different personality and lives in different environments, and myriad factors influence how an individual receives and accepts or rejects a dietary change message. To be a successful clinician, you need to be able to model your patients' cognitive structures, use those models to help you create effective messages, and delivery those messages in such a way that your patients not only listen to you but also take your advice. In the next chapter, I give you some tips and tricks on how best to state a message.

The Health Belief model

The Health Belief model, shown in Figure 19-3, attempts to predict health behaviors, using a core set of perceptions about the behavior itself and the disease/risk associated with performing or not performing that behavior. This model revolves around four major constructs:

- **Perceived susceptibility/perceived vulnerability:** How susceptible or vulnerable to a disease or negative health outcome a person believes himself to be. To take action, an individual must believe that he can get the disease and that he is not immune (if he is not, in fact, immune).

  For example, does the patient understand and believe that if he eats over 3,500 extra calories above his daily caloric needs that he will gain one pound of body fat?

- **Perceived severity:** How severe the patient perceives the disease or risk to be. To take action, an individual must associate the disease or risk factor with a negative enough outcome (such as pain, death, disability, significant economic ramifications, and so on) to warrant a change.

  For example, does he understand and believe that diabetes, if not properly treated, can lead to amputation of hands, feet, arms, and legs or even death?

- **Cost/benefit analysis:** To take action, an individual must perceive that the benefits stemming from the recommended behavior outweigh the costs (money, time, and inconvenience) of performing the recommendations. Further, the individual must perceive that changing the behavior is possible.

  For example, does he believe that the possible benefits of losing weight outweigh the costs (working out an extra 30 minutes every other day on top of his normal exercise routine and reducing his daily caloric intake by 20 percent), and the perceived distress associated with making these changes?

- **Cues to Action:** An individual must receive information that reminds or spurs him to take action.

  For example, would having a picture of fruits and vegetables on the refrigerator be a reminder for an individual on a diet to eat more of these food items?

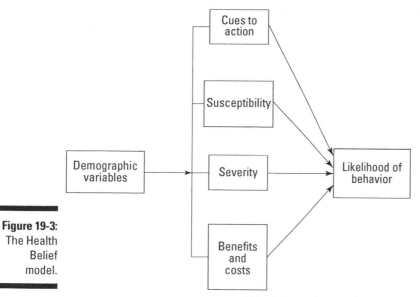

Figure 19-3:
The Health
Belief
model.

Suppose, for example, that your patient is at high risk for diabetes due to his current weight and dietary behaviors. Your goal is to help him lose 25 pounds and adopt a more healthy diet. Using the Health Belief model, you would provide information that gets him to acknowledge that he is at risk of developing diabetes (perceived susceptibility/perceived vulnerability); that getting diabetes puts his health in significant jeopardy (perceived severity); that persuades him that he has more to gain than lose by changing his diet (cost/benefit analysis); and that keeping a journal of how many servings of fruits and vegetables he eats in a day can help him achieve his weight loss goals (cue to action).

The Theory of Planned Behavior

The Theory of Planned Behavior, shown in Figure 19-4, suggests that intentions to perform a specific behavior are driven by three core factors acting in unison:

- ✔ **Attitude toward the behavior:** That is, an individual's acceptance or rejection of the need to adopt a behavior.

- ✔ **Subjective norms:** That is, the societal norms, expectations, and values surrounding the performance of the behavior.

✔ **Perceived behavioral control:** Very similar to self-efficacy (refer to the earlier section "Getting familiar with the terminology"), this refers to an individual's perceived ability to perform the behavior.

The main goal for the Theory of Planned Behavior is to raise intention to perform a behavior; however, actual behavior change is the ultimate endpoint for any type of patient counseling. So why don't researchers list that as the main goal for this theory? The idea is that if you can get a person to intend to do something, chances are he or she will do it. Sometimes that change may take a longer or shorter time, depending on the behavior — your goal is to get the client or patient to *intend* to do it and then let nature take its course.

Here's an example. Say that your task is to persuade a pregnant female to take prenatal vitamins to prevent a neural tube defect in her baby. She wants to take them because she feels that they are healthy for her and she needs them. Therefore, she has an attitude conducive to adopt a behavior. But that isn't the only factor that matters. Consider her subjective norms, or peer group influence. What do her family, friends, or husband suggest? If they are also supportive, she has an attitude and the subjective norms to support a growing intention to take the prenatal vitamins. But what if this woman absolutely cannot obtain prenatal vitamins, either because she cannot afford them or because her body is unable to digest, process, transport, or utilize folic acid? In this case, her perceived behavioral control results in her inability to take the vitamins.

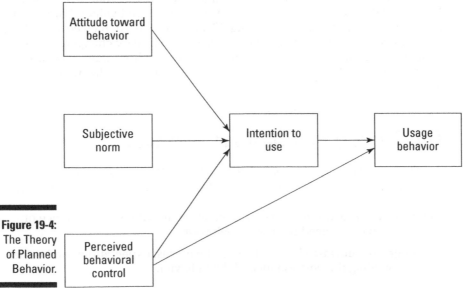

Figure 19-4:
The Theory of Planned Behavior.

Illustration by Wiley, Composition Services Graphics

Although some may argue that this is an *actual behavioral control* rather than a perceived behavioral control, the idea is still the same. If this woman does not have the ability, or perceived ability, to perform a behavior, getting her to intend to take prenatal vitamins will be difficult, despite the fact that she wants to take them and her social group is supportive.

Many theories or models look to alter the intention to perform a behavior among individuals because intention is pretty much required for an alteration in behavior to occur. If you take an action without first intending to do it, you have either been forced to take the action, or you do it by accident — neither of which produces a lasting change. The first (coercion) is illegal, and the other, being unintentional, won't be anything more than a one-time hiccup.

The Transtheoretical model

The Transtheoretical model, also known as the Stages of Changes model, states that change must be intentional, and it focuses on the decision-making capabilities of an individual. Designed to assist in the success of smoking cessation programs, this model has been used to promote other kinds of health behavior changes. More and more researchers are now looking to use this model with other health and wellness topics such as exercise, low-fat diets, alcohol abuse, weight control, and more.

In the Transtheoretical model, progress is made in five stages, shown in Figure 19-5. Each stage leads to the next:

- ✔ **Precontemplation:** In this stage, people don't intend to take action in the next six months. People may be in this stage because they lack information. Perhaps they haven't been informed about dietary recommendations and therefore are unaware of the consequences that can result if they don't adopt that recommendation. For example, a 55-year-old overweight male who eats fried chicken every day for dinner and is unaware that eating large amounts of fatty foods and cholesterol are bad for his heart is in the precontemplation stage. Lacking information about the dangers his diet poses to his health, he isn't thinking about reducing his calorie, fat, and cholesterol intake.

- ✔ **Contemplation:** People in this stage intend to change in the next six months. They are more aware of the pros and the cons of changing a behavior. Although people may actually get stuck in this stage, a situation called *chronic contemplation,* most people who get to this stage are truly contemplating changing their behavior.

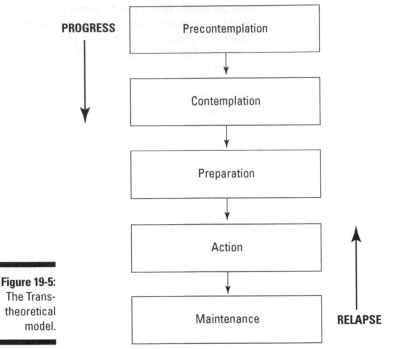

PROGRESS

Precontemplation

Contemplation

Preparation

Action

Maintenance

RELAPSE

Figure 19-5:
The Trans-
theoretical
model.

Illustration by Wiley, Composition Services Graphics

Going back to the earlier example, say that the man who eats fried chicken daily watches a television program on the benefits of reducing cholesterol on heart health. This program gets him thinking that perhaps he should eat less fried chicken so that he can lose some weight and increase the years he has left.

✔ **Preparation:** At this stage, people intend to take action within the next month. They have taken some noticeable steps to prepare to perform the behavior in the recent past and have chosen a plan of action, like joining a gym, going online to get recipes on salad making, or setting a time to take a multivitamin every morning. The man who eats fried chicken every day may prepare by planning to substitute grilled chicken for fried chicken every other day.

✔ **Action:** People in this stage have made significant changes in their lifestyles within the past six months to bring about the desired change. For example, the gentlemen who previously ate fried chicken every day has improved his diet by making significant reductions in how much fat and cholesterol he consumes daily.

Not all action is equal. To qualify for the action stage, the action must be significant enough to reduce the risk. The man in the example, for instance, isn't reducing his risk if he lowers his fat and cholesterol intake 1 percent or 2 percent only. He must be well into the double-digit range. He can't just decide to eat one fewer drumstick at every meal, for example.

✔ **Maintenance:** In this stage, people work to maintain their healthy behaviors and to prevent themselves from relapsing to their former bad eating habits. Returning to the gentleman in the example, he's now cognizant that he cannot eat fried chicken every day and has reduced his fat and cholesterol intake significantly. He's now healthier and feeling great. Instead of completely eliminating certain fried foods from his diet, he eats them once in a while but continues to eat his healthier diet. In so doing, he is able to maintain his healthier weight and keep his cholesterol levels in the acceptable range. Individuals in this stage are less tempted to relapse and become increasingly more confident as they continue their change.

Chapter 20

Communicating Health Information

. . . .

In This Chapter

▶ Uncovering health communication basics

▶ Understanding the science behind communicating

▶ Distinguishing between communication content and context

▶ Being aware of challenges when communicating

. . . .

Communicating information, particular dietary recommendations, is both a science and an art form. Persuading people to alter their dietary or other health behaviors, eliminate bad habits, and adopt new wellness routines is difficult, and not every health professional is successful. You can be the premier researcher in the world, producing the finest work, but if you can't communicate your information appropriately, then all your hard work loses much of its power to promote wellness.

Effectively translating dietary information to patients is a difficult yet essential skill for every clinician to master. The fact is that how you say something is just as important as what you say. In this chapter, I present the science behind communicating health promotional messages to someone — a valuable skill for future clinicians. Part of being a successful practitioner is being able to suggest health behavior change and then have your patient adopt those changes. This chapter gives you the foundational skills on message context (*how* to say something) so that you can be a more effective communicator of clinical nutrition.

Communicating Health Information: The Basics

If you're like most people, you take communication for granted, not giving much conscious thought to the factors that help you build an argument to compel someone to action. Chances are you didn't give much thought to the methodology you should use to persuade that person that your viewpoint was superior. You took information (message content) and probably hoped that the facts would speak for themselves. You were either successful or not.

As a clinical nutritionist, you'll find yourself doing the same thing: Only this time, your task is to persuade a patient to adopt your health behavior recommendations. What you will soon learn is that you'll be more successful if you concentrate not only on the content of your message but on the context as well.

Understanding how to frame a message in a way that empowers and inspires the listener to take action is a vital skill, and perfecting it is key to becoming a successful dietary clinician. In this section, I give you the information that will set you on the path of developing your own effective communication style.

Defining health communication

Before you can communicate health information, you first need to know what health communication is. You'll encounter plenty of definitions in various academic and professional circles, but here's the definition you need to know as it relates to clinical nutrition: *Health communication* refers to communication strategies you employ to affect the behaviors and decisions of individuals or groups as those decisions pertain to their health and well-being.

Health communication specifically looks to make the delivery of information more efficient and more effective. Health communication that is both more efficient and effective accomplishes the following:

- ✔ Improves health literacy
- ✔ Better tailors messages to the targeted recipients
- ✔ Improves access to health information
- ✔ Enables evaluations to be conducted in an effort to improve communication services

Introducing informed decision-making

Skilled researchers promote informed decision-making as the best tool to sustain optimal health in the community. The idea behind informed decision-making is that to make a responsible, informed decision on what treatment or course of action to take next, a person must have enough information on a subject to feel at least somewhat comfortable with the material being discussed.

To ensure that your patients have the information they need to make an informed decision, you must

✔ Make them part of the decision-making process

✔ Provide them with the best possible evidence and a clear set of choices based on that evidence

✔ Take into consideration their values and preferences related to the health decision and topic being discussed

Trying your hand with an example scenario

Keeping in mind the goals of health communication and the idea of informed decision-making, read the following hypothetical scenario. Then attempt to answer the questions posed at the end.

A husband and wife (both cancer free) come to see you to discuss how they can eat better in order to prevent cancer. They are of similar ages (he is 65 years old, and she is 63). Neither has any formal training or education beyond high school, and both read at a 7th-grade level.

They've scheduled this appointment because they want to change their diet. Watching the news the night before, they saw a report on how eating more vegetables and fruits can lessen cancer risk. They feel confident that they know how to cook and prepare the foods in their new diet, and they indicate that they have access to the foods they'll need (their home is near a grocery store) and enough money to buy more expensive produce. However, they claim that their children, whom they love very much and whose opinion they value very highly, are very much against their newfound healthy mindset.

How would you provide sound dietary information to this couple in a manner in which they can understand? How will you counsel them about amending their diet to lower their risk of developing cancer? Here are some things you should think about:

✔ **Applying the principles and goals of efficient and effective health communication, you would use communication strategies to inform and influence individual decisions that promote healthy outcomes.** In other words, you must deliver a message to this couple in a way that empowers them to accept and then implement your advice related to changing their behaviors.

✔ **Applying the principles of informed decision-making, you would provide patients with guidance to make the best possible healthcare decisions for themselves while at the same time allowing yourself to feel confident in the care options you are promoting to them.** You would give this couple enough information on the health outcome itself and their options regarding what they can do to help prevent this outcome from happening. If it has already occurred, you would provide information about what they can do to help treat the issue.

If you really want to be challenged, use the Theory of Planned Behavior (refer to Chapter 19 for information on this behavior model) to plan your response. The key is to help the couple get to the point where they develop the intent to change their diet. Be sure you address each variable in that model and how the diet itself or some key factor related to successfully adopting the diet (getting access to fresh, natural foods, for example, or changing their attitude so that they consistently *want* to choose healthy options over unhealthy ones) may benefit or burden them.

Grasping the Art and Science of Communicating

The best health communicators know that the effectiveness of a message and how efficiently it is delivered depends on the source of the information, the message itself, and the recipient. In this section, I explain these factors in detail and help you recognize the importance of the message's context. I also offer an example that illustrates how you can use this information to reach your audience.

Getting the nuts and bolts right: The content

Information can come from a variety of sources, but some have more weight, or authority, than others. For example, say that you read on a bubble gum wrapper that eating kale can prevent cancer; then at your next doctor's appointment, your physician tells you the same thing. Which source of information — the wrapper or the doctor — would you be more likely to accept advice from? Maybe both, but I would guess the physician.

The source of the health information affects the receiver's response to the information itself. If, for example, you suggest a dietary change to a friend with a statement like "I read about this health tip on the back of my gum wrapper. It suggests . . . ," chances are your friend wouldn't listen past "gum wrapper." Suppose, however, that you share the very same info, but instead of getting it from a gum wrapper, you read about it in a published, scientific article. She'll probably be much more receptive and inclined to give the suggestion more serious consideration.

In addition to the information coming from reputable sources, it must also be timely. Info that comes from questionable sources or is outdated undermines your authority.

Then, because such information, often published in scientific and professional journals, is often dry and hard for any but the experts to understand, you need to convey the information in a way that your listener can understand. The next three sections provide advice how to do just that.

Being content with your message's language

The next factor you have to consider is the actual message being delivered. Of particular importance is the language used. Many of the sources you will rely on as a clinician are often professional and/or scientific publications that can be challenging to understand. These kinds of works tend to rely on jargon that lay people may find confusing or off-putting. For that reason, you need to limit jargon or eliminate it altogether.

Also, the language of the message must be presented at a level appropriate for the receiver. The information given to an individual with an 8th-grade reading level, for example, must be written in language an 8th-grader can understand. The information cannot be written at a 12th-grade level; otherwise, the individual may have a difficult time comprehending the language and understanding its significance. For information about reading levels, head to "Health literacy" later in this chapter.

Knowing your audience: The receiver

The psychosocial mindset of the receiver (refer to Chapter 19) can greatly influence the reception of, and compliance to, the message. For example, if a receiver has very low perceived vulnerability of a disease (that is, she doesn't believe that she is at risk for developing the disease), no matter how well designed your message, altering this listener's behavior will be challenging.

When building a message, you need to tailor it to address the specific issues and mindset of the listener. With the patient who believes she's at minimal risk for a disease, for example, you would suggest that she is actually more vulnerable than she thinks she is, despite her perceptions to the contrary. This is where a large part of the art of communication comes in because you have to redirect her thinking without being perceived as attacking her point of view. (No one said clinical nutrition was easy!)

Know your audience! Always deliver a message that is at the appropriate reading level of the receiver and try to make a personal connection with the receiver. Trust me; you'll be more successful connecting with your audience if you do.

Engaging your audience

The best health communicators are keenly aware that sometimes *how* you say something is even more influential than what you say. Understanding this has led many researchers to develop very intricate, engaging materials that are theoretically sound and packaged into very effective messages. With a delivery that's appropriate to the audience, this information can be very impactful.

Say you have a perfectly designed message (message content) to deliver to a set of 10-year-olds on the benefits of eating cauliflower to help prevent cancer later in life. Your work is already cut out for you because what 10-year-old wants to sit and listen to some adult talk about cauliflower? If this message is perfectly designed to entice and engage the 10-year-old audience, chances are they'll probably adhere to the message. But deliver the message in a very distant, monotone, almost robotic style (message context), and your mission is going to fail, and fail miserably. You'd be lucky to have five seconds of your audience's attention.

The best messages are *engagingly persuasive;* that is, audience members feel directly involved in the message delivery process. They feel as if you are speaking to them individually because you care and because your message is important. That's the approach that's going to make your group of 10-year-olds eat their cauliflower.

As a health professional, you must make the message seem as though you've created it specifically for the receiver. Further, you must directly engage the receiver when you deliver the message. Otherwise, you run the risk of losing your listener's attention and becoming ultimately unsuccessful in persuading her to alter her health behavior or to make her more aware of a topic.

Working through an example

Message content, or the actual piece of information, must be factual, limited of jargon, and created with the appropriate reading level. Further, the message must personally connect with the audience to be effective.

Consider this example: You are charged with speaking to high school females on the dangers of malnutrition, specifically on how diets lacking in calcium can lead to early-onset osteoporosis. Your objective is to persuade your listeners to consume more milk to help prevent this disease.

Of the following two messages, which do you think would be most influential in altering the milk-drinking behaviors of these females?

✔ **Message 1** (Read this aloud in a monotone voice):

> Did you know that you will reach peak bone mass in your early 30s? After your mid-30s and going into middle adulthood, you will begin to lose bone mass. You can avoid this by fortifying your diet with calcium supplements or eating a diet high in calcium. Some foods that are high in calcium include dairy foods and cruciferous vegetables, like cabbage. Why should you start eating calcium-rich foods now? Calcium supplementation and proper diet in your teen-age years can help prevent osteoporosis later in life. If you don't get enough calcium when you're young, the post-30s bone degenerative process will hasten the process of osteoporosis.

✔ **Message 2** (Read this to yourself in an enthusiastic voice):

> Hey! What's going on, girls? Talking to you about getting older seems pretty crazy, right? Well, here's something weird to think about: Did you know that many older women have, or will have, a bone disease called *osteoporosis,* or adult bone loss? These women many times fall and break their hips, legs, arms, and so on. How does this relate to you? Many of these women were your age when they first put themselves at risk. That's right, your age. When you're a teenager, it's absolutely crucial for you to get enough calcium in the food that you eat. It's easy to do because some of the tastiest foods have tons of calcium in them. For example, eating your favorite breakfast cereal with milk, and fruit salad on the side is a great way to get the calcium you need. Plus calcium is fantastic for great looking, healthy hair and nails. So drink up!"

Which of the preceding messages do you think a group of high school females would be more receptive to? Probably Message 2. The language is more in tune with the girls' reading level and age group, and the content of the message includes references to other appearance benefits (great looking, healthy hair and nails) that Message 1 lacks and that teen girls may find more compelling because the benefit is more immediate.

Pay attention to any visual aids you use, as well. Of the two images in Figure 20-1, for example, which do you think would more likely sway a group of teenage girls? Probably the image on the left. Why? Because the girl in the figure is youthful and attractive. The image on the right, on the other hand, may be more effective for older women who may be more swayed by the progressively stooped posture of the woman in the image.

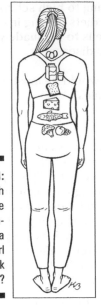

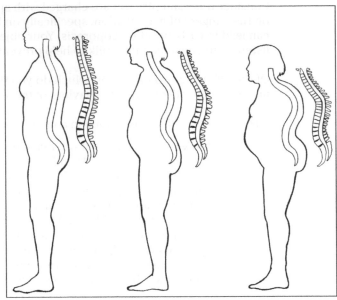

OR

Figure 20-1:
Which message best conveys that a teenage girl should drink more milk?

Even if you give Message 2 to the group of girls, a majority of them may have little desire to listen, let alone comply, due to a lack of perceived susceptibility. In that case, compelling them to improve their diets to include more calcium-fortified foods will be very challenging. For that reason, remember to always include psychosocial elements of your target audience in the message that you design and deliver. Augmenting your message to the needs of the audience can significantly impact how well your message is received. Using the health behavior models I introduce in Chapter 19 is great way to guide the design of a particular message.

Taking Your Communication to the Next Level

In the preceding sections, I cover the basics of communicating effectively, explaining the key components of any health message you deliver and offering examples that help you see how important it is to make sure you know and can reach your audience. Here I take you to the next level. The topics I discuss here can influence how your message is received and how effective it is.

As a dietary clinician, you can improve the effectiveness of your message if you understand that factors beyond your patients' control impact their perceptions of health information and their abilities to act on it. After all, no one lives in a vacuum. The environments in which you live and work affect the way you receive, react to, and act on information. Your environment also impacts the kind of information you hear — whether it's full and accurate, suspect, or even available at all.

To be a successful communicator, you must be aware of the following three major dimensions when you deliver information:

✔ The intrapersonal dimension

✔ The community dimension

✔ The political dimension

Each of these dimensions is multifaceted and can greatly influence both the way you deliver information and the way your patients receive it. Read on for the details.

Exploring intrapersonal influences

All people have their own histories, stories, and unique experiences that influence their opinions on given health topics. For the most part, these unique dispositions influence how people act and the decisions they make. These personal characteristics, like personality (which I outline in Chapter 19), can openly impact how and why people make, and subsequently act upon, health behavior choices.

Intrapersonal characteristics greatly influence how and why people behave as they do. These characteristics range from personality types that determine whether someone has an increased or decreased perceived vulnerability to a certain disease, or whether that same person believes he or she can adhere to a specific dietary recommendation, to personal likes and dislikes regarding taste preferences. To be a successful health professional counseling patients, you must take this information into consideration. (For details on health behavior theories, refer to Chapter 19).

Health communication researchers agree that messages that personally address the individual are more likely to be listened to and acted upon. In this section, I tell you how to create messages tailored to individuals or small groups.

Tailoring messages

One avenue health researchers are beginning to explore is *tailored messaging*. The idea behind tailored messaging is that the more personal a message is to a given individual, the more apt that individual is to listen and, more importantly, adhere to the message. Tailored messaging has proven to be an effective way to produce behavior change, particularly related to diet and exercise.

Although it's objectively impossible to tailor a message to every individual you'll advise, you can group individuals based on personality, demographics (age, race, ethnicity, or gender), health issues (diabetic status, for example), or any other grouping you find helpful.

Health literacy

Health literacy refers to an individual's ability to independently navigate the health service and information industry. Your recipient may fall in any of the following literacy levels:

- ✔ **Below basic:** People in this group possess only the most rudimentary literacy skills. To communicate with a patient in this category, you must use a 3rd-grade or below vocabulary.

- ✔ **Basic:** People at this level of literacy can perform simple literacy tasks and activities. If your patient falls into this category, you need to communicate using a 5th-grade or below vocabulary.

- ✔ **Intermediate:** At this level, people can perform moderately challenging literacy activities. With patients who fall into this category, you need to communicate in an 8th-grade or below vocabulary.

- ✔ **Proficient:** People can perform complex and challenging literacy activities. If your patient falls into this category, communicate with her using a 12th-grade or below vocabulary.

You can measure and assess health literacy in different ways, ranging from quick and easy surveys to more in-depth interviews. Whatever method you choose, in the end, the key piece of information is the literacy level of the recipient of your message. Knowing this, you can better tailor your message to your receiver.

A number of factors can influence a person's health literacy, such as access to information and cultural competency, for example, which you can read more about in the next section. Another is the person's actual reading level.

Understanding community complexities

Social and environmental factors influence how an individual receives, listens to, and adheres to (or not) information on a specific health behavior. Two variables to consider when assessing these influences are cultural competency and social norms.

Cultural competency

As cultures become more fluid and less static, society becomes more and more diverse. With the blending of diverse communities, the risk of a clash exists. *Note:* I use the term *clash* to describe different cultures melding together and to convey both the positive and negative components of this melding.

On the positive side, the cultures coming together learn about each other's people, language, and customs, and they discover how doing so enriches everyone. On the negative side are the issues that stem from one culture not fully understanding the other and ignorance that can result from that confusion. Many times, the negative side of cultures coming together produces a barrier in receiving a message or service.

To be most effective when you reach out to other communities, you must understand the culture of the population with which you're working. This skill is called *cultural competency*.

If you lack cultural competency, you may be unaware of and inadvertently create barriers between yourself and the people you are trying to communicate with. Consider these examples:

- ✔ **Certain words, phrases, gestures, or actions in one culture may mean something completely different or have no meaning in another culture.** You cannot assume something translates similarly among differing groups. For example, in many places, a thumbs up gesture signifies agreement or approval. In parts of the Mediterranean, Iran, and Afghanistan, however, it's an obscenity.

- ✔ **Body shape and size differ drastically among cultures.** Certain cultures value highly overweight women as a sign of healthiness and vigor. In Western societies, however, these same women would be seen as obese. As you suggest weight loss for health, you need to be careful about how you bring up the topic because you could easily cause offense.

Social norms

Social norms refer to the values and beliefs of a certain society that are widely practiced and accepted as normal. Social norms can be established by social groups and by society at large.

As someone who needs to communicate healthcare information, you must be acutely aware of the cultural or social norms through which the receiver hears the information. Many times efficacy or psychosocial issues (refer to Chapter 19) prevent the message from being delivered and/or received. Being sensitive to these unique circumstances can help you deliver a message successfully.

Looking at the influence of social groups

In some societies, for example, eating a high-fat, low-fiber diet is normal. In others, breastfeeding is taboo. So how do you recommend breastfeeding to women whose social network sees breastfeeding as taboo, or eating a low-fat, high-fiber diet to a person whose social network values a high-fat, low-fiber diet?

Such norms can directly affect the manner in which you communicate with your listeners. An individual's social circle can directly influence whether or not that person receives, listens to, or accepts or rejects a given message. In addition, the social norms can directly affect whether a person adheres to a behavior, even one that he or she personally wants to adopt.

Return for a moment to the husband and wife from the example at the beginning of this chapter (refer to the section "Trying your hand with an example scenario"). Both want to adopt a healthier lifestyle, but their children don't support them in this effort. In terms of social norms, the couple's children may have sway over their decision to change their diet.

Noting the influence of societal expectations

Just as social groups can influence health behaviors, social expectations exert an influence as well. Consider the difference between men and women in terms of intimate issues:

- ✔ **For women:** During their formative years, women have increased access to sexual education than do men. In addition, in the Western world, it is generally accepted that women be more in tune with their bodies than men. Discussions about sexuality or intimacy issues are much more common among groups of females than among groups of men.

- ✔ **For men:** Men are trained not to disclose pain or discomfort for fear of seeming unmanly. This masculinization of boys and men is creating a situation where men find discussing more intimate health issues hard. Chances are pretty slim that a group of middle-age men will sit around and have a discussion about incontinence (urination problems) or sexual dysfunction (impotence).

Reasons why this gender difference exists vary. However, the most important part to remember here is that certain topics are more sensitive for some groups than others. This sensitivity can most certainly relate to diet and nutrition as well. Take, for example, the issue of obesity. Non-obese individuals would probably take obesity-prevention outreach discussions less sensitively than obese ones. Sometimes, the state of overweight or obesity can bring self-esteem issues and, thus, an increased sensitivity in discussing these issues.

Assessing the political effect on communication

Just mention the word *politics,* and people tend to cringe, smile, shrug indifferently, or exhibit any combination of the three reactions. Whatever the response, as a health professional you must be tuned into the potential effect that the political landscape has on the way messages are developed, delivered, and disseminated. In particular, the following two issues are important:

✔ **The current areas of research and outreach:** The political climate tends to influence what and how much information is delivered about certain topics. In the United States, for example, the government is currently focusing resources on increasing physical activity among the nation's youth. Many funding opportunities are available for programs that focus on those goals and objectives related to that effort. In addition, much political discourse related to diet and wellness centers on physical activity.

To compensate for a lack of resources for research and outreach, try the following: Adapt your research, tie your endeavors to the area being funded currently, or solicit nongovernmental support.

✔ **Accessibility:** The ease with which people can access sources of information needs to improve among many sectors of society. Although some people have ample access to the Internet or libraries of books, for many others, these resources are luxuries they can't afford or don't have access to. Perhaps they lack private access, have no way to get to public places that offer those services, or they aren't allowed access.

To address this issue, look for available charitable services that exist in the area that can help provide resources to those most in need.

Part VI
The Part of Tens

For a bonus Clinical Nutrition Part of Tens chapter, head to www.dummies.com/extras/clinicalnutrition.

Part VI

The Part of Tens

In this part. . .

- Discover the top ten superfoods and how you can incorporate them into your diet

- Recognize the warning signs of eating disorders and how to distinguish among the different diseases

- Identify international resources to assist you in your studies or to gain insight on global efforts to combat nutritional issues

Chapter 21

Ten of the Greatest Superfoods

In This Chapter

▶ Foods that can make you healthy and strong

▶ Foods that can give you a longer and happier life

As people move further and further from more natural diets and toward more processed ones, the debate over wellness has centered on what effect an energy-dense diet has had on people's long- and short-term health compared to a nutrient-dense diet. Well, the results are in: People who eat an energy-dense diet instead of a nutrient-dense diet have an increased risk of developing obesity-related diseases, cardiovascular diseases, diabetes, some cancers, and more.

In this chapter I present some superfoods that can combat the effects of the more-processed diet. These foods are nutrient packed and can improve your health and your sense of wellness if you eat them regularly as part of a healthy diet.

Beans

Packed with fiber, beans are little power pills that are great for your heart. Fiber helps excrete excess cholesterol out of your body, thus lowering your risk of heart disease. Beans are also packed with protein and come in hundreds of different varieties. Be creative and try them all. Just don't eat too much, because they can cause a lot of gas! You've been warned.

Blueberries

Delicious and fantastic for your health, blueberries are full of vitamin C, fiber, *antioxidants* (substances in foods that help prevent or slow oxidative damage, which can lead to cancer), and potassium (which carries nutrients across cell boundaries to "feed" the cell). Some research suggests that these tiny blue pellets of goodness also provide relief from chronic inflammation.

You can eat blueberries in cereal, by themselves, as jam, on ice cream, in pies, and in a thousand other ways. One very popular way to eat blueberries is to freeze them and then put them on your favorite salad or breakfast cereal. (Frozen blueberries are just as nutritious as fresh ones, because the freezing process preserves the nutritional content.)

Broccoli

Broccoli is a fantastic source of fiber. It's available most of the year and is absolutely packed full of vitamins and minerals, including vitamins A, K, C, and B (in the form of folate). Some research also suggest that, because of its phytochemicals and calcium content, the nutrient-dense broccoli fights cancer and promotes healthy bone growth. (*Phytochemicals* confer taste and color to plants and have many claimed health benefits; be sure to read more about these chemicals in Chapter 6.)

Garlic

Almost every culture on earth uses garlic as a flavoring component, but it does more than just taste good. Garlic is also great for your blood pressure, and some research even suggests that it's a cancer fighter.

Garlic is also a great way to reduce the amount of salt you add to your food. The next time you need a little extra flavor, choose garlic instead of salt.

Honey

Research suggests that, due to its antimicrobial properties, honey can boost your immune system and help lessen symptoms of a cold and flu. According to some studies, eating local honey can help accustom you to potential allergens in the area. How? The bees pollenate flowers and create the honey from the pollen. Researchers speculate that, by eating honey made from local wildflowers, you can help lessen the effects of the regional allergens if you are susceptible to them.

As wonderful as honey is for older children and adults, *do not* feed honey to infants under one year old. Botulism spores in honey can cause an infant to develop *droopy baby syndrome,* a form of infant botulism that causes muscle weakness, constipation (one of the first signs of contamination), and a poor sucking reflex. If you suspect that your child has contracted infant botulism, seek immediate medical care.

Salmon

Salmon is so good for you that the American Heart Association recommends you eat more of it, along with other fatty fish, like mackerel and sardines, which are high in omega-3 fatty acids. Omega-3 fatty acids are protective against heart disease. Salmon is also high in protein and iron and low in saturated fat.

Salmon holds up to many different ways to serve it: Grill it, bake it, purée it into a dip, or eat it smoked on a bagel. You *must* try lox and cream cheese on a whole-grain bagel if you haven't had the pleasure yet. It's a fantastic breakfast!

Soybeans and Other Soy Products

A diet rich in soy offers a number of benefits, such as lowering cholesterol and, because of that, reducing the risk of heart disease. Soy is full of protein. It's also extremely versatile and can be served in a number of ways: tofu, oil, milk, the edamame served at your favorite Japanese restaurant, and more.

Females who have a known risk for breast cancer should be careful about how much soy they get in their diet. Some research has suggested that a link may exist between higher consumptions of soy and an increased risk of breast cancer. (The jury is still out on the link, however, so talk with your doctor if you have questions.)

Vinegar

Used for literally thousands of years, vinegar helps flavor and preserve food. It can also help with a whole host of health issues. Research has suggested that vinegar can

- **Relieve the sting of bug bites:** Dab apple cider vinegar on a cotton ball with a little water on the bug bite. Reapply every few minutes until the sting goes away.
- **Tone and firm up skin:** Vinegar applied to the skin can increase blood flow, evening out skin tone temporarily.

✔ **Keep your digestive tract cleansed, when taken daily (diluted, of course):** Vinegar helps breaks down proteins and other harder-to-digest foods.

✔ **Control foot odor:** Soak your feet in vinegar for about 15 minutes to kill odor-causing bacteria.

Walnuts and Almonds

Walnuts and almonds are filled with healthy fats and protein. In addition, they have qualities that help you fend off some chronic diseases. Walnuts, for example, decrease your risk of prostate cancer, and almonds can help alleviate chronic constipation. Odd, but true!

These and other nuts are good for you, but you have to eat smaller portions of these foods because of their high fat content. Added in your favorite cereal or eaten on their own as a snack, nuts are easy to integrate into your diet in a way that's well-balanced and healthy.

Yogurt

Yogurt is everywhere nowadays. From "fruit-on-the-bottom," Greek, kefir, and Icelandic style, you have scores of options to choose from at your local supermarket. Here's why yogurt deserves its place on the superfood list:

✔ **Its *probiotic* bacteria (the "good" bacteria) keep your gut healthy and you regular; these bacteria also provide constipation relief.** For more on why constipation is a health problem from a dietary perspective, head to Chapter 11.

✔ **The calcium and vitamin D content in the yogurt help prevent osteoporosis.** For more information on what osteoporosis is and how to avoid it, refer to Chapter 18.

✔ **It's a very versatile food.** You can eat it with cereal, use it in baking, dip vegetables and fruit in it, eat it plain, or whatever. Get creative.

✔ **It's a total nutrition food.** It has protein, calcium, sugars, some fat, and almost every other nutrient your body demands for healthy bone growth and development.

My favorites are the Scandinavian-styled yogurts. They are drinkable and delicious!

Chapter 22

Ten Things to Know about Eating Disorders

*T*he incidence of eating disorders, particularly in Western societies, has seen dramatic increases in recent years. Although most associated with late-stage adolescence and early adulthood, eating disorders can affect anyone at any age. The condition is so common that you probably know someone who is suffering with an eating disorder, even though you may not be aware this person is battling this health issue. Maybe you are battling it yourself. As a nutritionist, you will likely encounter people in your practice who suffer from disordered eating.

In this chapter, I discuss ten things that you should know about the three most common eating disorders (anorexia nervosa, bulimia nervosa, and binge eating disorder), from basic information on the topic to tools you can use to help prevent the disease to warning signs that the disease may present. Use this information as an entry point into this very complex problem.

Three Main Types of Eating Disorders Exist

Three main types of eating disorders exist: anorexia nervosa, bulimia nervosa, and binge eating disorder:

✔ **Anorexia nervosa:** This disorder is identified with very restrictive dieting, an excessive fear of gaining weight, and, eventually, a skeletal-looking frame due to the body's starving. It has the highest mortality rate of any eating disorder category.

✔ **Bulimia nervosa:** In bulimia, sufferers engage in binge eating episodes during which they feel a lack of control over their behavior, followed by a feeling of guilt that leads them to purge the food they just ate. To be diagnosed with bulimia nervosa, such episodes have to occur twice a week for at least three months.

✔ **Binge eating:** Binge eating disorder is defined as recurrent episodes of eating in a two-hour period what most people would eat in an entire day and lacking a sense of control over the eating during the episode.

Disordered Eating Is Different from Eating Disorders

Disordered eating differs from eating disorders. In *disordered eating,* there is some disturbance in eating behavior. For example, a person with disordered eating typically feels some level of dissatisfaction with his or her body size and shape and may exhibit behaviors such as an insistence on eating alone, chewing food but spitting it out to avoid swallowing, or employing other seemingly abnormal methods of eating.

An *eating disorder* is group of conditions where an individual is intensely preoccupied with his or her body weight and engages in abnormal eating behaviors (involving either insufficient or excessing intake) to a degree that threatens the person's health and, possibly, his or her life.

Generally, disordered eating is a precursor to an eating disorder. If left untreated, disordered eating can, and many times does, lead to more serious and potentially life-threatening health issues.

If you're like most people, you've had days when you just can't get your clothes to fit the way you want and feel stressed about it. Or maybe you've been skipping breakfast and lunch for the past few weeks because you're just not that hungry. Don't jump to the conclusion that you have disordered eating. Take a deep breath, relax, and determine whether your habit is something you can easily stop or resolve. If not, you may want to talk to someone about the behaviors that have you worried.

The Rate of Eating Disorders Is Increasing

In recent years, the number of individuals diagnosed with an eating disorder has increased. In the United States alone, 5 million people suffer from anorexia nervosa and bulimia nervosa, with women ages 18 to 30 years old making up the largest group of sufferers.

Although the increase could be due to a change in the language or diagnostic definitions, that's a hard sell. A change in the definition of a disease may include people in that category when before they wouldn't be, but the amount of people falsely defined would be small enough to have little influence on the overall number swell.

Men Suffer from Eating Disorders, Too

Eating disorders are typically reported among women. In fact, lifetime prevalence of anorexia nervosa is ten times greater in women than in men. Furthermore, more women than men report or are diagnosed with binge eating disorder. However, the perception that men rarely get these diseases is incorrect.

Although men reportedly are ten times less likely to have a certain eating disorder than are women, those numbers may not tell the whole story. Consider the following:

✔ Men are more apt to conceal their eating problems, thus leaving eating disorders in men largely undiagnosed or under diagnosed.

✔ Some say that up to one in five males suggest that they have some type of dissatisfaction with their body size and shape.

✔ If you compare the cases of eating disorders in homosexual men to the number of cases involving women, the rates are more comparable than are the rates between heterosexual men and women.

Hundreds of thousands of men worldwide suffer from an eating disorder. As a health professional, you must be aware that the same pressures that lead women to develop eating disorders can, and do, affect men. Bottom line: Although women still suffer from eating disorders at a higher rate than men, that tenfold gap is probably closer than the reported cases indicate.

Binge Eating Is Commonly Diagnosed among Adults

Binge eating disorder is the most common eating disorder. Approximately 3 percent of the U.S. population has been diagnosed with this disorder, and similar numbers are reported globally. Surprisingly, this disease is seen most often in 46- to 55-year-olds. Binge eating disorder is also the most common eating disorder among college-age adults (18- to 25-year-olds).

Binge eating, like all other eating disorders, is prone to underreporting, particularly among subgroups. So whatever number is given to you regarding how many people have these diseases, add a couple hundred, a couple thousand, or perhaps even tens of thousands to those total numbers, depending on the disorder and what subgroup you are researching.

You Can Be Overweight or Obese and Have Bulimia

You cannot be anorexic and be obese or overweight. In fact, one of the criteria for being diagnosed with anorexia is that you are consistently below normal body weight. With bulimia, the situation is a bit different. Overweight individuals can indulge in bingeing and purging cycles.

As I explain earlier in "Disordered Eating Is Different from Eating Disorders," bulimia is characterized by regular episodes of binge eating followed by episodes of purging. Because these episodes can occur relatively sporadically (a diagnosis requires them to occur an average of twice a week for at least three months), you can see how an individual could be overweight or obese and still meet the criteria for bulimia.

One Symptom Does Not an Eating Disorder Make

To be diagnosed with an eating disorder, a number of symptoms must be present. For example, to be diagnosed with anorexia nervosa, several of the following criteria must be met:

- ✔ You must be consistently below normal body weight
- ✔ You must refuse to gain weight to healthy levels
- ✔ You must have an intense fear of being fat or gaining weight
- ✔ You must have some sort of body image distortion issue
- ✔ For women, three consecutive menstrual cycles must be missed (called *amenorrhea*).

Now, if you are a thin person who was always underweight as a child and even into adulthood, and you do not exhibit any of the other symptoms, you do not have anorexia nervosa. Even if you start to worry about gaining weight, you are still not anorexic. To be properly diagnosed with an eating disorder, you must demonstrate a certain number of the diagnostic criteria.

Chances are you don't have anything to worry about. However, if you become overly concerned about your weight, continue to lose weight, or begin to display behaviors associated with disordered eating (refer to the earlier section "Disordered Eating Is Different from Eating Disorders"), have a chat with your physician. These conditions may indicate a situation that, if left untreated, could develop into anorexia.

Anorexia Nervosa Is the Most Deadly Eating Disorder

Eating disorders are mental illnesses, and, of all the mental illnesses, they have the highest death rate. Of all the different types of eating disorders, anorexia nervosa is by far the deadliest. Keeping your body below normal weight and the different methods with which this is accomplished — like intense exercise, vomiting, laxatives, outright starvation, and so on — is traumatic for the body. Many people with anorexia die of heart and other major organ failure due to the lack of body fat and the damage done by the complete lack of nourishment.

Excessive dieting can be considered an eating disorder. Consider these alarming statistics: 95 percent of all dieters regain their lost weight within a few years, and nearly one-third of regular dieters progress to pathological dieting. Further, of the pathological dieters, almost one-fourth develop some type of eating disorder.

Mental Health Treatment Is a Large Component of the Cure

Fifty percent of those diagnosed with eating disorders are also diagnosed with depression. To treat eating disorders, the recommended approach usually involves treating both the eating disorder and the underlying depression. This combination consists of individual psychotherapy, medication, information dissemination, family therapy, and, sometimes, hospitalization. The mental health component is probably the most important part of treatment for many sufferers.

One thing that makes treating eating disorders so difficult is that a person needs to eat food to survive, yet food is one of the root causes of the health issue the person is suffering from . . . quite the distressing situation.

You Need to Be on the Lookout for Warning Signs

Although many people associate eating disorders with teenage girls, they can affect anyone at any time. No one is impervious to the pressure to look a certain way. A few years back, for example, it was reported that up to 80 percent of 10-year-olds — *10-year-olds!* — reported being afraid to "get fat." And, as I mention in the earlier section "Binge Eating Is Commonly Diagnosed among Adults," binge eating disorder mainly affects middle-age adults.

Because these diseases know no age or gender boundaries, anyone can be affected at any point. Therefore, you need to be aware of your own feelings and behaviors regarding eating and on the lookout for those closest to you.

Chapter 23

Ten International Resources You Don't Want to Miss

*A*s diseases related to poor lifestyle choices — such as obesity, diabetes, some cancers, cardiovascular disease, and so on — have impacted countries around the world, an organized international response has sprung up to address them. In this chapter, I outline ten organizations that provide information, counseling, and sometimes goods and services to people who are most in need.

The Academy of Nutrition and Dietetics Foundation (ANDF)

Formerly called the American Dietetic Association Foundation, the Academy of Nutrition and Dietetics Foundation (ANDF) is the world's largest charitable organization devoted exclusively to nutrition and dietetics. Its membership includes experts in nutritional sciences who seek to expand the discussion of nutritional diseases globally and to help bring about an end to such health concerns.

Specifically, the ANDF makes available to its members a directory of resources for international food, nutrition, and dietetic professionals. This directory fosters collaboration between scientists and helps students and other professionals seeking financial assistance and resources. For more information, go to http://www.eatright.org/foundation/default.aspx.

Australasian Society for Parenteral and Enteral Nutrition (AuSPEN)

Just like the British Association for Parental and Enteral Nutrition (BAPEN), explained in the next section, the Australasian Society for Parenteral and Enteral Nutrition (AuSPEN) is a charitable association that aims to increase knowledge of the problems stemming from malnutrition. This multidisciplinary society explores the field of clinical nutrition in its efforts to end malnutrition and other nutritional diseases in the Southwest Pacific, specifically in Australia and New Zealand. For information on AuSPEN, go to http://www.auspen.org.au/.

The British Association for Parenteral and Enteral Nutrition (BAPEN)

The British Association for Parenteral and Enteral Nutrition (BAPEN) is a charitable association that aims to increase the public's awareness of problems that stem from malnutrition. It also strives to provide access to nutritional care to individuals who are most in need.

Comprised of several professional organizations, including national organizations of patients in need, physicians, dieticians, nurses, and pharmacists, BAPEN aims to improve nutritional care. Sounds good to me. For more information, go to http://www.bapen.org.uk/.

Irish Society for Clinical Nutritional and Metabolism (IrSPEN)

The Irish Society for Clinical Nutritional and Metabolism (IrSPEN) is dedicated to making screening for and treatment of individual and community nutritional issues, particularly malnutrition, a primary focus of the global community. For information, go to http://www.irspen.ie/.

Ireland spends about $2 million per year treating diseases and health issues related to poor nutrition. For this reason, a pressing need exists for efforts in research and outreach to be expanded to help curb and eventually prevent the effects and thus the costs of these diseases.

The Nevin Scrimshaw International Nutrition Foundation (INF)

The goal of the Nevin Scrimshaw International Nutrition Foundation (INF) is to assist developing countries with nutrition research and outreach to combat issues surrounding hunger, food access, and malnutrition.

The INF conducts three major activities: providing fellowships for continuing education in the field of nutritional sciences, conducting original research in nutrition, and spreading information on nutritional research and policy. For more information, go to http://inffoundation.org/.

The Nutritional Barometer

The Nutritional Barometer lists the resources provided by the world community to the approximately 40 countries where over 90 percent of the globe's malnourished children live. The information provided in *The Nutritional Barometer* illustrates the status of childhood malnutrition, identifies who is most in need, and lists the resources available to assist in lessening the health problems caused by poor diet during childhood.

The Nutritional Barometer is produced by Save the Children and World Vision. Its purpose is to assist with programs created to reduce the number of children stunted by severe malnutrition by 40 percent, a goal outlined in the World Health Assembly's 2025 proposal. (Being *stunted* refers to a lack of physical growth during adolescence due to malnutrition early in life.) For more information, go to http://www.savethechildren.org.uk/resources/online-library/nutrition-barometer.

Nutrition Education and Consumer Awareness Group

The Nutrition Education and Consumer Awareness Group (http://www.fao.org/ag/humannutrition/nutritioneducation/en/) grants technical assistance to the Food and Agriculture Organization (FAO) of the United Nations. The organization's services help develop outreach efforts and design policies to promote public awareness and knowledge about healthy dieting and overall wellness.

The FAO leads international efforts to end nutritional diseases. Specifically, malnutrition and food security issues are at the forefront of its programs. For more information, go to http://www.fao.org/home/en/.

UNICEF

UNICEF, an international organization within the United Nations, has a multitude of programs aimed at protecting children's rights. The organization's primary focus is the health and welfare of children worldwide, and its humanitarian outreach extends to the remotest parts of the world and to people, especially children, who are most in need.

One of the organization's goals is to reduce food insecurity around the world, and it lobbies governmental agencies to adopt certain food policies to secure access to food. In addition to addressing childhood nutrition, UNICEF also offers education services, HIV/AIDS treatment, and services to protect children from abuse and violence. For more information, go to http://www.unicef.org/.

Vitamin and Mineral Nutrition Information System (VMNIS)

Created by the World Health Organization (WHO), the Vitamin and Mineral Nutrition Information System (VMNIS) is a database of micronutrients. This database contains international, national, regional, and sometimes even local information on the nutritional status of member nations. The WHO uses this data to help direct resources globally to fight hunger and malnutrition. In that way, the VMNIS helps shepherd efforts to curb micronutrient deficiencies worldwide. For more information on VMNIS, go to http://www.who.int/vmnis/en/.

World Public Health Nutrition Association (WPHNA)

The World Public Health Nutrition Association (WPHNA) is open to any individual who advocates on behalf of bringing about a higher level of awareness to the issues surrounding world hunger, food access, and malnutrition. WPHNA also certifies, via an application and testing procedure, members who work in public health nutrition.

The WPHNA has members in more than 50 nations and provides a forum in which members can collaborate with each other. The organization is very inclusive and welcoming. Definitely check it out if you plan to pursue any type of nutritional science degree or profession. Go to http://wphna.org/.

Index

About the Author

Michael J. Rovito, PhD, is the founder and executive director of the Men's Health Initiative and a lecturer in the Department of Health Professions at the University of Central Florida. His work specializes in health behavior change, men's health, and community health promotion. He has published works on topics including perceptions of testicular and prostate cancer, masculinity, and roles of men in society. His future work is focused on promoting health equity for men and boys in society and advocating for healthy lifestyle policy.

Dedication

This book is dedicated to my wife, Kathy. I think God gave you an extra helping of patience when He found out that you and I started dating. You are without a doubt my favorite person and best friend. Much love to you.

Author's Acknowledgments

I'd like to thank my parents, Patti and Mike: You two are living testaments to a small town American dream story. When others would have given up, you kept going. Kerri, Tara, and I are successful because of the limitless love you showed us, the endless hours you worked to put food on our modest table, the guidance you gave us to make the right choices and to keep our path to success true, and the faith you had in each of us to make our own decisions about the kind of lives we wanted to lead. I can count on one hand people I know who are fortunate enough to have had this experience.

I also acknowledge mine and Kathy's Shiba Inu, Lola. This little girl lay at my feet while I typed this book. You brought much joy to our lives. You deserve a treat. Good girl!

Publisher's Acknowledgments

Acquisitions Editor: Anam Ahmed

Editor: Tracy L. Barr

Technical Editor: Valerie Schulz, MMSc, RD, LD/N, CDE

Art Coordinator: Alicia B. South

Project Coordinator: Rebekah Brownson

Illustrator: Kathryn Born, MA

Cover Image: © Amy Whitt / jupiterimages

Printed and bound by CPI Group (UK) Ltd, Croydon, CR0 4YY

27/10/2024

14580404-0001